CLINICAL PSYCHOLOGY IN SINGAPORE

An Asian Casebook

CLINICAL PSYCHOLOGY IN SINGAPORE

An Asian Casebook

Edited by

GREGOR LANGE AND JOHN DAVISON

with DEBORAH AMANDA GOH

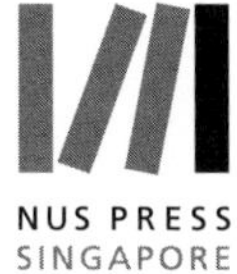

NUS PRESS
SINGAPORE

Published by:

NUS Press
National University of Singapore
AS3-01-02, 3 Arts Link
Singapore 117569
Fax: (65) 6774-0652
E-mail: nusbooks@nus.edu.sg
Website: http://www.nus.edu.sg/nuspress

ISBN: 978-9971-69-854-6 (Paper)

National Library Board, Singapore Cataloguing-in-Publication Data

Clinical psychology in Singapore : an Asian casebook / Gregor Lange and John Davison, editors.
– Singapore : NUS Press, [2015]
pages cm
Includes bibliographical references and index.
ISBN : 978-9971-69-854-6

1. Clinical psychology - Singapore - Case studies. 2. Psychotherapy - Singapore - Case studies. 3. Clinical psychology - Practice - Singapore.
I. Lange, Gregor, editor. II. Davison, John, editor.

RC467
616.89 -- dc23   OCN897851342

Designed and typeset by: Pressbooks.com, PDF rendering by Prince XML.
Cover illustration by: Clara Tan
Cover design by: Nelani Jinadasa
Printed by: Markono Print Media Pte Ltd

CONTENTS

PREFACE

The practice of clinical psychology is deeply embedded within its cultural context. Nowhere is this more relevant than in Singapore, a microcosm of Asia, a juncture of East and West, and home to people of diverse ethnicities and religions. The country is remarkable for its economic dynamism and its dramatic shifts in intergenerational cultures. Whether psychologists are treating Kevin, an 11-year-old with devastating encephalitis, or Julia, a reluctant Chinese teenager unable to grasp the seriousness of anorexia nervosa, or Mr Tan, admitted to the psychiatric ward to give his household some respite from his dementia, they must constantly adapt their work to find the best fit with the expectations, ideals and traditions of the people who live here.

This casebook arose from our experiences teaching psychology at the National University of Singapore. We were frustrated with the non-Asian teaching resources that had limited relevance for Singaporeans and noticed how our students lit up when we shared our own experiences of working with local clients. Students were more engaged when we were evaluating situations more directly relevant to their daily lives—as when assessing the level of risk for the national serviceman who was hearing voices. They were also keen to gauge whether a Chinese uncle's superstitions were normal or pathological, and to discuss the therapeutic challenges of involving two working parents and their domestic helper in behavioural therapy for a disobedient son.

Rather than an exemplar text or a 'how-to' guide, this casebook provides a snapshot of how psychologists in Singapore weave clinical psychology into their local practice. It aims to contribute to this evolving and dynamic profession by helping Singaporean clinicians, students, researchers and the public engage in a meaningful dialogue on the future of clinical psychology in Singapore.

The division of the cases by age—children and teens, adults, and the elderly—provides a natural grouping that occurs across mental health services, psychology professions and university modules. The broad spectrum of chapters within each of these age groups reflects the growing diversity in the current practice of clinical psychology in Singapore. Each chapter focuses on a different client, issue and treatment, along with the different settings in which clinical psychology takes place. The casebook includes clients with common mental health problems such as depression, panic disorder and autistic spectrum disorder, as well as more unusual problems like pyromania, exhibitionism and frontal-lobe epilepsy.

These case studies are authored by clinical psychologists and neuropsychologists working in Singapore and are based on real Singaporean clients and families. The authors themselves vary in their training, experience, clinical roles and clinical styles, as well as their age and ethnicity, but they all share a dedication to evidence-based practice. Their willingness to let us into their consultation room allows us to see how they assess and work within the context of a client's presenting issues, developmental background and culture, and within the Singaporean health system. The authors describe their successes and also depict how they grapple with tensions in the therapy room and with cultural and ethical issues. They provide recommendations for others in the field, and raise important questions for us to ponder.

The settings our authors work within range from the Institute of Mental Health to the Singapore Prison Service, the Ministry of Social and Family Development, specialist hospital services, university training clinics and private practice. Several authors describe developing specialist services that extend to client groups who have been previously unheeded. This includes the work of Nenna Ndukwe at the Functional Gastrointestinal Disorder Psychology Service at the National University Hospital of Singapore, Ranjani Utpala at the Eating Disorders Programme at the Singapore General Hospital, and Julia Lam and Munidasa Winslow of Promises Healthcare for addictions and mental health. As clinical psychologists are increasingly required to provide specialist roles, many authors, such as Jade Jang, emphasise the importance of specialist training for psychologists to avoid "missed diagnoses and misdiagnosis".

Significant challenges arise even before clients walk in the door: Singaporeans have to cope with the considerable stigma attached to mental health issues and 'doctors of the mind', and endure the pressure to save face in circumstances of difficult personal or family situations. Kenji Gwee, Nenna Ndukwe and several other authors highlight the significance of empathising with the client's frame of reference and the importance of psycho-education. The authors also show how intervention can lead to remarkable changes when clients and their families build a more informed understanding of present issues and engage actively in psychological services.

Other tensions occur within the therapy room. Ranjani Utpala, Jeffrey Ong and Eunice Yap highlight the importance of finding a balance between enacting the expert role that Singaporeans often expect and engaging in the collaborative empowerment of clients that is required for psychological change. Others discuss the challenge of not knowing 'how hard to push' their clients to express their emotions, particularly if they do not share the same culture. Similarly, Adaline Ng queries the effectiveness of assertiveness training when confident expression of opinions may be frowned on in local contexts.

Many of the authors describe the challenges of engaging family members in assessment and therapy—a seeming paradox in a nation that self-identifies with collectivism and family cohesion. They reflect on a variety of factors that may limit family involvement, including attempts to save face and deflect blame, the conviction that the psychologist is an expert who is best placed to 'fix' the client, as well as the time pressures that families face when they have two working parents. Authors such as Clare Kwan illustrate the crucial role of "stepped care" services for mental health and contemplate how we can better incorporate families, educators and communities into our treatments.

Other themes relate to working within the Singaporean system. Joy Low worked with a boy in a welfare home whose behaviour was too difficult to be managed at home or at school, and Tan Li Jen and Chew Qian Ru Charis treated another boy struggling with PSTD following severe child abuse. These authors share insights into the often unseen vulnerable populations in Singapore. They reflect on how psychologists can collaborate with other disciplines and multiple systems of care and provide recommendations of how Singapore can progress with child welfare issues.

Paul Fisher and Joy Lim report on the limitations of the traditional, Western medical model for working with challenging behaviours in dementia. They convey the innovative approaches of person-centered care at a large local hospital, a model which extends from the therapy room to all care staff and throughout the hospital system. On a different front, a number of chapters are set within the forensic system of Singapore. Clients here are often motivated primarily by a court mandate for therapy, but their presentations vary remarkably: an average guy-next-door type arrested for obscene sexual acts (Kenji Gwee); a 20-year-old charged with ten counts of mischief for fire setting (Ho Wei Tshen and Chu Chi Meng); an Eurasian teenager with ADHD that was perhaps contributing to his marijuana use (John Davison); a woman besieged by her own gambling and related offenses (Julia Lam and Munidasa Winslow), and a woman with borderline personality disorder and a past punctuated by instability, broken relationships, drug use and self-harm (Adaline Ng). Whilst therapy for these clients was mandatory, psychologists convey the positive aspects of this context: the structure and safety of the prison system, the opportunity for intensive therapy, the fear of further incarceration as a motivating factor in participation, and the prospect of treating clients who in other circumstances would rarely have the chance of psychological intervention.

Most authors stress the importance of adapting assessment and therapy for the Asian setting and their clients' individual beliefs. Tay Sze Yan and Kenji Gwee portray how psychological formulations and treatments can be moulded for a Chinese immigrant with a poor level of education and literacy. Jasmin Kaur and Adaline Ng both provide examples of how their therapy is integrated with the Buddhist faith of their clients, and Catherine Cox warns that clients' antagonism towards Western treatments and hospitals can lead to non-compliance in treatment and potentially dangerous outcomes. Desiree Choo and Ranjani Uptala emphasise the importance for psychologists to reflect not only on their clients' cultural values, but also on how their own beliefs (e.g., child-rearing and discipline) can inadvertently impact on therapeutic relationships and clients' prognoses.

Several authors are wary of applying foreign measures to their clients. Some report limitations in local research and resources. Elaine Sum and Iliana Magiati question the validity and reliability of a diagnosis of autism when relying on Western diagnostic tools, and encourage caution and more comprehensive assessments. Whilst most authors rely on foreign norms, some agencies have developed their own translated tests and now have local normative data. Simon Collinson reports that Singapore now has the most comprehensive age and education stratified neuropsychological data available in Asia for older adults. This gives psychologists more confidence in the challenging task of assessing poorly educated and elderly Singaporeans.

This is an exciting time for clinical psychology in Singapore. Despite the continuing stigma attached to mental health disorders, Singapore's mental health services and clinical psychology practices are evolving quickly. We see increased government recognition and funding, the introduction of new postgraduate clinical programs, and an improvement in the breadth and specialisation of services. This growing sophistication makes it a valuable time for us to publish these first accounts from grassroots experience and to engage actively in the evolution of our profession.

The dynamic development of Singapore's mental health services is paralleled in other Asian countries. The cases will resonate with clinicians and clients in many cities and regional centres that share some of the cultural and societal challenges, familial tensions and personal achievements described here. Moreover, as Asians play an increasing role in international communities, psychologists and health systems around the world must develop their competencies in assessing and treating them. This casebook bears relevance for working with Asian clients across the globe.

This book provides useful first-hand accounts of disorders and their treatment for students at the undergraduate level. Those in postgraduate clinical or counselling courses will gain a detailed insight into assessment, formulation, and therapy within a local context. Clinicians may use this text to reflect on their own psychological practice or to assist with their supervision of other clinicians. We also hope that the general reader who picks up this book will be better able to appreciate the hopes and struggles of people with mental illness, its impact on their families, and the role of clinical psychology in the wider society.

John Davison and Gregor Lange, the editors

ACKNOWLEDGEMENTS

This casebook is dedicated to the clients who have provided its heart and soul. We would like to acknowledge the journey they embarked on and wish them well in the future. We are also grateful to our authors, who have willingly narrated their own clinical practice, publicly reflecting on their successes, but also on their challenges, tensions and questions. We acknowledge their dedication to their clients and the evolving profession in Singapore, and their commitment to completing these chapters on top of their intensive workloads.

We are thankful for the National University of Singapore (NUS) Faculty of Arts and Social Sciences (FASS) Staff Research Support Scheme, which provided funding for our research assistant, Deborah Goh, who provided perceptive research and meticulous editing. We also thank Kelly Ann Zainal, Tan Sze Ying, Si-Ning Yeo and Elvis Tan who kindly assisted with background research, proof reading and indexing for this project.

Christine Chong, Peter Schoppert, and NUS Press were enthusiastically committed to this ambitious project from the start.

Lastly, our family and friends for their invaluable support and encouragement. In particular, we thank Barbara, Zoe and Anya for their boundless love and patience; Margaret McClure and Graham Davison for their intellectual insight and practical help; and Chris McMorran, a great colleague and friend, who has provided ongoing inspiration and support.

CONFIDENTIALITY

The cases included here are based on actual case histories or a composite of cases. Ensuring client confidentiality is of utmost concern and essential for publishing any client-related information. We consulted with experts from the Centre for Biomedical Ethics, Yong Loo Lin School of Medicine, National University of Singapore about the process of de-identifying cases and ensuring confidentiality in client related publications. All of the cases were based on actual clinical experiences. Various demographic characteristics (names, occupations etc) and clinical details have been changed to protect the anonymity of clients and their families. Any resemblances to actual people is purely coincidental.

INTRODUCTION: CLINICAL PSYCHOLOGY IN SINGAPORE

GREGOR LANGE AND JOHN DAVISON, WITH DEBORAH AMANDA GOH

Singapore is a dynamic small island metropolis of 5.4 million inhabitants. Its population consists of Chinese (74.2%), Malays (13.3%), Indians (9.1%), and others (3.3%) (Statistics Singapore, 2013), who share a large diversity of cultures and religions, languages and dialects. This young nation approaching its 50th birthday in 2015, has rapidly transformed from a developing country to a first-world nation. Its fast-paced evolution is occurring across all domains of life, from business, infrastructure and education, to public and private healthcare services. Changes in these domains have resulted in dramatic shifts in Singaporeans' way of life and given rise to a unique context of mental health needs and prospects. Within this realm, the profession of clinical psychology is relatively new, but is quickly finding its feet.

Overview of Psychology Services in Singapore

Although Singapore has already achieved first-world standards in many areas (including medical healthcare) other areas—the mental health services in general and clinical psychology in particular—are still in earlier stages of development. Whilst these services are developing considerably—with heightened government recognition and funding, new postgraduate clinical programs, and increasing breadth and specialisation of services—there remains considerable stigma and misunderstanding of mental health disorders in Singapore by both the general public and clinicians.

Aware of this discrepancy, the Singapore government is in the process of expanding on strategies proposed in the country's first National Mental Health Blueprint (2007–12). The Blueprint provides a foundation for policies aimed at bringing local mental health services on par with international standards of best practice. It emphasises a comprehensive approach towards addressing the mental health needs of the entire population, from persons who are mentally healthy, to those who are at risk, as well as individuals with existing mental health conditions. Primary aims of the Blueprint include raising awareness of mental health care across all ages, improving community-based services, increasing the numbers of clinical psychologists, psychiatrists, and other allied health professionals and encouraging their collaboration, as well as developing and strengthening evidence-based practices among various clinical psychology services in Singapore (Table 1).

TABLE 1. MENTAL HEALTH BLUEPRINT — EIGHT KEY VALUES	
1	Mental health encompasses both mental well-being as well as the absence of mental disorders
2	Mental health is an integral part of general health
3	Mental health promotion and care must be both evidence-based and cost-effective
4	Those with mental disorders should preferably be given appropriate services within the community
5	Services should be available to everyone
6	The mentally ill should not be discriminated against
7	The needs and views of the mentally ill should be considered when planning, delivering and evaluating services
8	Mental health care and promotion is a multi-sectoral effort

Clinical psychology is a young and evolving discipline in Singapore. The authors of this casebook bear witness to the increasing breadth of settings and roles for psychologists: their employers range from the Institute of Mental Health, to the Singapore Prison Service, the Ministry of Social and Family Development (MSF), specialist hospital services at the KK Women's and Children's Hospital (KKH) and the National University Hospital (NUH), university-training clinics and private practice.

INTEGRATED MENTAL HEALTH CARE: CLINICAL PSYCHOLOGY PRACTICES IN SINGAPORE

As clinical psychology gains greater recognition as a profession in Singapore, the unique skills of clinical psychologists are becoming better understood and utilised. In addition to their traditional roles in mental health settings, psychologists are increasingly recognised for their provision of services in specialist areas of rehabilitation, medical care, neuropsychology and forensic settings. Furthermore, the roles and responsibilities of the clinical psychologist have expanded a long way from the traditional domains of assessment and psychotherapy. Psychologists commonly provide consultation and training for staff, engage in clinical supervision of other psychologists or clinicians, carry out research and auditing, and play advisory roles for government bodies or other organisations.

The practice of clinical psychology is centred on 'evidence-based' services. Clinical psychologists' expertise in human behaviours and emotions as well as in research methods and statistics places them in an ideal position to develop and evaluate psychological services. In Singapore, clinical psychologists are starting to get involved in performing key functions for new programs to promote mental health and in developing rehabilitative and intervention programs. Programs involve reaching out to clients with psychosis or schizophrenia and providing support to families and caregivers through public education (Ee, 2004) and early intervention programs (Chong et al., 2005). Others, such as the KK Women's and Children's Hospital's postnatal depression program, help women who have or are at-risk of postnatal depression through screening, intervention, and follow-up care. Mental disorders among the elderly (dementia, depression, delirium and psychosis) are addressed by Changi General Hospital's community-based psychogeriatric program. Support groups run by other organizations include psycho-educational support groups for cancer patients and caregivers at the National University Cancer Institute Singapore (NCIS) and dialectical behavioural therapy groups for helping adolescents better manage emotions at the Institute of Mental Health (IMH). These examples of the involvement of clinical psychology all share a common theme: improving mental health promotion and mental well-being.

Mental Health Promotion

Mental illness in Singapore is often neglected because of misunderstanding, misconception, discrimination and stigma. A study based on the 1996 Singapore Mental Health Survey found that only 37% of Singaporeans were willing to seek professional help if they experienced an emotional or mental health problem (Ng et al., 2003). Moreover, the most recent 2010 Singapore Mental Health Study identified a large majority (84%) of Singaporeans with comorbid mental and physical disorders who were not using mental health services (Chong et al., 2012). Untreated, these mental illnesses may become chronic, social or occupational impairments, and even engender suicidal behaviour (Phua, Chua, Ma, Heng & Chew, 2009); Phua et al. (2009) highlighted the fact that mental illnesses contribute 11% to Singapore's chronic disease burden. Mental health problems can also place significant strains on family relationships as a majority of clients with serious mental health conditions (e.g., schizophrenia) are reliant on care from their families (Tan et al., 2004).

A number of factors contribute to low service use and poor treatment rates. Firstly, the stigma of having a mental illness or attending mental health services remains high in Singapore and mental illness is commonly perceived as bringing shame to the family (Foo, Merrick & Kazantzis, 2006). Secondly, barriers to seeking professional help include a mistrust of psychological services and professionals and once again, the desire to "save face" (Kee, 2004). Ang and Tan (2004) also identified a lack of awareness of the availability of psychological services as a restricting factor to mental health care in Singapore. Last but not least, another major concern for Singaporean families may be the significant financial costs associated with mental health care for clients and their families. According to Chong (2007), many of the mentally ill in Singapore do not have adequate cover under their Medisave accounts, a national healthcare savings scheme that draws from an individual's own income. Furthermore, Medishield, a basic medical insurance scheme aimed at defraying long-term medical expenses, only recently began to cover treatment of psychiatric conditions, and then only for conditions diagnosed after 1 March 2013 (Ministry of Health, 2007).

TABLE 2. MENTAL HEALTH PROMOTION

Focus	Sample programme	Goals
Outreach in Schools	Children's One-stop Psycho-Educational services (COPE)	Help secondary school youth to manage their emotions
Outreach at Workplaces	Treasure your mind (TYM)	Raise mental health awareness of working adults
Outreach in the Community	Nurture your mind (NYM)	Promotion of mental well being in community settings
Public Education	Dementia and Depression public education plan	Promotion of knowledge of dementia and depression

Clinical psychologists are thus positioned to play a crucial role in promoting an understanding of mental health problems, raising awareness of the value of psychological services, and improving access to them. This may be carried out through general mental health promotion campaigns and outreach at schools, workplaces, and the community through the Health Promotion Board, the provision of community and inpatient programs by public hospitals, and, as many of our authors are doing, through assessment and therapy with individuals and families in public and private practice. Some examples of additional programs and initiatives are outlined in Table 2.

Developing Manpower—Clinical Psychology Training in Singapore

The development of current and new mental health services requires the ongoing recruitment of clinical psychologists. As a relatively new profession in Singapore, the number of practising clinical psychologists remains significantly lower than what is required for population needs. Until recently, postgraduate psychology courses were unavailable, so psychologists in training had to pursue formal training overseas. More commonly, and to address the shortage of clinical psychologists, a significant number of practitioners received 'on-the-job training' and supervision. This meant taking on mental health care roles straight out of their undergraduate major in Psychology, or after having obtained a related master's degree without further clinical psychology training involving supervised clinical placements and coursework.

To address this gap in formal training, and to raise the standard of psychological knowledge and practice, two local universities recently created postgraduate programs in clinical psychology: the National University of Singapore (NUS) and James Cook University (JCU); both were initiated in conjunction with Australian universities (Melbourne University and JCU respectively). These local training programs are closely aligned with Australian training guidelines and curriculum and rely predominantly on Western research and textbooks. Furthermore, many psychologists working in Singapore have been trained in Europe, North America and Australasia. As such, clinical psychology in Singapore continues to have strong foreign, and particularly Western, influence. Whilst these academic roots are predominantly foreign, the *practice* of clinical psychology occurs within its unique cultural landscape, and is provided primarily by Singaporean clinicians for Singaporean clients and their families.

JCU has been offering postgraduate programs in clinical psychology since 2004; to date 50 students have graduated with a master's degree (32) or clinical doctorate (18). NUS more recently started offering two master's programs in 2008: an NUS only program and a joint degree program (JDP) with the University of Melbourne. To date 95 students have graduated from the NUS master's program, while 36 are currently enrolled. NUS is currently reviewing options for doctoral level clinical psychology program.

At both schools, most of the clinical psychology students are women, with males typically accounting for less than 20% of any given cohort (pers. comm. with program coordinators; *see* Table 3). It is not unusual to have a gender difference in this profession, with more females choosing this career. However, such a low proportion of male clinical psychologists may act as a barrier for accessing psychological services if clients would prefer to be seen by a male.

TABLE 3. GENDER OF CANDIDATES ENROLLED IN NUS CLINICAL PSYCHOLOGY PROGRAMMES 2008–14	
Females	80 (82.5%)
Males	17 (17.5%)
Total	**97 (100.0%)**

Note: Data available for NUS programmes only

Both the JCU and NUS programs are self-funded, with fees ranging from 58,005 SGD for a two-year master's to 87,024 SGD for a doctoral program (fees as of 2014). These are significant costs for aspiring clinical psychology students, and probably affect what demographic of students applies for the courses. Fortunately, a number of scholarships are available on a case-by-case basis as outlined in Table 4 (data available for NUS programs only). Just over half (57%) of NUS candidates were able to obtain scholarships between 2008 and 2014. The greatest number of scholarships was provided by Ministry of Health Holdings (MOHH) (23.7%) and the Institute of Mental Health (IMH) (16.5%). As the number of available scholarships varies from year to year, there is some uncertainty about how much funding is available for future students. Scholarship recipients are usually required to serve a bond with their sponsoring organisation for a period of two and a half to four years. Scholarships thus increase the likelihood of candidates remaining in Singapore upon graduation, and contribute to the manpower required locally. They also provide an important channel for more equitable selection of trainees, ensuring that this profession is not only available to individuals with affluence or those who belong to certain ethnic groups.

Despite the introduction of programs by NUS and JCU and the scholarships available, there continues to be an unmet demand for highly qualified and experienced clinical psychologists. To meet this demand, more training and professional development opportunities are required. This includes increasing and improving on existing master's programs and the implementing of more doctoral level programs to ensure higher level skills and the ability to take on specialist positions and leadership roles. Furthermore, the fast development of the profession and services in Singapore will benefit significantly from ensuring that senior and highly trained psychologists are available to provide mentorship and clinical supervision (*see* later). These services are vital in assisting other mental health clinicians to reflect on and develop their own skills and for ensuring patient best practices.

TABLE 4. SCHOLARSHIP DISTRIBUTION TO NUS CLINICAL PSYCHOLOGY STUDENTS (2008—14)	
Ministry Of Health Holdings (MOHH)	23 (23.7%)
Institute of Mental Health (IMH)	16 (16.5%)
Ministry of Social and Family development (MSF)	2 (2.1%)
National Healthcare Group (NHG)	3 (3.1%)
Singapore Prison Service	3 (3.1%)
National Council of Social Services (NCSS)	2 (2.1%)
Workforce Development Agency (WDA)	1 (1.0%)
Tan Tock Seng Hospital (TTSH)	1 (1.0%)
Singapore General Hospital (SGH)	1 (1.0%)
Ministry Of Education (MOE)	1 (1.0%)
Ngee Ann Polytechnic	1 (1.0%)
Health Manpower Development Plan (HMDP by Singhealth)	1 (1.0%)
Self-funded	42 (43.3%)
Total	**97 (100.0%)**

Regulation and Registration of the Clinical Psychology Profession

There is currently no formal or legal regulation for setting up a clinical psychology practice in Singapore. The statutory regulation of the profession is imminent and will be a positive development. This process requires that psychologists must be registered to practise; this protects the title 'psychologist' and provides reassurance to the public of a psychologist's competence and fitness to practise. It also creates a system of accountability to ensure that the service provided is of a certain standard. Regulation can also stipulate ongoing professional development requirements and outline criteria for training and supervision to ensure psychologists consistently provide high levels of quality training, practice and service delivery.

The Singapore Psychological Society (SPS) was founded in 1979 with a mission to "advance psychology as a science and as a profession in Singapore" and ensure high standards of professional practice. In order to accomplish this, SPS maintains a register of psychologists where psychologists' qualifications and experience are verified. This is consistent with practices of other international psychology associations, like the American Psychological Association (APA) and the Australian Psychological Society (APS) that have a register for clinical psychologists. The SPS currently has 236 members, of which only 59 (25%) are clinical psychologists (SPS, 2014).

One of the key challenges for the SPS is that registration is currently not mandatory and no formal licensing procedures exist for clinical psychologists. Furthermore, only a small number of services require SPS registration as a prerequisite for their psychologist employees. Accordingly, there is little incentive for clinical psychologists to register. Because of the absence of a mandatory register for psychologists in Singapore, an accurate number of clinical psychologists is not available. In a recent study of senior clinical psychologists providing supervision in Singapore, 59% of participants were registered with SPS, 30.8% were registered with the Australian Psychological Society, 20.5% indicated that they were neither registered nor licensed as a psychologist in any country, and a small proportion was registered elsewhere (Law & Lange, unpublished).

While the SPS is striving to work towards a national register and act as the body overseeing the quality of psychology services, the Ministry of Health (MOH) has independently started its own process of accrediting and licensing allied health professions through the Allied Health Professionals Act (2011). Occupational therapists, physiotherapists and speech-language therapists have recently been regulated under this Act, with other allied health professions, including clinical psychologists, expected to be included in the coming years.

Mental Health Research

Singapore is ideal for research as there are discrete, homogenous ethnic groups, in a concentrated geographical area. Conducting and disseminating mental health research and examining the practices of clinical psychology in Singapore are essential to improving existing mental health services. The authors of this casebook have provided references to local research and resources pertaining to their cases. While the availability of research varies for different presenting issues, authors consistently report limited availability of local data on many mental health problems, assessment tools, and therapy outcomes. Whilst publication of local research is increasing, Singaporean psychologists will have to continue relying on clinical research and normative data from overseas.

<table>
<tr><td colspan="2" style="background:#555;color:#fff">TABLE 5. CULTURAL SPECIFIC THEMES</td></tr>
<tr><td>Cultural Themes</td><td>Adaptations</td></tr>
<tr><td>Language</td><td>A language-appropriate service refers to not only the use of clients' preferred language but also to understanding the meaning of particular uses of language (e.g., English or Hokkien dialect), and how it is used by different groups such as children or the elderly.</td></tr>
<tr><td>Persons</td><td>Person factors include characteristics such as race and ethnicity. Matching clients with therapists has been shown to be related to remaining in treatment longer (Coleman, Wampold, & Casali, 1995).</td></tr>
<tr><td>Metaphors</td><td>Infusion of cultural metaphors, symbols, and overarching cultural concepts can align therapy with existing client belief systems and heuristics. For instance, cultural sayings can be used in therapy to more clearly convey meaning or insights to clients.</td></tr>
<tr><td>Content</td><td>Attending to the cultural content of a mental health treatment can enhance alignment with client worldviews.

For example, some Singaporeans having a more collectivist belief system and practices might benefit from not pathologizing these and not emphasising aspects such as individuation or differentiation.</td></tr>
<tr><td>Concepts</td><td>Unique cultural concepts, such as "face" or being "kiasu" (Chinese idea of being afraid of "losing out") should be understood and respected in therapy.</td></tr>
<tr><td>Goals and methods</td><td>Customs and cultural values should be considered in setting treatment goals and establishing suitable procedures to reach those them.</td></tr>
<tr><td>Context</td><td>Consideration of context allows clinicians and clients to examine broader issues, such as the social and economic realities that may include acculturative stress, migration, availability of social supports, or pressures for couples to both work.</td></tr>
</table>

Note: Adapted from Bernal & Sáez-Santiago (2006)

However, there has been increasing interest in establishing local evidence-based measures and norms. For example, Collinson et al. (2014) conducted a study that provides normative data from over 1,000 Singaporeans aged 55 and older on the Singapore adaptation of the widely used Repeatable Battery for the Assessment of Neuropsychological Status (RBANS) test. More normative studies are needed to afford psychologists more confidence in using psychological assessment and therapy tools.

A large proportion of clinicians are trained overseas, and consequently incorporate Western frameworks into their practice. Limited research exists as to whether these clinical models and theories of mental disorders and therapies can be applied to local clients. Singaporean clinicians would thus benefit from research that addresses these issues, and evaluates the differences in various cultural groups' experience and expression of psychological distress. Also of value would be the study of factors influencing ethnic groups' access to and engagement in psychological services. As agencies and clinicians are increasingly required to provide data on the efficacy and efficiency of their services, this push for evidence-based practices can provide a positive opportunity for psychologists to do 'in-house' research—assessing what works or not in their local setting and adjusting their practice accordingly.

The last few decades have seen significant inroads into research on cross-cultural adaptation of psychological assessment and treatment. A commonly highlighted finding is the advantage of treatment adapted to specific ethnic groups and cultures. (Smith et al., 2011). Bernal & Sáez-Santiago (2006) have identified eight common cultural themes that provide a useful framework for the alignment of psychological services to culturally diverse clients (*see* Table 5). Each of these themes emerges throughout the case studies in this book as authors describe various factors that impact on their work with their clients.

FUTURE DIRECTIONS OF CLINICAL PSYCHOLOGY IN SINGAPORE

Clinical psychology is a discipline that has been evolving significantly in Singapore over the last ten years, but still requires significant development, regulation and support. We can identify five important future directions:

Clinical Training

More places in local postgraduate clinical psychology courses need to be offered to meet the increasing demand for mental health professionals. This is in line with the Health Manpower Development Plan (HMDP, 2008), as outlined in the Singapore Mental Health Blueprint. Scholarships play a valuable role in supporting students' access to these courses. In addition to grades and experience, selection of scholarship candidates should consider demographic factors relevant to needs of the local population by prioritising students who are from cultural minorities, have different language skills, or are male. Lastly, additional doctoral level clinical programs are important to provide a higher level of training, expertise and additional competencies beyond those obtained at the master's level.

Clinical Supervision

Supervision is a key element in the training and promotion of the professional development of clinical psychologists. Clinical supervision involves meeting regularly with another professional (normally with training in the skills of supervision) to discuss casework and other professional issues in a structured way. The purpose of supervision is to help a clinician learn from their experience, develop their skills, and ensure best practice for their clients and service. There is a need for more clinical supervisors to train new graduates and to supervise less experienced clinicians. Increased supervision will also ensure an appropriate process for addressing many challenging clinical, ethical, and professional issues (e.g., managing at risk clients, or preventing therapist burnout), and for maintaining self-care for students and clinicians practising in this challenging profession (Law & Lange, unpublished).

Clinical supervision needs to be a recognised and essential activity, implemented as part of a clinician's regular workload. Organisational or government funding could help overcome existing challenges, including limited funding and the number of supervisors as well as recognition of the benefits of supervision for both clinicians and patients, and the risks of not providing supervision. To ensure a high level of quality and safety in clinical supervision practices in Singapore, we may learn from psychology boards in other developed nations, such as Australia and the UK, who have outlined board-approved standards, competencies and training required for clinical supervisors (Law & Lange, unpublished).

Registration or Licensing

Registration for both clinical psychologists and clinical supervisors should be established. Many overseas psychology boards now require the formal registration of clinical psychologists and training for supervisors to ensure best practices. This would also provide a framework for training, continuous professional development, as well as overall quality assurance.

Culturally Adaptive Practice

Awareness and sensitivity to local culture allows clinicians to best meet the needs of their clients. Assessments as well as therapy practices need to be adapted whenever possible or relevant. Working on reducing stigma and reaching out to clients most at need or members of minority groups or marginalised communities is important. Mental healthcare systems and clinical psychologists play an ongoing role in this process. For example, through the Healthy Mind Hub, the governmental Health Promotion Board is working towards preventative mental healthcare by promoting mental resilience and positive mental well-being.

Culturally Sensitive Research

Clinical psychologists are trained as scientist-practitioners and have the opportunity to conduct local research, examine the epidemiology of mental disorders, and assess how interventions may be adapted to different clients in the local context. Singapore provides many exciting opportunities for clinicians to conduct such research. For example, frameworks such as those proposed by Bernal & Sáez-Santiago (2006) and Smith et al. (2011) could be empirically tested; normative data could be developed for commonly used assessment tools, and treatment outcomes for typically utilised interventions could be studied.

CONCLUSION

The profession and discipline of clinical psychology is going through dynamic change with many exciting opportunities in training, practice, governance, and research. Our casebook strives to contribute to an understanding of how clinical psychology fits into the unique Singaporean context. We aim to discuss how individuals enter the mental healthcare system, how intervention is adapted to a local setting, what challenges clients and their therapists face, how their treatment outcomes are evaluated, and how clinical psychology services can be tailored to local needs.

This introductory chapter provides the context for the varied and complex case studies that follow. The following chapters give a snapshot of clinical psychology *in practice* in Singapore. This book is therefore a unique resource, offering insights into the practices and principles of clinical psychologists contextually placed within the local mental health services. Each chapter emphasises not only the diversity and challenges faced by clinical psychologists in Singapore but also the creative ways in which they leverage the cultural and social context to help their patients.

PART 1.

CHILD AND FAMILY

CHAPTER 1.

BETTER DEAD THAN FED

Eating Disorder (Anorexia Nervosa)

RANJANI UTPALA

INTRODUCTION

Julia, a 16-year-old Chinese girl, was reluctantly brought to an outpatient psychiatrist by her mother, Anne, and subsequently referred to a psychologist. A year before presentation, Julia had started complaining about her weight and food intake. She had begun cutting "junk food" from her diet and restricting her consumption of carbohydrates, sugar and fats. As Anne worked daily from 7am to 8:30–9pm, Julia remained unsupervised in her absence. About six months prior to presentation, a neighbour informed Anne that she often caught sight of Julia sprinting up and down the stairs of their HDB block after school. Over the next few months, Anne noticed that while the intensity of her daughter's exercise regime increased, her appetite decreased and she was rapidly losing weight. When finally assessed, Julia had been amenorrheic for four months, was 158 cm tall and weighed 38 kg (BMI 15.2), which placed her in the "underweight" category (*see* Table 1.1).

During her intake session with the psychologist, Julia was adamant that she did not have an eating disorder, and did not need treatment. She "knew" that she was fat because she had not reached her ideal weight of 32 kg and felt that her mother was overreacting to her weight loss. Julia's breakfast consisted of a glass of diluted milk (one part milk, three parts water) and lunch was a piece of fruit. A light dinner was usually eaten at home under her mother's supervision. Her exercise regime included 100 sit-ups, 100 crunches, 100 leg presses and 100 leg-ups twice a day. Additionally, she was running about 5 km daily and taking the stairs to her apartment on the twelfth floor at least twice a day. She acknowledged having very low levels of energy, feeling tired most of the time, and falling asleep in class. While Julia had some awareness of her restricted diet, she felt disgusted by how "greedy" she could be when, for example, she treated herself to a spoonful of low-fat yogurt.

TABLE 1.1. BODY MASS INDEX (BMI) BY AGE (YEARS)								
Weight status	Percentile	BMI by age (years)						
		12	13	14	15	16	17	18
FEMALES								
Severely Underweight	<3rd	≤14.4	≤14.8	≤15.1	≤15.4	≤15.7	≤15.9	≤16.1
Underweight	3rd – <5th	14.5–14.8	14.9–15.2	15.2–15.5	15.5–15.8	15.8–16.1	16.0–16.3	16.2–16.5
Acceptable weight	5th – <90th	14.9–23.4	15.3–24	15.6–24.6	15.9–25	16.2–25.4	16.4–25.7	16.6–25.9
Overweight	90th – <97th	23.5–27.5	24.1–28.3	24.7–28.9	25.1–29.4	25.5–29.7	25.8–30	26.0–30.3
Severely Overweight	≥ 97th	≥27.6	≥28.4	≥29	≥29.5	≥29.8	≥30.1	≥30.4
MALES								
Severely Underweight	<3rd	≤14.4	≤14.7	≤15	≤15.3	≤15.6	≤15.9	≤16.1
Underweight	3rd – <5th	14.5–14.8	14.8–15.1	15.1–15.4	15.4–15.8	15.7–16.1	16.0–16.3	16.2–16.6
Acceptable weight	5th – <90th	14.9–24.3	15.2–25	15.5–25.5	15.9–26.1	16.2–26.5	16.4–27	16.7–27.4
Overweight	90th – <97th	24.4–29.2	25.1–30	25.6–30.6	26.2–31.2	26.6–31.7	27.1–32.1	27.5–32.4
Severely Overweight	≥ 97th	≥29.3	≥30.1	≥30.7	≥31.3	≥31.8	≥32.2	≥32.5

BMI-for-age chart developed by Health Promotion Board, Singapore (2002).

BACKGROUND

Julia was born full-term, the elder of two children, and her physical, cognitive and psychosocial development was within normal limits. Prior to the onset of the eating disorder, she had no significant medical or psychiatric history. Her parents, Anne and Trevor, separated when she was two because of Trevor's infidelity, ongoing substance abuse, and gambling. During the three-year separation, Anne and Trevor often reunited. Julia's younger brother, Shane, was conceived during one of these reconciliations. However, the couple was divorced at the time of his birth, when Julia was five. Neither Anne nor Julia reported any significant distress throughout that period.

As a child, Julia was well-liked by her peer group and had many friends. When she was between eight to nine years old, she was enrolled in the school's Trim and Fit (TAF) club. While this surprised Anne as she felt that Julia was "cute and chubby, not fat", she considered it an opportunity for her to learn about diet and exercise as she had gained some weight since commencing primary school. Julia reported some teasing by classmates for belonging to the "FAT" club (TAF spelt backwards), but by the end of primary school, she had been out of the program for over a year. She made a smooth transition into secondary school and was a high achiever, receiving grades of 85 or more in her examinations. Her favourite subjects were mathematics and science, and she took up dance and piano as co-curricular activities.

Despite Anne having full custody of both children, Shane lived with his father for the better part of five years. Julia developed a close relationship with her mother for the first eight to ten years of her life, and was happy Shane didn't live with them. Anne reported that Julia felt rejected by her father's clear preference for Shane; she denied this but became withdrawn and sullen when discussing her relationship with her father. When Julia was nine, Anne met her current husband, Chris, and married him two years later. This transition was particularly hard for Julia as they moved in with Chris and she now had to "share mum".

ASSESSMENT

The clinical psychologist's assessment comprised a 60-minute interview focused on Julia's eating behaviours; her body concept, beliefs about weight, fear of fatness and

> **Fact Box 1.1. Changes in Diagnostic Criteria from DSM-IV-TR to DSM-5**
>
> - Removal of "refusal to maintain weight" as this implies intention on part of the patient which can be hard to assess;
>
> - Amenorrhea criteria removed: this allows for a broader group of people including males.
>
> - Pre-menarchal and post-menopausal females to be diagnosed accurately as well as those women who exhibit all other AN symptoms but continue to menstruate.
>
> - DSM-5 includes ability to state if person is in partial/full remission. Partial remission: if full criteria were met previously and Criterion A is no longer met, but B and C are still present. Full remission: full criteria met previously but not presently.
>
> DSM-5 allows for classification of severity of the disorder based on BMI.

weight gain; her experience of the illness and perception of her current state; risk assessment; and motivation and goals for treatment. During this session, Julia made little eye contact, spoke very little, gave monosyllabic responses and was initially difficult to engage. However, she opened up when the therapist shifted the focus from her eating habits to her frustration at being "unfairly dragged" to therapy by her mother. She displayed a low level of motivation, and declined to complete self-report measures such as the Eating Disorders Questionnaire (EDE-Q; Fairburn & Beglin, 2008), the Eating Attitudes Test (EAT-26; Garner, Olmstead, Bohr, & Garfinkel, 1982). Such measures can be helpful as they provide additional information about ED symptoms and behaviours that a client might not openly discuss. Further, they can also be used as outcome measures to evaluate progress of therapy.

While Julia reported fleeting thoughts of suicide, she had never harmed herself intentionally and denied any current intention to do so. At most, she would pinch herself when she was feeling very distressed. She was thus assessed to be at low-risk for self-harm. This level of risk changed significantly over the course of treatment and will be described in detail in the treatment section. There was no risk of violence to others or from others towards her. However, establishing medical safety was paramount and Julia was reviewed regularly by the physician-in-charge who admitted her to hospital when she became medically unstable.

DIAGNOSIS

Based on the Diagnostic and Statistical Manual, fifth edition (DSM-5; American Psychiatric Association, 2013), Julia met the criteria for Anorexia Nervosa (AN), Restricting Type, Severe, which are as follows:

Criterion A: Significantly low body weight

With a BMI of 15.2, Julia was considerably underweight and had not gained any height during adolescence, contrary to what is expected of a typically developing youth.

Criterion B: Intense fear of gaining weight or becoming fat, or persistent behaviour that interferes with weight gain

Despite having a very low weight, Julia was highly fearful of gaining weight and felt that she needed to lose more weight. She restricted her food intake and exercised excessively in order to avoid putting on weight.

Criterion C: Disturbances in perception of weight and shape

Julia was absolutely certain that weighing over her subjective target of 32kg meant that she was fat. Despite being severely underweight and malnourished—her body had stopped functioning at its full capacity, resulting in amenorrhea—Julia could not grasp the seriousness of her low weight and the extent of her illness. Severe weight loss can result from a medical condition or major depressive disorder (MDD). However, individuals with MDD do not express a conscious desire for weight loss, nor do they exhibit distorted body perceptions associated with AN. MDD was therefore ruled out as a differential diagnosis for Julia. No medical problems were discovered that could better account for Julia's weight loss.

FIGURE 1.1. INTEGRATIVE FORMULATION

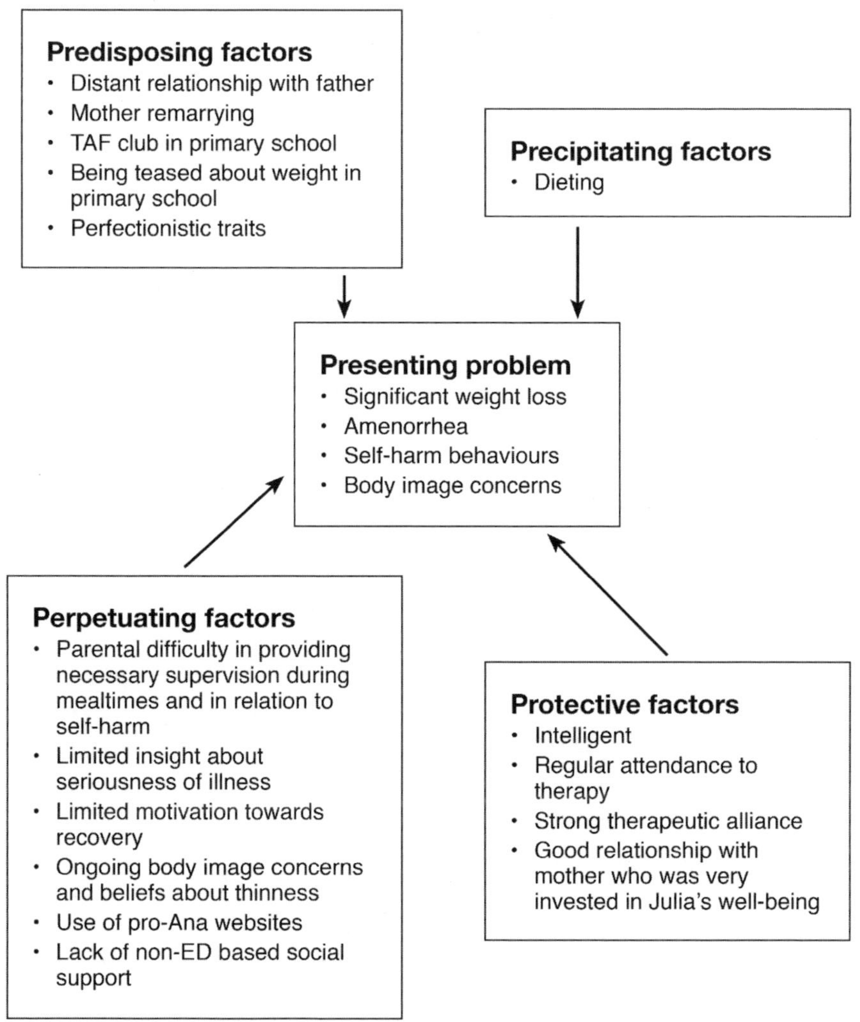

Figure 1.1 depicts the case formulation and how various factors are linked to the presenting problems.

Following the psychologist's intake assessment, family-based treatment for anorexia nervosa (FBT-AN; Lock, Le Grange, Agras & Dare, 2001) was suggested as a means of intervention, as recommended by the current best practice guidelines of the National Institute for Health and Clinical Excellence (NICE, 2004). However, Trevor did not want to be involved in Julia's treatment. Anne and Chris were unable to take time off work. On top of that, Anne believed that it was the responsibility of trained professionals, rather than the family, to help Julia. She insisted that Julia receive individual therapy.

Because of her low level of insight and motivation, Julia struggled to identify recovery-based goals for treatment. During the first therapy session, she told the therapist that she was only attending the session to "get mum off my back". The therapist used Julia's frustration as the focal point of therapy to build rapport, provide validation and enhance motivation.

The First Admission: Building Rapport and Acknowledging ED

Julia was initially seen as an outpatient for two sessions, after which she was admitted to hospital due to a drastic weight loss of 2 kg within two weeks. As an inpatient, Julia reluctantly engaged in mandatory therapy sessions that were primarily aimed at providing supportive therapy. As she was closely monitored in the hospital, Julia was unable to restrict her food intake or engage in exercise. She found these limitations highly distressing and was emphatic about losing weight upon being discharged.

> **Fact Box 1.2. What is Family-Based Treatment (FBT)?**
>
> FBT draws from several family therapy models and is currently the best established treatment for adolescents with AN. This treatment approach (popularly known as the "Maudsley method") is a manualised program in which the therapist empowers parents to team up and implement various behavioural and psychological strategies required for weight restoration, provided that the adolescent is medically stable. FBT-AN is based on the principle that hospitalization is not a cure for AN. Rather, parents are seen as the primary resource in the treatment of their child's illness. The treatment program aims to assist parents in the process of helping their child recover at home by leveraging parental love and understanding of their child and family, together with the consultant expertise of the therapist (Eisler, Lock & Le Grange, 2010).

Therapy sessions focused on her adjustment to the ward environment and the management of challenges she faced in the ward (e.g., eating at meal times, comparing herself to patients who remained thinner than herself while she gained weight). The therapist used empathic validation to allow her to process the loss and grief that she was feeling and encouraged her to explore aspects of herself that were not weight-related. Although she initially struggled with this, Julia was able to identify that she wanted to excel in dance and academic work, particularly her dream of studying overseas. Helping Julia to broaden her perspective and identify goals and values allowed her to think of life outside the eating disorder ("ED").

About a month into the admission, Julia began acknowledging that she had an ED and became more open to discussing her challenges. Although she found it challenging to finish all her meals in hospital, she felt comforted by the fact that she did not have a choice in the matter. The psychologist used "externalizing ED" as a method of helping Julia make a distinction between her own and the ED's voice. Julia was able to identify that there was a part of her that did not allow her to make healthy choices about food and exercise. Despite this, she saw ED as a friend who offered safety and comfort. In order to help her gain a more balanced perspective of ED, Julia was encouraged to write a letter to ED both as a friend and an enemy. While she wrote a long letter to ED as her friend, she was unable to write to ED as an enemy.

Towards the end of the admission, Julia began to have meal outings with her mother and struggled to eat under her mother's supervision. On each of the visits, she would refuse to eat, preferring to come back to hospital to have her meal. In therapy sessions, Julia said that the ED voice was very strong at mealtimes and knew that if she made a fuss, her mother would back down.

The psychologist met with Anne to discuss strategies to put into place on meal outings. However, Anne was unable to supervise Julia during meals and consequently, Julia was unable to fully overcome ED at mealtimes, especially outside of the hospital. In an effort to facilitate discharge planning, FBT was once again offered to Anne as part of the treatment plan; however, Anne declined due to Julia's strong objections. Subsequently, Julia was discharged after ten weeks in hospital during which she gained about 8 kg; her weight was 44 kg and BMI was 17.6.

The Second Admission: Talking about Safety

Post-discharge, Julia did not attend therapy and was next seen by the psychologist about four weeks later when she was admitted to hospital following an intentional overdose of 30 paracetamol tablets. She had also lost about 3 kg.

During this admission, Julia was more open in therapy as she was shaken up by her overdose. She had not intended to kill herself but simply wanted to "sleep forever" as she was tired of fighting the ED's voice. Julia told the psychologist that she had been engaging in self-harm behaviours for about a year. She had initially started pinching and hitting her stomach and eventually began cutting her upper thigh and stomach with a razor blade, and spoke of visiting pro-ED websites where she learnt new ways to self-harm through disordered eating. Julia's use of pro-ED websites was brought to Anne's attention but Anne did not think she could monitor Julia's internet use.

The focus of weekly therapy sessions during this five-week admission was on Julia's self-harm. The therapist worked with Julia to conduct a detailed behaviour chain analysis of the environmental and intrapersonal factors preceding and following the overdose. Other strategies that were used included teaching Julia emotion regulation as well as distress tolerance skills such as sublimation techniques (using drawing or writing to overcome urges) and self-soothing (doing her nails or mum's hair). Julia responded well to the traffic light system, which involves using the colours "red", "yellow" or "green" as a way of communicating her current level of risk. Rather than voice her feelings, Julia would communicate her level of distress to ward staff and parents by using a colour card. "Red" meant that she needed supervision as she could not guarantee her own safety, "yellow" meant that she was having thoughts of hurting herself but felt confident that she could rely on her own skills to manage, and "green" meant that she was safe. She identified as being "red" once during her admission and it took her close to an hour to move from "red" to "green", during which time she was closely monitored and used activities to distract herself (writing in her journal, drawing and doing her homework).

At discharge Julia had gained about 4 kg and weighed 45.5 kg. Although she continued to restrict her food intake during the day, Anne supervised dinner times and Julia maintained her weight for about a month post-discharge. During this time, she was very distressed by her increased weight and sessions focused on exploring her body image concerns. Exercises included building pictorial collages of her notions of beauty, identifying people in media she looked up to for reasons other than physical beauty and exploring the difference between "body as form" vs "body as function". Media literacy work was undertaken as a way of helping her dissect the reality of what is portrayed in the media. During one of the sessions, she was asked to use clay to sculpt her body as she saw it. During this exercise, Julia recalled that her aunt had recently described her as looking "well fed" and said "I'd rather be dead than well fed!" She then proceeded to draw incisions on her "clay body" and eventually decapitated it. Julia was weeping inconsolably at this stage and said that she was "red". Her mother was contacted but as she was unable to attend to her, Julia was escorted to A&E. Although she had calmed down significantly by the time she was seen and denied thoughts of suicide, she was admitted to the ward.

The Third Admission: I'm a Celebrity, Get Me Out of Here

During a week-long admission aimed at stabilizing her mood, Julia finally wrote her "ED as my enemy" letter. Among other things, she wrote "you have made me a celebrity in a place where it doesn't matter if you are a celebrity or not. You have destroyed everything that is important to me and I can't do the things I love because of you." At the therapist's request, Julia completed the Anorexia Nervosa Stages of Change Questionnaire (ANSOCQ; Rieger, Touyz, Schotte, Beumont, Russell, Clarke et al., 2000), which assesses the patient's readiness to change; Julia's responses showed that she was in the "pre-contemplation" stage. Figure 1.2 shows a diagrammatic representation of the stages of change model.

Following this admission, Julia was seen for about 17–20 outpatient sessions. Initial sessions focused on developing a safety plan that included things she could do, places she could go and people she could call when feeling unsafe. Julia assembled a 'survival tool kit', which was a physical box that contained flashcards with the traffic light cards, affirmations, distraction strategies, her goals, red paint to use to draw on her body (because she liked to see blood), etc. Although she continued to have thoughts of self-harm, Julia was able to effectively use her tool kit and adhere to her safety plan for almost two months.

FIGURE 1.2. STAGES OF CHANGE MODEL BY PROCHASKA AND DICLEMENTE (1983)

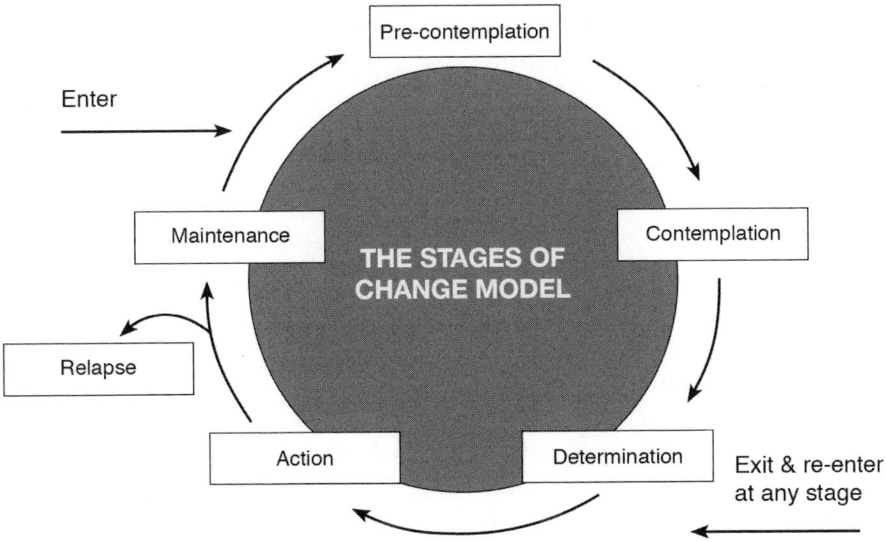

Adapted from http://johnnyholland.org.

In addition to safety planning, motivational enhancement therapy was undertaken and included activities like values identification (80th birthday reflective exercise), decision-making (pros and cons of ED vs recovery) and extending identity beyond ED (exploring non-ED Julia's wants). The pace of therapy was slow, matching Julia's ambivalence regarding change, and sessions often involved expressing empathy and validation for her struggles.

After eight weeks, Julia's mood and affect in session were visibly different. She became more sullen and withdrawn and did not engage as well in therapy. During one session, she disclosed that although she did not have active thoughts of suicide, she had recommenced cutting her upper thighs and stomach as a way of regulating her emotion. A behavioural chain analysis revealed that a few weeks prior when she showed her mother the "red" card, Anne had said, "You can't always depend on me" and this triggered Julia. The next four to five sessions focused on Julia's relationship with her mother, the sense of rejection and abandonment she felt when she heard "you can't always depend on me" and when Anne had remarried.

Anne was invited to a session during which she expressed her confusion about why Julia was "still sick" when her weight was stable. She was highly critical of Julia and felt that the self-harm behaviours were merely attention-seeking and the problem with food was "just in her head". Despite the high level of criticism, Anne was genuinely worried about Julia's health and future. Anne was seen individually to explore her frustration and to give her psycho-education about eating disorders. Anne expressed her fear that she was losing Julia because of the ED and she was taken through the externalization of ED exercise to help her separate her child from the ED. Lastly, a relationship repair session allowed each of them to express their individual wishes and limitations. Once Anne renewed her commitment to supporting Julia during times of crisis, the relationship started to mend.

About a month after these sessions, during which Julia and the therapist continued to work on her ED symptoms, in particular, distorted perception of her body and decreasing levels of exercise, the therapist resigned from her role and informed Julia that she would be leaving in two months. The plan was for her care to be transferred to another psychologist on the team, but Julia struggled with the departure of her psychologist and the loss of the therapeutic relationship. She only attended two sessions after this. In what turned out to be the last session, Julia was silent and cried throughout the session, while the therapist sat with her in silence for the most part. The last thing Julia said as she walked out was "I can't say goodbye to you."

Although follow-up therapy was recommended for Julia, she did not attend appointments to see the psychologist and failed to attend her psychiatric reviews once she stopped seeing the psychologist. Anne was aware that Julia was not seeking treatment because she did not want to and could not be persuaded otherwise. Anne stated that she would monitor Julia's eating as well as mood and take her to A&E if she was concerned for her safety.

DISCUSSION

Julia initially presented as an outpatient, but was admitted to hospital due to significant weight loss within a short period of time. At the time of her first admission, Julia was severely dehydrated, bradycardic (low heart rate) and, at the age of 16, was at risk of having a stroke. Medical complications secondary to AN are numerous and can be potentially life-threatening. Some early signs that life-threatening starvation has begun include loss of menstruation in postmenarcheal females, hypothermia (low body temperature), hypotension (low blood pressure), osteopenia and/or osteoporosis, dry and flaky skin, lanugo, and cardiac dysfunction (Crow & Swigart, 2005). Chronic medical consequences as a result of starvation include impact to the central nervous system, the cardiovascular, renal, gastrointestinal and endocrine systems. Therefore, careful and regular medical assessment is a critical component of treatment of an eating-disordered patient.

The most frustrating aspect of working with Julia was the lack of family involvement, especially for an evidence-based treatment for an illness known to have poor prognosis. The National Institute for Health and Clinical Excellence (NICE, 2004) guidelines recommend that "family interventions that directly address the eating disorder should be offered to children and adolescents with anorexia nervosa". Family-based treatment for AN (FBT-AN) was initially developed for treatment of anorexia nervosa in adolescents (Lock et al., 2001) and has since been adapted for treatment of bulimia nervosa (Le Grange & Lock, 2007). Provided that the adolescent is medically stable, parents are seen as the primary resource in the treatment of their child's illness. FBT empowers parents to help their child recover at home by implementing behavioural and psychological strategies aimed at weight restoration and maintenance (Eisler, Lock & Le Grange, 2010).

Although the family was offered FBT, they declined as they were unable to attend FBT sessions because of work commitments. While this may have been the case, cultural factors may also have been at play. Asians tend to place high importance on the expertise of professionals (Lin & Cheung, 1999) and this was apparent in Anne's beliefs about "trained professionals" helping Julia. An FBT clinician resists the expert stance and works to empower parents to take charge of their child's recovery. However, Anne might have felt overwhelmed by this prospect.

Fact Box 1.3. The Holistic Health Framework in Singapore

After the Trim and Fit club (TAF) was discontinued, weight management programs in schools now sit under the umbrella of the Holistic Health Framework (HFF) initiative. HHF has expanded the focus from physical health to include social and mental health well-being of students; one of its principles is to promote inclusion and ensure that overweight students are not singled out. Membership of HHF is not compulsory but schools do continue to run weight management programs based on HHF principles.

Furthermore, since mental illness is seen by Asians as reflecting poorly on the family (Leong & Lau, 2001), it is possible that a family-based approach might have been interpreted by Anne as blaming the family. Although the therapist emphasized that FBT is not about attributing blame, in collectivistic societies people tend to be reluctant to discuss personal problems with those outside of their reference group (Baeollo & Mori, 2007), and it is possible that Anne did not feel comfortable being open with the therapist about her concerns.

As Julia's parents were unable to commit to FBT, the prognosis for Julia from the outset was poor. Given the ego-syntonic nature of AN, Julia had very limited insight into the seriousness of her illness, which was worsened by her ongoing use of "pro-ana" websites that provided tips and advice from other sufferers. The use of such websites among the ED population is prolific (Wilson, Peebles, Hardy, & Litt, 2006) and adolescents exposed to these websites are likely to have higher levels of body dissatisfaction, decreased quality of life, and longer durations of EDs (Borzekowski, Schenk, Wilson, & Peebles, 2010). Julia's continued use of these websites and Anne's refusal to restrict this behaviour were maintaining factors that were detrimental to her recovery. This highlights the importance of clinicians assessing internet usage and providing parental education about associated harm, and to work actively with parents to discourage use of harmful sites.

As a child, Julia had been slightly overweight and was enrolled in the Trim and Fit (TAF) club at school. The TAF program was an MOE initiative, which ran from 1992–2007, aimed at reducing the risk of childhood obesity. The program was successful in meeting these aims as prevalence of overweight students decreased from 11.7% in 1993 to 9.5% in 2006 (The National Bureau of Asian Research, 2008). However, there was stigma attached to being in the program (Ho, 2010). In a study of 4,400 Singaporean females aged 12–24 years, of the 7% of the sample who were at risk of developing eating disorders, one-third reported having been part of TAF and about 60% of these participants were teased about their weight (Ho, 2010).

Eating disorders share common risk factors with obesity, such as dieting, body dissatisfaction and weight-related teasing. While the vast majority of school-based obesity prevention programs have historically targeted behavioural factors (e.g., healthy eating and exercise), possible psychological contributors are often not targeted (Haines & Neumark-Sztainer, 2006). There are empirically supported reasons for integrating eating disorders and obesity prevention work and such an integrative approach needs to be undertaken to ensure that participants are not harmed (Stice, Shaw, & Marti, 2007). In Julia's case, the ego-syntonic nature of AN was further exacerbated by the "thin is in" message that she received from the media and through her experience in TAF club. Although she was teased only minimally about her own admission, she spoke of the experience leaving her with a fear of fatness and a belief that you have to be thin to fit in.

Julia's deliberate self-harming (DSH) behaviour was yet another factor that contributed to the complexity of her presentation and effective treatment. Self-harming behaviour is a common comorbidity among ED patients with evidence that 22.2% of outpatients with AN engaged in self-harming behaviours and 11.3% had attempted suicide (Sansone & Levitt, 2004). While the exact relationship between ED and DSH is unclear, treatment interventions should first aim to reduce the frequency of self-harming behaviours, explore their function and help the client reframe them as ego-dystonic (Sansone, Levitt, & Sansone, 2004). Hence, much of the initial therapy conducted with Julia focused on safety planning and reducing her levels of self-harm.

Therapy ended in an unplanned and abrupt manner due to Julia "dropping out" of treatment upon being informed of the therapist's resignation from the clinic. While patient dropout is a common phenomenon in psychotherapy, most people tend to dropout early in treatment (Mueller & Pekarik, 2000). The therapeutic relationship has long been acknowledged as an important factor in psychotherapy, with a strong alliance between the therapist and client being indicative of positive outcome and a client's continuation in treatment (Saunders, 2000). Although it was initially quite difficult to engage Julia in sessions, a strong and secure alliance was eventually established and this was largely due to the fact that Julia reported feeling understood and accepted by the therapist. When termination was initially addressed, Julia reported that she was losing the one person who accepted her unconditionally. It was apparent that she struggled with the loss of this relationship but there was limited opportunity to process this loss because of the abrupt end to their sessions. A strong countertransference was identified by the therapist, who felt unsettled by the way therapy ended. The therapist reflected on whether termination had been addressed appropriately and what could have been done better. Supervision played a key role in helping the therapist process these issues; finally, writing this case study has been cathartic in helping the therapist to reflect on the journey undertaken with Julia.

Now recognized as the third most common illness in adolescent girls, superseded only by diabetes and asthma (Maine & Bunnell, 2010), eating disorders have become a major public health issue due to significant psychological and physical morbidity, as well as high mortality rates (Johnson, Cohen, Kasen & Brook, 2002). In Singapore, the prevalence of young females at risk of developing an ED is 7.4%, which is comparable to the West (Ho, Tai, Lee, Cheng & Leow, 2006). This is not surprising given that Singaporean Chinese women exhibit lower levels of body satisfaction, greater eating disorder psychopathology, and more concern about their weight compared with their Australian counterparts (Mond, Chen & Kumar, 2010; Soh, Touyz, Dobbins, Surgenor, Clarke, Kohn et al., 2007). While there are no Singaporean epidemiological studies exploring the prevalence of eating disorders or anorexia nervosa, Kok and Tian (1994) reported that Singaporean adolescents exhibited greater body dissatisfaction and a higher drive for thinness compared with American undergraduate students. In another Singaporean study, Wang, Ho, Anderson & Sabry (1999) found that only 36% of Chinese Singaporean female youth were satisfied with their present weight and most respondents perceived thinness to be the ideal body shape. High levels of ED pathology among Singaporeans have been reflected in a four-fold increase in number of patients presenting with AN between 1994–2002 (Lee, Lee, Pathy & Chan, 2005). However, given that only 22–30% of people with ED seek and receive psychiatric treatment, this increase may be an underestimation (Johnson et al., 2002; Stice & Shaw, 2004). Locally, this may be due to a lack of education about eating disorders or due to a reluctance to discuss personal problems outside the family unit or social circle (Chen, Mond, & Kumar, 2010).

This case highlights the challenges of working with an adolescent with AN complicated by low mood, low motivation and self-harming behaviours. In addition to the complexities inherent to treatment of eating disorders, the challenges to implementing an evidence-based approach have been described. This case study emphasises the importance of developing a therapeutic alliance with a client with poor insight and motivation and addressing termination issues.

DISCUSSION QUESTIONS

1. The Trim and Fit Club initiative received a lot of criticism for the messages that young people received. How can we strike a balance between the important messages of prevention programs aimed at reducing the risk of obesity while being mindful of psychological factors that might contribute to development of eating disorders?

2. What factors might have impeded Julia's family members from attending therapy? What strategies could be used by Singaporean psychologists or services to increase the engagement and commitment of family members for family-based treatments for anorexia?

3. How do you think the media impacts on young people, specifically in terms of body image, weight and shape beliefs?

4. Do you think parents, clinicians and educators should include discussions about the media in their interaction with children/adolescents? If yes, what issues do you think they need to raise? If no, why not?

5. Is there a possibility that students in the Holistic Health Framework program may be singled out as children with mental or social problems? How can schools run prevention programs without causing harm or creating opportunities for teasing?

CHAPTER 2.

A HARD START TO LIFE

Encephalitis and Challenging Behaviours

JOY LOW

INTRODUCTION

Kevin was an 11-year-old boy living at the Institute of Mental Health (IMH). He was awaiting transfer to Rainbow Children's Home for long-term residence and had been referred to the Ministry of Social and Family Development's (MSF's) Clinical and Forensic Psychology Branch (CFPB) for a neuropsychological assessment of his cognitive and academic abilities. At the point of his referral in 2013, Kevin had presented with a host of behavioural difficulties. He had displayed aggression towards others by poking their eyes, was noncompliant to instruction, frequently threw temper tantrums, was extremely hyperactive, and engaged in repetitive behaviour like tearing paper. Because his many problems were causing serious disruptions at school and his residence, multiple clinicians and organisations had been working together to coordinate the best form of care for him.

BACKGROUND

In Kevin's early years, there was little evidence for significant concern about his development. However, at the age of four, he suddenly developed a high fever and was rushed to Temasek Hospital, whereupon he was diagnosed with acute necrotising encephalitis (ANE), a devastating and rapidly progressive neurologic disorder that occurs in children after common viral infections.

Kevin experienced the typical symptoms of ANE, which include a high fever, upper respiratory infection, and convulsions. Shortly after being admitted, he fell into a coma. He only regained consciousness eight days later—one of 70% of ANE patients to survive these acute symptoms. He was, however, left with permanent and severe mental delay. Magnetic resonance imaging (MRI) brain scans showed abnormality in Kevin's left hemisphere: in his thalamus, cerebral peduncle and midbrain. Although his condition had stabilised over time, Kevin's challenging behaviours manifested to the point that his parents found him unmanageable. He was thus admitted to children's homes on multiple occasions. A typical children's home in Singapore involves a high staff to child ratio, with staff ranging from caseworkers to counsellors as well as house parents. The homes generally also have relatively low levels of security, and a variety of reasons for admission including child abuse or neglect.

A year later, Kevin was admitted to a government hospital for vasculitic rash, and diagnosed with possible cutaneous vasculitis (a disorder that destroys blood vessels). He was again admitted for non-accidental injury in October 2008 and April 2009, following short periods at home. Cuts and bruises found on his body were allegedly inflicted by both parents attempting to manage his behavioural difficulties. Within the ward, staff found Kevin's behaviour difficult to control, as he would hide under beds and attempt to abscond.

As a result of suspected physical abuse by his parents, Kevin was referred to the MSF's Child Protection Service (CPS). Due to concerns about potential physical abuse should he continue to remain at home, Kevin was removed and placed in various children's homes. However, the children's homes also had difficulties managing Kevin's challenging behaviours. At the age of eight, these were extensive and they included physical and verbal aggression towards staff and other residents, inappropriate touching of others, defecating in rooms, and refusing to put on his clothes especially when sleeping at night. Kevin was also reported to be hyperactive and easily distracted, which made it more difficult for the staff to manage him. He was admitted to the Institute of Mental Health (IMH) on multiple occasions for psychiatric assessment and review. During his IMH admission, he was diagnosed with conduct disorder (CD), attention-deficit/hyperactivity disorder (ADHD), and intellectual disability. While these diagnoses described Kevin's main presenting problems, they were also thought to be directly caused by his underlying ANE condition and symptoms. Shortly after his discharge from IMH, Kevin took up long-term residence at Rainbow Children's Home.

Kevin came from a family of four: his parents, himself and a 10-year-old sister. His father worked as a taxi driver while his mother was a homemaker who reported a history of poor physical health. The family primarily spoke in Mandarin at home.

Although Kevin had initially been enrolled in a mainstream primary school, his academic performance had generally been below average. He would disengage from class activities and did not socialise with his classmates. He also hid under the desk and had occasional outbursts in class. A teacher aide had been assigned to look after him, but proved ineffective in controlling his disruptive behaviour. He was subsequently transferred to a special school.

ASSESSMENT

A neuropsychological assessment was administered to establish a profile of Kevin's current cognitive strengths and weaknesses in light of his challenging behaviour. This was aimed at helping the professionals involved to better understand his treatment needs and the best way to communicate and care for him. In addition, the comparison with his previous assessment scores was aimed at finding out whether there were significant improvements in his cognitive skills over the past three years.

Kevin had undergone neuropsychological assessment at Temasek Hospital three years before the current assessment. The results indicated that he had significant difficulties in all aspects of attention and executive functioning. His ability to process information quickly was lower than expected for his age. However, this was most likely a result of poor attention: when he engaged well on a task, he could process information more quickly. His visual skills were a personal strength, while his ability to express himself verbally was a weakness. Kevin's literacy and numeracy skills were also extremely poor.

Fact Box 2.1. What is a Clinical Neuropsychologist?

Clinical neuropsychologists address neurobehavioural problems related to acquired or developmental disorders of the nervous system. The types of problems are extremely varied and include such conditions as dementia, vascular disorders, and other neurodegenerative disorders, traumatic brain injury, seizure disorders, learning disabilities, neuropsychiatric disorders, infectious disease affecting the CNS, neurodevelopmental disorders, metabolic disease and neurological effects of medical disorders or treatment.

Neuropsychologists apply specialised knowledge in the assessment, diagnosis, treatment and rehabilitation of individuals with neurological, medical, or neurodevelopmental disorders across the lifespan. Paediatric neuropsychologists provide clinical services to children and adolescents (and their families). They are skilled in clinical assessment and treatment of brain disorders. Essential skills include specialised neuropsychological assessment techniques, specialised intervention techniques, research design and analysis in neuropsychology, professional issues and ethics, culturally competent approaches in neuropsychology, and an understanding of implications of neuropsychological conditions for behaviour and adjustment. Competence in clinical neuropsychology requires the ability to integrate neuropsychological findings with neurologic and other medical data, psychosocial and other behavioural data, and knowledge in the neurosciences, and to interpret these findings with an appreciation of social, cultural and ethical issues. Preparation in clinical neuropsychology begins at the doctoral level and specialized education and training is completed at the postdoctoral level.

Overall, Kevin's general cognitive functioning fell within the mildly intellectually disabled range, and his adaptive functioning was significantly lower than his peers. It was hypothesised that the combination of ANE, the Mandarin-speaking family background, a history of non-accidental injury, his multiple placements, and the disrupted school performance were likely to have impacted on Kevin's lowered scores at the time.

During assessment sessions at IMH, Kevin did not present like a typical 11-year-old. He engaged in minimal conversation, typically responding with poor enunciation in one-word answers or short phrases. Kevin did not maintain much eye contact, tending to look down at objects in his hands or around the ward. He was right-handed but had a weak pencil grip. In addition, Kevin was easily distracted. Nonetheless, he responded well to prompts including brief praise, tapping on his arm to redirect his focus, and making eye contact. He was relatively compliant in completing all tasks and was fairly determined to complete tasks that he found challenging.

Kevin's odd behaviour quickly presented itself during his assessment sessions. At the commencement of each session, he would ask for paper, without which he refused to participate in any task. Upon receiving the piece of paper (printed with a picture), Kevin would fold it into parts and neatly tear it into equally sized pieces. With the torn pieces of paper in hand, Kevin would carry out the tasks set before him. During breaks, he would attempt to piece the paper back together, akin to a jigsaw puzzle. At the end of each session, Kevin was rewarded with another piece of paper, with which he would repeat the same actions (folding and tearing). It was hypothesised that underlying anxiety and the need for tactile stimulation contributed to his obsession with paper and his subsequent compulsion with tearing/reassembling. In addition, Kevin occasionally requested to be scratched on his body (back, toes, fingers). This was consistent with reports from IMH and school staff, which served to further support the hypothesis that Kevin's behaviours were indications of his need for tactile stimulation.

A variety of standardized neuropsychological measures were used to assess his different functional domains. They included his current cognitive functioning, executive functions, basic literacy and math, behaviours, and adaptive functioning (Table 2.1).

Overall, Kevin's general intellectual functioning was extremely low for his age. His verbal cognitive functioning (ability to understand, reason with, and express verbal information) was also extremely low. It was likely that his Mandarin-speaking family background, disrupted school performance and multiple placements affected the development of his age-appropriate verbal reasoning abilities. On the other hand, while Kevin's visual perceptual reasoning (ability to perceive and reason with visual information) abilities were below expected levels for his age, they were not as impaired as his verbal reasoning skills. In addition, he had made significant gains over time when compared to his assessment results from three years ago at Temasek Hospital. This indicated that Kevin was better at understanding visual than verbal information.

TABLE 2.1. NEUROPSYCHOLOGICAL MEASURES ADMINISTERED FOR KEVIN'S ASSESSMENT

Neuropsychological Test / Questionnaire	Subtests / Form Administered
Wechsler Intelligence Scale for Children, 4th Edition (WISC-IV)	Core subtests + Arithmetic
Wide Range Assessment of Memory and Learning, 2nd Edition (WRAML2)	Design Memory
Delis-Kaplan Executive Function System (D-KEFS)	Trail Making Test and Verbal Fluency
Wechsler Individual Achievement Test, 2nd Edition (WIAT-II)	Numerical Operations and Word Reading
Behavior Rating Inventory of Executive Function (BRIEF)	Parent and Teacher forms
Child Behavior Checklist (CBCL)	Parent form
Teacher Rating Form (TRF)	Teacher form
Adaptive Behavior Assessment System, 2nd Edition (ABAS-II)	Parent and Teacher forms

During the assessment, Kevin demonstrated adequate hand-eye coordination. His response speed, however, was compromised when the task depended on handwriting abilities, because of his weak pencil grip. Moreover, Kevin had a tendency to be easily distracted. He was unable to focus on the instructions for a task, much less concentrate on a task for longer than ten minutes without prompting. His focus improved only slightly when prompted. Kevin also could not perform more than one task at a time. His difficulties with attention generally affected his performance on all tasks. For example, Kevin struggled with tasks that relied on his working memory (ability to hold and manipulate information in his mind) and general memory, as he was often not paying attention to the original information in the first place.

Assessment of Kevin's higher-level abilities was limited by his difficulties with attention, basic language, and sequencing. It was also evident from his current assessment and school records that Kevin's academic achievement was far below expected levels for his age. On top of his widespread cognitive difficulties, Kevin was a boy who struggled with completing everyday tasks independently. This was based on observations and interviews with Kevin's teachers, IMH staff, and reports from the children's homes. He particularly struggled to communicate effectively with others and to care for himself independently. These difficulties tended to manifest in environments that were unfamiliar and unstructured (e.g., public places).

Finally, it was clear that all the professionals who dealt with Kevin were concerned about his challenging behaviours. Rainbow Children's Home staff tended to be most concerned with his habit of poking the eyes of staff and peers. During the first month of admission to his current children's home, it was estimated that he poked the eyes of other people about six times every day. This was in addition to other aggressive, noncompliant, or problematic behaviours seen within the Home.

Overall, Kevin had significant difficulties across many of his cognitive domains. Many of his difficulties stemmed from deficits in basic functions, such as attention, weak finger grip and coordination, and low intellectual functioning, which affected the other aspects of his functioning.

DIAGNOSIS

Kevin was diagnosed by the IMH psychiatrist with conduct disorder, ADHD, and intellectual disability. Due to his severe and pervasive aggression and noncompliance, Kevin met clinical criteria for conduct disorder. His inattention and hyperactivity were also evident, and disruptive enough to his daily functioning to warrant an ADHD diagnosis and corresponding medication. Finally, his cognitive and adaptive functioning were clearly below expected levels for his age; he met the criteria for intellectual disability. Some may argue that these diagnoses were secondary to ANE and thus purely descriptive of what was already known as the symptoms of his condition. Nonetheless, these diagnostic labels were useful in enabling mental health professionals to have a standardised means of communicating his presenting problems and treatment needs. While multiple comorbid diagnoses made the prognosis of Kevin's case difficult, they also highlighted the need to delineate the clusters of his problem behaviours to provide targeted management and treatment.

INTEGRATIVE FORMULATION

Predisposing

Kevin was diagnosed with ANE at the young age of five. As a result, he developed severe neurological and behavioural difficulties. Kevin's parents could not manage him and resorted to harsh physical methods. As a result, Kevin was admitted to multiple children's homes, but even then his behaviours continued to be unpredictable and challenging.

Precipitating

When faced with difficulties in managing Kevin's behaviour, his parents used very harsh physical disciplinary methods. This resulted in the CPS's involvement in ensuring Kevin's ongoing safety.

At home, Kevin's main presenting problem was his habit of poking others in the eye. It was hypothesised that Kevin relied on others' eye contact to assess whether he had their attention or not. Poking their eyes was thus his attempt to redirect their focus towards him. This was consistent with his past behaviour of breaking others' spectacles. Over time, these behaviours were reinforced when others reacted to them and fulfilled his desire for attention. It was also noted that Kevin's poking behaviour extended to other situations where he found it difficult to express his needs or wants (presumably compounded by his poor verbal and social skills).

Kevin's obsession with paper (the anxiety of losing a piece of paper and the self-stimulating function of paper tearing) precipitated other problem behaviours. This included Kevin's refusal to bathe, taking a piece of paper into the toilet, and not participating in group mealtimes.

Perpetuating

Kevin's unresolved neurological condition and poorly understood behavioural patterns continued to perpetuate the difficulties of managing him. His parents' level of understanding and insight about Kevin's behaviours remained low. As they lacked the knowledge and commitment to resume full-time care of Kevin, allowing him to return to his home was not an option. Kevin's history of poor positive attachment with consistent caregivers was also thought to exacerbate his current behavioural difficulties.

Protective

Despite his widespread difficulties, Kevin demonstrated some personal strengths. He was able to meet his basic day-to-day requirements (e.g., attending school, interacting with teachers), although he required much time and guidance. In addition, Kevin had made significant progress in his visual reasoning skills within the past three years. In addition, his parents maintained some level of interaction with him, especially Kevin's father, who regularly visited him at the children's homes.

PROGNOSIS

Because of the permanent nature of his acquired brain injury, it was unlikely that Kevin's neurological condition would be resolved. The possibility of Kevin being at risk of hurting himself or others without constant supervision meant that the chances of him achieving independent living as an adult were also low. Factors that could improve the prognosis of his treatment included placement in a secure and therapeutic environment, multidisciplinary involvement in his care, and ongoing assessment and review of his behavioural patterns.

TREATMENT

As Kevin moved to Rainbow Children's Home, it was important to establish and maintain consistency in his education and caregiving environments, so that the most effective behavioural strategies and interventions could be implemented and reviewed. Based on Kevin's current neuropsychological profile of strengths and weaknesses, behavioural strategies were formulated and given to Kevin's caregivers and teachers.

Fact Box 2.2. Who is Responsible for Persons with Poor Prognosis in Terms of Independent Living?

In Singapore, the responsibility of care for children below the age of 16 years lies with their parents or legal guardians. This would similarly apply for any child with significant intellectual and adaptive difficulties. For families where the biological parent is unable to assume full-time care of the child, the Family Child Protection and Welfare Department of MSF may intervene to provide assistance and support. Interventions may include placement of the child in a welfare home that can better cater to the child's specialised needs. Typically, a multidisciplinary team of professionals would be involved to provide holistic care to the child within the welfare system.

Beyond the age of 16, there are a few organisations that provide assistance to adult individuals who require significant amounts of support in their day-to-day functioning. There are short- and long-term residential care options, including adult residential homes, community group homes, and hostels. One such organisation would be MINDSville@Napiri (MV). MV is a multiservice centre that integrates four services under one roof—a group home for adults with intellectual disability; a Children's Wing, and MINDS third Training and Development Centre (TDC). The Home is a facility within the compound dedicated to the care of adults with intellectual disability who are unable to care for themselves independently. This program provides accommodation, nursing care, supervision and rehabilitation for persons with intellectual disability, aged 18 and above.

Additional organisations provide peripheral support, such as special education, employment assistance, and transportation. The Disabled People's Association (DPA) and SG Enable websites provide more information.

For example, establishing consistency and predictability in Kevin's daily routine was important. Minimal changes to Kevin's daily schedule were ensured, and pictures were used to show him the order of events in a day. A reward chart was also used to encourage his participation in activities.

A multidisciplinary approach in Kevin's care was critical. Follow-up with the hospital regarding his current neurological condition and medication regime was deemed important. Open and regular communication between Rainbow Children's Home and Kevin's special school was strongly encouraged to maintain consistency in intervention approaches and to facilitate the exchange of valuable ideas for implementation.

Kevin was prescribed a cocktail of psychiatric medication aimed at managing his challenging behaviours and improving his functioning at school. Despite his heavy medication, however, Kevin still continued to exhibit significant aggressive and challenging behaviours. This raises the question of the ethics and evidence-base of medication use in children to manage aggressive behaviour.

A case conference was held with Kevin's IMH psychologist and medical social worker (MSW), school psychologist and form teacher, child protection officer (CPO), and Rainbow Children's Home social worker and psychologist. Feedback of the current assessment results was provided, and intervention plans discussed. Follow-up support was provided to Rainbow Children's Home in the form of group discussions with its staff every month. The sessions involved care staff, the Rainbow Children's Home psychologist, nurses, and teacher aides. The initial focus was identifying Kevin's high-risk scenarios and triggers towards his aggressive behaviour. With regard to Kevin's poking behaviours, the A-B-C (antecedents, behaviour, consequences) model was applied to understand the function of his behaviours. It was identified that he tended to poke (or even threaten) others when they turned their attention away from him.

Rainbow Children's Home staff were also supported with strategies that were largely based on attachment and behaviour modification principles. Broader strategies emphasised the importance of building a positive relationship with Kevin so as to establish a secure and trusting caregiving environment. Practical means of ensuring such an environment included introducing elements of positive parenting training into their interactions with Kevin, such as having the staff initiate affection (e.g., a pat on the shoulder, side hugs), identifying one or two consistent attachment figures within the home for Kevin, practicing strategies to encourage desirable behaviour (e.g., praise, rewards), and teaching him new skills and behaviours (e.g., role modelling, incidental teaching, behaviour charts). Behaviour modification strategies were emphasised on immediate rather than delayed reinforcements. In this sense, a token economy (e.g., collect minimum number of stars to exchange for a prize at the end of the month) was substituted for daily behaviour charts and rewards.

"Thinking out of the box" was paramount when it came to devising behavioural strategies for Kevin's case. Other specific behaviour modification strategies that attempted to address his poking behaviour included physically distracting him with toys or tasks that involved the use of his hands (e.g., paper tearing). When preventative measures were ineffective, however, some level of physical restraint was used to prevent his escalation to poking, namely by holding both his hands. However, this resulted in Kevin getting frustrated and throwing a tantrum. As such, staff attempted lightly holding both his hands while singing melodies that were improvised on the spot. This appeared to work significantly well, and staff were able to de-escalate and soothe him quickly during similar situations. Subsequently, this strategy was so effective and consistently used by staff, that Kevin was also able to recognise these as cues for his inappropriate behaviour and even apologised to the staff on several occasions.

Nevertheless, it was emphasised that preventative strategies were preferred over reactionary measures (e.g., time out after the problem behaviour was already completed). Therefore, the Home's staff were encouraged to stay alert and attuned to Kevin's current emotional and behavioural state and to remain vigilant and note any indicators of distress before his behaviours escalated. Intervention continued for several months as poking others remained one of his most challenging behaviours, especially since it posed the risk of physical harm to the other staff and residents. In addition, Kevin's poking behaviour had also extended to other forms of physical aggression over time, including poking others' private parts and slapping their faces.

In addition to his aggressive behaviours, there was also concern about Kevin's obsessive-compulsive traits. Initially, Kevin was obsessed with tearing and reconstructing paper. His fixation was so significant that it interfered with his mealtimes and showers. Staff could not understand the function of such behaviour, although they hypothesised that Kevin's paper tearing alleviated his anxiety and fulfilled his need for tactile stimulation. Having no paper was therefore thought to be distressing for Kevin and likely to trigger his aggressive behaviour. Staff arranged to give him a piece of paper at set times each day. Additional paper was given as a reward for complying with instructions (e.g., taking his medication).

At this point, intervention was ongoing and continued to address the challenges that Rainbow Children's Home staff faced in caring for Kevin every day. Due to the unpredictable nature of his behaviours, intervention strategies had to be flexible and systematic. As a result of the permanent and severe nature of his neurological condition, Kevin is likely to remain institutionalised in the long term, and require significant amounts of structural and specialised support from the social welfare system. Collaboration between multidisciplinary professionals and agencies would ensure that Kevin's current needs would always be prioritised.

DISCUSSION

Acute necrotising encephalopathy (ANE) in childhood is a rare type of encephalopathy characterised by multiple, necrotic brain lesions showing a symmetric distribution pattern (Mizuguchi et al., 1995; Manara, Franzoi, Cogo, Battistella, 2006; Mizuguchi,

Yamanouchi, Ichiyama, & Shiomi, 2007). These brain lesions occur mainly in the bilateral thalamus, brain stem, tegmentum, and cerebellum. Cases were first studied in Japan, but have since been found in several other countries (Manara et al., 2006). It is unknown what the prevalence of ANE is in each population, but only a few case studies have been documented in the literature to date. The prognosis for ANE remains poor, although there has been some success in early treatment (Manara et al., 2006). The literature pool about ANE is extremely limited and culturally biased. It will require many more years of intensive studies and research for this condition to be better understood and evidence-based interventions to be established.

Children and young people in children's welfare homes have complex mental health needs. These vulnerabilities stem from pre- and post-care experiences and may include trauma, attachment and developmental difficulties (Golding, 2010). Frequent changes of placement, lack of advocacy and poor inter-agency communication hamper the delivery of proper services to the child. This has a negative impact on educational and social development, and deprives the child from access to therapy for current mental health issues (Golding, 2010). Unfortunately, research statistics on Singapore's welfare homes are currently unavailable for public dissemination.

Consistent across international research is the finding that children in the welfare system face many barriers in their journey towards receiving services. The parent or caregiver may find the process of applying to the right service too onerous, or lack the means of transport or time to bring the child to services. Caregivers may also find it difficult to communicate to the therapist when both speak different languages or have different cultural beliefs. While it is not uncommon for children with outwardly and obviously problematic behaviours (e.g., aggression, self-harming) to be identified by the healthcare system for psychological services. This places children with more covert problems (e.g., depression) at a disadvantage as they are less likely to receive such services. Finally, subjecting children to multiple placements is also problematic. These children are less likely to receive mental health services and more likely to face difficulties in building trusting relationships (Beck, 2006). Case notes may also be misplaced or delayed in the move (McAuley & Davis, 2009).

Any agency faces multiple issues when it takes in a child: (i) the focus of the intervention; (ii) the viability of the current placement; (iii) the possibility of securing a long-term caregiver; (iv) the child's educational needs; (v) the child's health and mental health needs. A multi-agency collaboration involving healthcare, education, and social care provides improved communication and information sharing, as well as tailored interventions along with considering the holistic needs of the child and the caregiver (Golding, 2010). In Singapore, for example, steps are being taken to reach such a multi-agency accord. The Youth Level of Service/Case Management Inventory (YLS/CMI) and Child and Adolescent Needs and Strengths (CANS) have been adapted to local norms and are currently used as a unified guideline to inform intervention plans for children and young people.

In summary, this complex case emphasises the need for interventions to span multiple agencies and professional disciplines. The role of the clinical neuropsychologist was to conduct ongoing assessment, formulation, and development of effective behavioural strategies for use with Kevin's caregivers and teachers. Kevin is likely to remain institutionalised in the long term, and his potential to achieve independent living remains low. As a client of both the medical and social welfare system, Kevin's case requires long-term input by mental health professionals, medical care workers, social workers, and home care operations staff to maximise his care.

In addition, because of Kevin's unique medical, social and cultural profile, it was difficult to find systems of care that catered to such a specific set of needs, especially in the international literature. Instead, highlighting Kevin's case study should support the importance of ongoing consultation and collaboration between multiple systems of care to provide seamless and intensive support for this special child. It may also stimulate the state to recognize the demands for long-term placements (e.g., residential treatment facilities) for such children with complex needs.

DISCUSSION QUESTIONS

1. Kevin had a hard start to life and has required involvement from a range of health and welfare providers. What value does the clinical neuropsychologist add to assessment and therapy with people such as Kevin?

2. In the face of limited and culturally biased literature about ANE, what are the advantages and disadvantages of diagnosing a child with ANE in Singapore?

3. In Kevin's case, his regular reviews with the psychiatrist involved monitoring and adjusting his psychiatric medication. What might be some of the ethical considerations involved in a heavy medication regime for a child with special needs?

4. With the understanding that cases like Kevin's require intensive resourcing from the welfare and medical system, how could we consider increasing support for parents so that children with special needs can remain in their homes?

5. Discuss the existing community resources and policies in Singapore that provide specialised care for children with special needs. What needs to be improved or added to ensure a broad safety net for such a population?

CHAPTER 3

DISORGANISED BOYS NEED ORGANISED WORLDS

ADHD and Oppositional Defiant Disorder

JOHN DAVISON

INTRODUCTION

Aaron Reed was a 17-year-old boy referred by his mother to a clinical psychology private clinic. He had been released from prison four months earlier, after serving an 11-month term for marijuana possession. Although he would be on probation for two years, a past diagnosis of ADHD had allowed him to escape community service. Instead, he was required to attend regular sessions with a psychologist who would assess his current difficulties, provide treatment as necessary, and him his transition into the community.

Since his release Aaron had moved in with his mother and repeated his GCE 'O' Levels. His parents, an Australian father and Chinese mother, had separated when he was 12 and maintained little to no contact with each other. Aaron attended the first assessment session with his mother and the second with his father. He presented as confident and excitable and described himself as an "entertainer"—he was talkative, frequently joked, and showed off his "prison build". He was also restless throughout the session: frequently changing his position, checking his cellphone and getting distracted by noises outside the room.

Aaron's mother and father had different perspectives on his current situation. Mrs Lau (maiden name) felt that her son did not need therapy; her only concern was his fulfilment of the court mandate. She was quick to excuse his past drug use, minimise his troublesome behaviours (both past and present), and dismiss his past diagnosis of ADHD. Mr Reed, on the other hand, was concerned about Aaron's academics, fluctuating moods and impulsive aggressive behaviours. However, his wife, Aaron's stepmother, refused to let Aaron to live with them until he proved to be "back on track".

Aaron and his father's main concerns related to his studies and social life. Aaron was easily distracted and found it difficult to pay attention in class. He walked around class and joked with his peers, was impudent to his teacher, impulsively kicked chairs over and tripped his peers up. Whilst he enjoyed his role as "class clown", he reported being stressed about his studies and worried about being expelled. Within a month of returning to school, he had been suspended for three days for swearing at a teacher, given several detentions for being disruptive in class and for not following instructions, and gotten into two "standoffs" with peers, which had almost escalated to physical fights. He claimed to have been provoked and was simply maintaining a stance learnt in prison to "show no fear". He refused to allow anyone to consider him a "wuss" or think that they could "mess [him] around".

The transition from prison to living at a new home with his mother had been daunting. Whilst prison was by no means a place of comfort, Aaron had become accustomed to its routines and rules. Rather than the euphoria he expected with his new freedom, he felt lost without the structure of prison life. He was also overwhelmed by the new responsibilities of living more independently, becoming reacquainted with friends and family, and deciding on what to study.

Aaron's academic performance was variable. Whilst he excelled in Math, he was falling behind in his other subjects, and had recently failed a number of tests. In addition to being easily distracted at school, he was finding it difficult to study at home: he had no desk in his room, he could not stay focused for long periods of time, and his mother failed to monitor his studying. Despite Aaron's determination to do well at school, he was losing confidence. This was exacerbated by his fear of failing. He had set goals to reduce his classroom problems: avoiding talking to anyone or making friends, and studying for as long into the night as possible. However, he was finding these expectations difficult to maintain, and was becoming increasingly frustrated with himself, his peers and his teachers.

Aaron and his parents reported no concerns about drug use since his release from prison. When interviewed separately, he admitted meeting up with older friends from prison who still used drugs, and sometimes feeling tempted to join them. However, he claimed to have no intention to use drugs in Singapore. Serving as deterrents were his twice-weekly urine tests, an ankle monitor which traced his whereabouts, and an instant five-year prison sentence if were caught in possession of drugs again.

BACKGROUND

Aaron was an only child with no stepsiblings. Mrs. Lau reported that Aaron's developmental milestones were normal. Since his early years, he had displayed high levels of energy, was very talkative and had difficulty sitting still. His father compared Aaron to his ex-wife, noting that they were both messy and disorganized, and were disposed to expressing their emotions strongly, embarrassing him with their verbal and emotional outbursts. Such behaviour became especially problematic once Aaron started primary school: he often walked around in the classroom, interrupted his teachers and peers; he was disorganized and had trouble completing his homework. His school performance was inconsistent, with grades ranging from top of the class to failing.

In secondary school, Aaron's behavioural problems increased and his teachers became less tolerant: he was expelled from two schools—both times for fighting with peers in class. At 12 years of age, following his first expulsion and failure in one of his PSLE examinations, he was referred by his school for psychological assessment, and diagnosed with attention deficit hyperactivity disorder (ADHD), combined type.

While no psychotherapy was offered Aaron, he was trialed on Ritalin, a psychostimulant. However, Aaron was non-compliant with both the Ritalin ("it dulled me—I lost my personality") and the Chinese herbal medicines his mother recommended "to help him relax". Instead, at age 16, he began using marijuana together with friends from school, asserting that "it helped me relax and gave a great buzz". This quickly developed to more regular use ("a few times a week"). His parents were not aware of his drug use until six months later, when the police arrived unexpectedly at his father's door, and detained Aaron immediately.

Because his parents "always argued" he preferred it when they lived separately. He idealised his father, his "best friend", with whom he could share anything. When his father remarried when Aaron was 15, Aaron entered into a conflictual relationship with his stepmother, who "couldn't handle [him]" and "didn't want him in the house". He also spoke critically of his mother. He was frustrated with "the negative vibe" of their home, her unpredictable moods, her laxness in disciplining him (she was "too lenient") and her indifference to what he did and him in general. In fact, during her son's assessment, Mrs. Lau had declared that "parenting is not disciplining", had endorsed his past marijuana use ("In any other country it wouldn't be a problem"), and had supported his aggressive behaviour ("If someone doesn't like you, spite them!").

Aaron's recalled his prison sentence, which he found boring and lonely, with both rancour and gratitude. He also found it challenging to know whom to like and trust. However, it also gave him the opportunity to reflect on his life goals and family relationships; for example, he had resolved to improve his relationship with his stepmother. He claimed to have had a few minor physical confrontations, but no traumatic physical or sexual experiences.

ASSESSMENT

As Aaron was diagnosed with ADHD when he was 12, his latest assessment was not primarily diagnostic but aimed at identifying his presenting problems, and strengths and weaknesses; and at screening for comorbid problems that are often evident in teenagers with ADHD. While a diagnosis of ADHD is relatively stable, the severity and expression of ADHD symptoms can change throughout adolescence and adulthood.

Two 90-minute clinical assessment interviews were conducted. These served to a) detail Aaron's current presenting problems and background, b) assess his parents' parenting skills and perspectives, and c) build rapport to increase the likelihood of their involvement in Aaron's treatment. In addition, with Aaron and his mother's consent, a phone interview was conducted with both his probation officer and his form teacher. These calls aimed to assess Aaron's behaviour across different settings and from multiple perspectives, in order that the psychologist might gauge the severity of his difficulties and understand the rationale behind the court referral.

Achenbach's ratings scales (Achenbach & Rescorla, 2001) were used to screen for both ADHD symptoms and other emotional and behaviour issues and competencies. Aaron completed the Youth Self Report (YSR) and his parents separately completed the Child Behaviour Checklist (CBCL). Aaron and his father both gave high ratings for attention problems, which fell in the clinical range. These included items such as "can't sit still, restless, hyperactive" and "inattentive or easily distracted". His father also noted some rule-breaking behaviours (borderline range), such as "disobedient at school" and "teases a lot". In contrast, his mother's scores fell within the normal range, consistent with her minimising of his problems in the clinical interview.

Direct behavioural observations can be particularly important when assessing ADHD; they allow psychologists to assess the severity of reported problems, identify the contexts these problems occur in and determine if ADHD symptoms occur across two or more settings. As Aaron had already been diagnosed with ADHD the psychologist deemed a school observation unnecessary. A phone call to his teacher provided adequate information about his behaviour. Aaron also showed good insight into his classroom difficulties and an openness to sharing them.

Neurocognitive assessments, such as the Continuous Processing Test (CPT) can also supplement a diagnostic assessment of ADHD, although there is no consistent

Fact Box 3.1. Singapore Treatment Studies

Although there have been only a handful of studies published on ADHD and disruptive behaviour disorders in Singapore, there is a broad range of treatment studies currently underway. These range from a randomised controlled trial on the efficacy of an ADHD intervention involving a brain-computer interface; an observational study of Traditional Chinese Medicine (TCM) treatment for children with ADHD; an interactive web-based game for helping angry children and youth, and an intervention based on improving nutrition and social skills for children with conduct disorder and hyperactivity (Institute of Mental Health, 2013).

See Institute of Mental Health website: http://www.imh.com.sg/

cognitive profile that defines people with ADHD (Hale et al., 2010). The CPT was not used for Aaron's assessment because the primary reason for referral was not diagnostic.

Although no prison reports were available, Mr. Reed supplied the psychologist with a copy of the psychological report from Aaron's assessment at age 12. This provided not only confirmation of his past diagnosis of ADHD, but a measure of his cognitive abilities. Aaron had been found to demonstrate above average intelligence and did not have a learning disorder. As intelligence is relatively stable over time (assuming no neurological trauma), further IQ testing was not deemed necessary.

Aaron presented with a low risk of self-harm. Whilst his self-confidence was not high, he was not depressed, had no suicidal ideation or intent, and did not report any past or present self-harm. His risk of harming others was moderate, but not a major risk: while frustration with his peers had led to increasing incidents of physical confrontation at the time of his assessment, and he had been in fights prior to his incarceration, he had shown adequate restraint since his release. Aaron claimed that he did not enjoy or drink alcohol. However he was at moderate risk of drug use because of his regular marijuana use for six months before imprisonment, his impulsivity, his current socialisation with ex-inmates, and limited parental monitoring. Protective factors for abstaining from drug use included his strong intention to abstain and the terms of his probation.

DIAGNOSIS

Whilst a comprehensive diagnostic assessment was not undertaken, Aaron's presentation was consistent with his previous diagnosis of ADHD, Combined Type. He met the DSM-5 criteria for symptoms of inattentiveness and hyperactivity-impulsivity across multiple settings; these were clearly impacting on his social and academic functioning. Like many boys with ADHD, he concurrently met criteria for oppositional defiant disorder (ODD). His symptoms of ODD included "angry/irritable mood" and "argumentative/defiant behaviours" but not "vindictiveness".

Whilst Aaron reported irritable moods and often felt low and frustrated at school, he did not meet the criteria for depression. He was able to enjoy himself outside of school, and reported no problems with his appetite, sexual interest or energy level.

Although Aaron used marijuana frequently before his sentencing, it is unlikely that he would have met the criteria for substance abuse or dependence in the past. However, as no assessment was completed (or released) this potential past diagnosis remained unclear.

INTEGRATIVE FORMULATION

Predisposing Factors

Consistent with the neurodevelopmental model of ADHD, Aaron presented with symptoms of hyperactivity, impulsiveness, inattention and disorganisation from an early age. Although none of Aaron's family members had a known diagnosis of

ADHD, his mother presented with some traits that paralleled his ADHD symptoms. Aaron's ADHD symptoms predisposed him to difficulties in academic settings, social relationships and emotional regulation throughout his life, and peaked at times of stress.

Aaron's parents often found his ADHD symptoms difficult to handle; parenting was challenging and resulted in frequent conflict both with Aaron and between themselves. Aaron's difficulty in controlling his own frustration and anger further increased the likelihood of conflict, both at home and with his teachers and peers. His parents learnt ways to minimise these conflicts at any cost: a *coercive family process* developed in which, when faced with difficult behaviour they were quick to give in rather than discipline him (Patterson, 1982). Over time, they learnt to ignore and accept his misbehaviour and only engaged in limited monitoring of his activities.

Aaron's parents' separation, their ongoing discord and his continual change of schools resulted in an unstructured environment, inconsistent discipline, and minimal supervision. These probably limited Aaron's opportunity to develop adequate self-control and conflict resolution skills. Consequently he found it difficult to maintain relationships, socialized with and was easily influenced by with delinquent peers, and got into trouble at school.

As a result of his frequent conflict with others, Aaron developed an expectation that all social interaction would lead to contention and negative reactions from others. Thus he would always gear himself up for antagonism from his teacher, peers and family members. This defensive stance was reinforced by the aggressive mentality he had developed from his prison stint.

Aaron compensated for his impulsiveness and inattention by establishing a personality as an entertainer. While this helped him make friends and maintain a positive sense of self, his fluctuating self-control sometimes led to conflicts and rejection from friends and teachers who are less tolerant of his brand of humour. His inattention and disorganisation also made it difficult for him to remain on task and cope with his responsibilities. It was a constant challenge for him to stay focused on his academic work and perform consistently at school.

Precipitating Factors

Aaron's presenting problems were precipitated by his release from prison and his move into his mother's house. This represented a shift from a structured environment with clear rules and a stable routine to an environment with limited structure, inadequate monitoring and increased personal responsibility and independence. Furthermore, Aaron was faced the challenge of attaining his GCE "O" Levels, re-establishing social relationships with family and peers, and monitoring his impulsive and risky behaviour. This transition accentuated his difficulties in attentional control, organisation and regulation of his emotions and behaviours, and triggered his presenting problems.

Perpetuating Factors

A number of cognitive, behavioural, systemic and contextual factors perpetuated Aaron's presenting problems. His inattention and disorganisation made it difficult for him to concentrate on processing new information in class and keep up with his homework. His response was to "not bother" in school—resulting in boredom, limited learning, and increasing incidents of misbehaviour.

Aaron had a limited repertoire of skills for controlling his own impulsivity and hyperactivity and dealing with the consequences of his actions. His negative expectations of interactions with others and his struggles to control his frustration made him defensive and easily provoked. This led to his peers being wary when interacting with him, which fuelled Aaron's frustration, and led to either escalating conflict or his avoidance of others—a vicious cycle.

Aaron set high standards for himself, which motivated him to pursue his goals at school. However, he was ill-equipped to deal with unfulfilled goals, partially because they were unrealistic. He also exhibited cognitive distortions that probably perpetuated his disruptive behaviour. For example, he used "all-or-nothing thinking" ("If I don't get agro with them, I'm a wuss"), "mind-reading" ("My teacher thinks I am stupid and just wants to piss me off"), and had an external attribution bias—blaming others for his disruptive behaviour.

Mrs. Lau's "hands-off" parenting provided limited structure, monitoring, discipline and emotional support for Aaron. This created a difficult environment in which Aaron had to compensate for his own disorganisation. Moreover, his mother's mood swings frustrated and saddened him. He did not know how to respond to her and often avoided her completely. This coping strategy reinforced his low mood and his negative relationship with her.

Protective Factors

Aaron maintained a strong relationship with his father and kept in frequent contact with him. His parents supported his therapy and his father was willing to be actively involved if required. Aaron was motivated to attend therapy, and despite being belligerent on occasion, was able to communicate openly and candidly with the therapist. In spite of his problems at school, his intellectual capacity was above average and he was motivated to learn. During his time in prison he had identified areas in his life that he wanted to improve on. These included achieving academically, improving his relationship with family and staying out of prison. He claimed to have completely resisted any urge to use drugs since his release. His court mandate provided additional motivation to be compliant with therapy.

PROGNOSIS

The prognosis of ADHD can be daunting, because it is associated with social, academic, emotional and behavioural problems. For Aaron, potential negative outcomes were failing at school, being expelled for misbehaviour, experiencing escalating relationship difficulties, and at worst, a return to prison if his behaviour led to violence or drug use. Factors that could improve his prognosis included regular attendance and compliance with therapy, his parents' involvement in therapy, continued avoidance of illegal drug use, clear communication among his therapist, psychiatrist, family members, and school, and possibly, the use of medication to control his ADHD symptoms.

Whilst there is no quick-fix or cure for ADHD, a good proportion (half to two thirds) of youth with ADHD will not meet criteria for ADHD as adults as they learn to compensate for their symptoms, or as their symptoms lessen or change (Brassett-Harknett & Butler, 2007). Psychological treatment for ADHD and disruptive behaviours with and without medication has a strong, growing evidence base (Kapalka, 2010). It was thus expected that Aaron would benefit from cognitive behavioural therapy (CBT).

TREATMENT

Aaron's court mandate did not define the focus, duration, or frequency of his treatment sessions. After Aaron's assessment and formulation, the psychologist proposed weekly CBT sessions in conjunction with brief parent psycho-education and medical consultation.

At the time of writing, Aaron had attended ten therapy sessions over a period of 20 weeks. Both of his parents were encouraged to attend his earlier therapy sessions. While his mother declined to attend, she consented to making 'update' phone calls. His father, with Aaron's consent, attended a total of four sessions. Aaron missed ten sessions throughout the course of therapy because of forgotten appointments and exam stress. His mother's lack of enforcement of his regular weekly attendance also contributed to his non-attendance.

Aaron's goals for therapy included becoming less stressed and more organised in his studies, avoiding expulsion from school or a return to prison (because of drug use or fights), and maintaining better relationships with his family. Whilst his mother's only concern was that he complete the court mandate, his father hoped that Aaron would pass his examinations and gain more control over his anger and disruptive behaviour—in which case he might invite Aaron to live with him again.

To develop these goals with Aaron and his parents, the psychologist focused on both Aaron's strengths and difficulties. During their discussions, positive terms such as "self-control" and "high energy" were used instead of "impulsivity" and "hyperactivity". Aaron's presenting problems were reframed to highlight skills that could be strengthened to improve his life in specific ways. For example, his poor control of his emotions was reframed as a skill to be developed, which would reduce his risk of expulsion and help him relate better to his family and friends. His disorganisation and inattention were reframed as practical skills that could help him achieve at school and attain his goal of qualifying for university. Aaron was also referred to a psychiatrist for a medical consultation. However, he and his mother were quick to decline the ADHD medications prescribed.

An initial focus of therapy was the development of a plan to deal with situations that might put Aaron at risk or lead to expulsion from school or prison. Aaron admitted feeling tempted to use marijuana when meeting with his fellow ex-inmates, but was confident that he could abstain from drugs. The psychologist encouraged him to avoid these peers when he was feeling vulnerable, and Aaron role-played ways of saying "no" with his own witty one-liners. The psychologist monitored his drug use and intentions each session, and also informed his parents and probation officer of any concerns.

Another risk issue that arose later in therapy was unprotected sex. Aaron had recently become involved with a past girlfriend and his impulsivity, limited sexual experience, and the lack of boundaries, made him likely to engage in unsafe sex. Psycho-education was provided about the risks associated with unsafe sex (e.g., sexually transmitted diseases, pregnancy), safe sex practices, and the importance of planning ahead to compensate for impulsive urges. Aaron and the psychologist role-played ways of talking about these issues with his girlfriend. While he was willing to discuss these issues candidly and appreciated this information, he was adamant that he would never use a condom.

To help normalise his difficulties and maintain a healthy self-concept, Aaron's ADHD symptoms were discussed as strengths and weaknesses that fell along a continuum—similar to any sensory or motor skill. He learnt to label and rate his moods (frustration was from 0 = "cool" to 10 = "extremely pissed off"), and then identified situations that triggered these moods (boredom in the classroom or seeing someone "giving me the eye"). Using the CBT 5-part model (Greenberger & Padesky, 1995), he learnt to be aware of early warning signs of these moods developing (e.g., foot tapping, beginning an internal monologue of swear words, or giving someone "the eye").

Once these triggers and warning signs were identified, Aaron and the psychologist brainstormed techniques to break the cycle impulsive actions that led to conflict. These included "Stop-Think" (a verbal cue to pause before acting impulsively), self-statements ("It ain't worth it."), distraction from urges to misbehave (writing a letter to his girlfriend), and simple relaxation techniques. These coping strategies were practiced during his therapy sessions, and Aaron was encouraged to experiment with them at home and at school, and to evaluate their effectiveness in lowering his frustration and helping him circumventing conflict.

Whilst Aaron wanted to retain his "agro", he was confident and willing to experiment with other coping techniques, particularly in the classroom setting. In clinical sessions the psychologist would help him reflect on situations that had arisen during the week (e.g., cursing the teacher), and retrospectively role-play them, practising new and less aggressive ways of communication. They also brainstormed for positive outlets for his high energy during school. Whilst the teacher refused his request for breaks during class, he was able to take a walk between classes and started attending the gym regularly.

Aaron was confident in his intelligence, but worried about his school performance as the clear structure and schedule of prison contrasted starkly with his current situation. This insight was used to encourage him to develop his own external structure to compensate for both his unstructured home environment and his own attentional difficulties at school. Aaron developed an individualised learning plan, within and without the classroom. However, techniques for developing his learning in class, such as reducing distractions (cell-phone off) and re-focusing attention on his teachers by using his watch as a visual cue were met with limited success. He remained convinced that the three-hour classes were too long and the teachers too boring, and resorted to studying alone outside of class to catch up.

Aaron found more success improving his study patterns. He started studying in the library instead of at home and used his smartphone to create a daily study schedule. He developed self-monitoring skills (e.g., using a "self-alert" on his smart-phone which buzzed every 15 minutes), cueing him to check his alertness, ask himself, "What should I do next?", and respond proactively. If his energy level was either too low or high, he would do push-ups before returning to his task. His parents paid for individual tuition three times a week, which he found more beneficial than the classroom environment. These skills and support helped him feel more confident in his ability to study, and considerably reduced his worry and sense of helplessness about his studies.

After ten sessions of therapy, and with his GCE "O" Level examinations looming, Aaron and the psychologist agreed to "pause" therapy and to resume follow-up sessions in two to three months' time. They had already recognised a number of positive changes in Aaron. Post-therapy completion of the CBCL and YSR indicated his rule-breaking behaviours had lessened (both in normal range) and his attention problems had improved (although still in the clinical range). Aaron reported abstaining from all drug use (confirmed by his probation checks). He had developed a greater awareness of his impulsivity and frustration, and had learnt effective skills of self-regulation. While classroom interactions were still a challenge, and he displayed a defiant attitude towards teachers and peers, his greater restraint was rewarded by a lack of suspension from school. And despite considerable difficulty learning in the classroom, he had developed and maintained a positive study regime. He failed English in his mid-term examinations, but passed all other subjects, and scored within the top five of his class in Math, Physics and Chemistry.

Unfortunately, little had changed in Aaron's home environment and his relationship with his mother, possibly because these had not been the primary foci of therapy. Aaron still felt considerable frustration and anger towards his mother. While he had developed positive coping strategies for his moods, he also recognised that future intervention would be beneficial, potentially even in facilitating his moving in to live with his father. His father was also supportive of prospective intervention. His probation officer reported no concerns and encouraged him to resume therapy soon to fulfil his mandate.

DISCUSSION

To date, there are no epidemiological studies specifically addressing the prevalence or demographics of ADHD or ODD in Singapore. However, a recent systematic review indicated that prevalence rates of ADHD in Asia (based on 15 Asian studies) average about 4–5% of school-aged children, consistent with international rates (Polanczyk et al., 2007). This equates to about two students in an average class of 40 students in Singapore. A diagnosis of ADHD is one of the most common reasons for referrals to Singapore's mental health community teams—usually resulting from concerns that students' poor attention and associated externalizing behaviours are having a negative impact on their academic development (Woo et al., 2007; Ang et al., 2012).

Recent research indicates that about 70–80% of adolescents, as well as one third to half of the adults diagnosed with ADHD will continue to meet diagnostic criteria later in life. A sizeable proportion of the remainder will experience residual symptoms that cause significant impairment (Ramsay & Rostain, 2007). The difficulties experienced by Aaron—his oppositional behaviour, drug use, risky sexual behaviour and difficulties in academic and social relationships—are common among teenagers with ADHD (Barkley, 2006). Indeed, boys with ADHD are more likely than not to fulfil criteria for ODD (Brassett-Harknett & Butler, 2007).

Fact Box 3.2. Nutritional and Herbal Supplements for ADHD

Many people in the general population are sceptical of using prescription drugs for ADHD and prefer nutritional and herbal interventions. However, research studies have clearly shown that supplements are neither safer nor more effective, and many are not backed by sufficient research to support their efficacy or document their adverse effects. St John's Wort, vitamin therapies, de-leading and iron supplements appear to be ineffective in improving ADHD symptoms, and may even cause toxicity or death (Kapalka, 2010). However, some compounds show more promising effects on ADHD, including caffeine and Omega-3. The latter is currently being researched in Singapore.

Substance abuse can cause serious problems and complicate treatment for clients with ADHD (Bardo, Fishbein & Milch, 2011). The psychologist originally assumed that this would be a key focus of therapy for Aaron, in light of his lax home environment and his difficulties in self-control. However, the Singaporean government's strict regulations and probationary terms acted as sufficient deterrents to his relapse, and allowed treatment to focus on other pertinent goals.

Psychosocial treatment has been shown to be increasingly effective for children, teens and adults with ADHD and associated problems. Studies have demonstrated how children diagnosed with ADHD can improve their ability to learn, exercise self-control and interact with peers (Barkley, 2006). However, longitudinal studies generally show that regardless of treatment, youth with ADHD are still more likely to present with more academic, social, psychiatric and behavioural problems than their counterparts without ADHD (Molina et al., 2009). Thus, whilst Aaron showed considerable positive change over the course of treatment, he is still likely to face difficulties in the future, particularly during developmental transitions or times of stress. This highlights the important role clinicians play in encouraging youth with ADHD to develop positive relations with the mental health system, and plan ahead for transitions such as entering National Service, tertiary education, or the workforce.

Studies to date have provided some clear recommendations for the treatment of ADHD. Because of the pervasive and multidimensional impact of ADHD, therapy should be multimodal, preferably within a multidisciplinary team. The National Institute for Health and Care Excellence (NICE) guidelines for ADHD recommend psycho-education, parental training, psychological treatment, and drug treatment for patients with severe impairment or showing little response to psychosocial interventions (National Institute for Health and Care Excellence, 2013).

Psychosocial intervention should target a range of domains, such as self-control, social skills, problem-solving skills and the appropriate expression and handling of emotions. There are some well-developed manualised treatments available (for examples, *see* Barkley & Murphy, 2006; Solanto et al., 2008). These include step-by-step psycho-education and specific skills development, which are available through individual or group therapy, or self-help books.

The prognosis for treatment is improved if clients readily accept the ADHD diagnosis and recognise the need for change (Kapalka, 2010). For Aaron—and many teenagers with ADHD who have developed defiant or oppositional behaviours—therapeutic engagement can be difficult and requires more than simply adapting a manualised treatment (i.e., a treatment that follows a standardised process for all clients outlined by a manual). In Aaron's case, the psychologist fostered his involvement by acknowledging the family's unwillingness to accept an ADHD diagnosis. He normalized Aaron's difficulties by reframing them as specific strengths and weaknesses rather than symptoms of a disorder. He also ensured that the therapy focused on Aaron's primary concerns: stress about his studies, his anxiety about being expelled, his frustration with his relationships, and his determination to maintain communication with his father.

Aaron's tendency to "get pissed off" was addressed openly in therapy—for example by asking Aaron directly, "How will I know if you are pissed off at me?", and by encouraging him to share his frustrations when they were expressed during therapy sessions. The collaborative nature of CBT was also helpful in helping both Aaron and the psychologist to avoid a pattern of defensiveness or judgment against one another. Although Aaron was aggressive to his father, he also idealised him, and this may have provided a positive template for his relationship with the psychologist as an older male who could play a supportive role in his life.

Effective therapy with people with ADHD requires therapists to recognise how a person's symptoms of ADHD can influence the course of therapy and the therapeutic relationship. Difficulties in organising and planning usually lead to non-attendance, with drop-out rates sometimes in excess of 50% (Kapalka, 2010). Inattention and hyperactivity can lead to difficulty in focusing and boredom during a session. Aaron and the psychologist attempted to compensate for these difficulties by using text reminders for sessions, involving his father, using an agenda on the whiteboard for each session, turning their phones off during sessions, and providing brief "drink breaks" when Aaron was restless. This helped in-session, but did not succeed in modifying his irregular attendance throughout therapy.

Aaron's impulsivity during his sessions led to comments that were often uncensored and surprisingly honest. This offset his defensiveness and actually made it easier to assess his real emotions and thoughts. However, the therapist also learnt to be sensitive about what questions were asked in his parents' presence and to clearly communicate confidentiality issues with all parties, so that Aaron would not feel too exposed or regret his own comments.

Parental psycho-education and training is usually an important component of therapy for children and teenagers with ADHD. Although Aaron's mother's parenting style and his home environment was considered an important perpetuating factor for his presenting problems, it was difficult to engage her in therapy in order to address these issues directly. This highlights the need for clinicians to adapt ADHD treatment models to each client—selecting components that best fit a person's individual and contextual strengths, and maintaining realistic expectations for therapeutic outcomes.

Whilst Aaron's frequent non-attendance probably moderated the success of his therapy, he did not drop out of therapy, and was not averse to returning to it. Ideally, with ongoing therapy and experience, Aaron will have the opportunity to develop a more comprehensive perspective on ADHD. Acceptance of his difficulties could lead to a stronger sense of identity and self-esteem, to improved relationships, and an ability to generalise the skills he had gained to tackle other problems in the future.

1. Aaron's case demonstrates how ADHD is a pervasive disorder that impacts many domains of life. In teenagers, this might include academic problems, oppositional behaviour problems and risky behaviours such as drug and alcohol use or unsafe sex. As a psychologist, how would you have decided on goals for therapy with Aaron and what would have been your therapeutic focus?

2. Interestingly, a local study with a large sample size (n= 2,574) found that of all the CBCL and Teacher's Report Form (TRF) scales, scores on the Attention and ADHD scales best discriminated children and adolescents who were referred to the Child Guidance Clinic at IMH from those who were not referred (Ang et al., 2012). These findings differ from studies in the USA and Netherlands, in which items such as 'Unhappy, sad and depressed' best discriminated referrals (Achenbach & Rescorla, 2001; Verhulst et al., 1989). What factors do you think might contribute to this cultural difference?

3. In Singapore, clinicians are required by law to report client drug use to the legal authorities. How do you think this could impact on confidentiality, assessment and treatment with clients who are using drugs?

4. The diagnosis of ADHD is a controversial issue, and even more so with the recent publication of the DSM-5, which has expanded its criteria to allow 1) ADHD symptoms to be present before age 12 (instead of before age 7 in the DSM-IV); and 2) fewer symptoms (5 instead of 6) required to attain a diagnosis for those over 17 years of age (American Psychiatric Association, 2013). What are some advantages and disadvantages of expanding these criteria for ADHD diagnosis?

CHAPTER 4.

MISSED DIAGNOSIS AND MISDIAGNOSIS

Anxiety and Autism Spectrum Disorder

JADE JANG LEONG YEOK

INTRODUCTION

Bang! The toilet door smashed into John's face, shattering spectacle lenses into pieces that cut into his eyes. He was rushed to the hospital, underwent two eye surgeries and had his eyes taped shut. Even after he could open his eyes a few days later, he could not see anything—it was a terrifying experience for a ten-year-old. He cried, screamed, and struggled with the medical team whenever they reviewed him, but over the next few days he slowly regained his vision.

Things changed after his discharge. John refused to sleep with the lights off, and insisted on having a nightlight in his room and one of his parents accompany him until he fell asleep. He was so fearful of the dark that he avoided unlit areas of his home. When he needed to use the toilet at night, he would switch on all the lights one by one until he reached it. He had frequent emotional outbursts and would cry and scream if his parents did not accede to his requests. While his parents were not religious, they played religious prayer chants on the advice of their older relatives in a bid to calm him down. The plan backfired when he developed fear reactions to these chants.

He began having nightmares almost daily for several months on end. He would scream and shout in his dreams but awake with no recollection of having done so. He also became more irritable and more insistent on his preferences. He would shout and throw tantrums more frequently. His parents found it difficult to understand these behaviours as he kept his thoughts to himself.

As he refused to return to the school where the injury had occurred, John's parents arranged for a school transfer. John found it hard to adjust to his new school. He especially did not like the toilet in his new school as it was dark and he was afraid that "monsters would chase after him". His fears were further heightened after an occasion when the toilet lights were turned off while he was inside. From then on, he refused to go to the school toilet unaccompanied. For John, going to the toilet was like having a heart attack—his heart would pound wildly and he would have difficulty breathing, and even a few months later, he would still rush in and out of the toilet when he needed to relieve himself.

John's fear of the dark and related emotional issues persisted for more than a year after his physical recovery, prompting his ophthalmologist to refer him to a psychiatrist. The psychiatrist's initial impression was phobia of darkness (i.e., achluophobia) with features, but not a full diagnosis, of post-traumatic stress disorder (PTSD). John was subsequently referred to a psychologist for psychotherapy.

As the psychologist began looking into his history and background, she started to uncover other concerns. Since young, John's parents had had to grapple with his strong opinions and insistence on his own views, as well as his passiveness during social interactions. Even with his immediate family whom he was most comfortable with, he rarely initiated social interactions and tended not to share his thoughts and interests with them. His poor conversation skills and poor eye contact, as well as rigidity in thinking, further affected his social interaction and communication. On top of this, and prior to his accident, John had already displayed numerous fears that his parents felt were irrational, too persistent and too intense.

BACKGROUND

John came from an intact family with two younger siblings—a brother two years younger and a baby sister. His father was a professional and his mother was a homemaker. His family did not have a history of developmental or mental illnesses. John attended a mainstream primary school and performed well academically, obtaining 1s and 2s in all subjects.

John was born full-term, had no pre- or post-natal issues, and met his usual developmental milestones. However, his parents noted that he was a sensitive child who would insist on having his own way. He often reacted in an extreme manner to seemingly small and irrelevant events, and found it difficult to regulate his emotions when upset. For example, John's parents shared that he had once gotten very upset when they insisted on purchasing a piece of furniture he had a "bad feeling about".

His parents first noticed his limited interest in interacting with his peers when he was about two and a half years old. He preferred to play with older children and adults, and did not befriend his peers easily. He did not seek out friends at primary school, and while he would play chess with a few classmates during recess, he was otherwise passive and did not engage much with them. Although he identified some classmates as his friends, his parents felt that their interactions were quite superficial.

John was restless and always fiddling with something, even when working on his schoolwork. In Primary 1 and 2, his teachers complained that he would walk around and talk unnecessarily during lessons. Even at Primary 4, he was occasionally reprimanded for restlessness or for talking out of turn. He was not afraid of airing his opinions and had engaged in minor arguments with teachers and classmates whose opinions were contrary to his.

John's fears encompassed numerous things. His fears were often specific to a particular person, animal, or object, but he had difficulty explaining why these

Fact Box 4.1. Considerations for Diagnosis of ASD

DSM-5's (American Psychiatric Association, 2013) move from previously separate Autistic Disorder, Asperger Disorder, and pervasive developmental disorder-not otherwise specified (PDD-NOS) to a single continuum of Autism Spectrum Disorders with different levels of severity, recognises ASD as a 'spectrum' disorder where one may fall anywhere on the wide spectrum of each area of functioning. For example, in terms of difficulties with social interaction, one may be actively avoidant, aloof, or overly involved. In terms of cognitive functioning, one may be found anywhere on the spectrum between intellectually disabled to intellectually gifted.

People with ASD also commonly present with uneven ability profiles and may even have very significant discrepancies in their different areas of functioning (e.g., Geschwind & Levitt, 2007; Joseph, Tager-Flusberg & Lord, 2002). For example, a person with ASD may have exceptional language reasoning abilities, but poor social chat and conversation skills; another may have superior cognitive ability, but very poor self-care and social awareness. Hence, in persons with ASD, we cannot assume that one's overall functioning is adequate simply from observing his or her functioning in a specific area (a commonly made assumption). Each area of functioning needs to be explored individually.

In attempting to rule out ASD, one cannot simply look for the absence or presence of behaviours but at the quality of a person's functioning. The authors of the Autism Diagnostic Observation Schedule, Second Edition (ADOS-2; Lord, Rutter, DiLavore, Risi, Gotham, Bishop, 2012) manual cautioned about the need to consider the baseline frequency of behaviours. As described in the ADOS-2 manual, some behaviours are expected to occur at high frequency (e.g., eye contact, vocalisation, facial expression), others rarely occur (e.g., stereotyped speech, echolalia), and still others present with great variability (e.g., gestures). Consequently, a few observations of odd behaviour are enough to warrant concern whereas a moderate frequency of "prosocial" behaviours does not indicate the absence of abnormality.

frightened him. For instance, John reported being afraid of a particular tree near his home. He was adamant about not going near it as "bad things would happen". If his parents insisted on walking past it, he would close his eyes and have them hold his hands to guide him past it. His parents had a difficult time understanding why, compared to his peers, John presented with such persistent and intense fears, which seemed to have no apparent triggers and were not the result of bad experiences.

ASSESSMENT

These assessments, in combination with interviews with his parents and observations of his behaviour during sessions, were useful in identifying characteristics consistent with an ASD diagnosis. Even though John had a good command of language, he was observed to have limited social initiation and response. He related better with people whom he was familiar with or with whom he shared similar interests. He engaged well in conversations relating to his interests in chess, solar systems, or mathematical puzzles. Otherwise, he did not initiate conversations and when spoken to, answered directly and without elaboration. He also tended to avoid topics that he perceived to be in his areas of weakness. Overall, it was difficult to involve him in small talk. John also lacked interest in others, had difficulties in developing and maintaining relationships, and had poor social awareness. He related better to adults than with his peers and did not have any close friends. When he was young, he preferred to play on his own and had to be coaxed to join other children in their play.

John displayed deficits in nonverbal communicative behaviours. His eye contact tended to be brief and inconsistent. He also had difficulties in adjusting his behaviours to suit different social contexts. His facial expressions were usually exaggerated and occasionally incongruent to the situation. For example, he smiled when his parents were scolding him. As he was less attuned to social cues, such as facial expressions and emotions, others would perceive him as being aloof, direct, and tactless.

Since young, John exhibited unusually strong interests in a restricted range of topics. At one point in time, he had been fascinated by escalators and would insist on stopping to observe their movements for more than five minutes each time. He displayed extensive knowledge of solar systems. He was also very familiar with the Mass Rapid Transit (MRT) system and would frequently ask to go on train rides. His most current special interests were chess and mathematical puzzles. In addition, John was sensitive to certain tactile and visual stimuli. When in lower primary school, John's low tolerance for noise had resulted in him covering his ears during recess as he found the sounds in the canteen too overwhelming. After his eye injury, his parents noticed that he would sometimes cry and hit himself when he woke from his afternoon nap. He was also very sensitive to certain tastes.

John's preference for routines and resistance to change were also quite evident. When he was a toddler, he was very particular about how and where things were kept. He needed to know at the beginning of a day or week what his schedule would be;

he did not take well to last minute changes and would react with angry outbursts. Nonetheless, he was fairly compliant if told in advance what would be happening.

John's initial presenting concerns and symptoms were consistent with either a phobia or anxiety. However, further clarification revealed that he also presented with several features associated with Autism Spectrum Disorder (ASD): difficulties with social interaction and communication, fascination with specific, narrow interests (i.e., chess), and rigid thinking. Comprehensive diagnostic assessment was conducted to determine if he met the diagnostic criteria for ASD. John's parents were interviewed using the Autism Diagnostic Interview-Revised (ADI—R; Rutter, Le Couteur, & Lord, 2003)—a semi-structured diagnostic interview conducted with caregivers that focuses on a child's developmental history, social interaction, communication, and patterns of behaviours. John was administered the Autism Diagnostic Observation Schedule (ADOS; Lord, Rutter, DiLavore, & Risi, 2000)—Module 3, which is a semi-structured, standardised assessment of one's communication, social interaction patterns, and play.

A cognitive assessment is another important component in the assessment of ASD as it provides insight into a client's language abilities, and information to rule out differential diagnoses. It also aids the psychologist in evaluating the suitability of the client's schooling arrangements. Results of the cognitive assessment using the Wechsler Intelligence Scale for Children—Fourth Edition (WISC-IV) indicated that, compared to his peers, John's cognitive functioning was well above average. This suggested that while he would require support for his other ASD-associated challenges, he should be able to cope with the academic demands of mainstream education.

As part of the clinical assessment to clarify John's presenting issues, the Spence Children's Anxiety Scale (SCAS) was administered to both John and his mother. This scale sought to assess the severity of anxiety symptoms in the following six domains: generalized anxiety, panic/agoraphobia, social phobia, separation anxiety, obsessive compulsive disorder, and physical injury fears. As compared to his same-aged peers, John's endorsement of the SCAS indicated elevated levels of anxiety in relation to separation anxiety and physical injury fears. His mother's responses indicated that he had elevated levels in terms of overall anxiety and all other domains with the exception of obsessive compulsive disorder.

DIAGNOSIS

Comprehensive diagnostic assessment revealed that John displayed impairments in social interaction, social communication, and had certain stereotyped patterns of behaviours. In terms of social communication, he had poor social awareness, displayed limited social initiation and response, lacked an interest in others, had deficits in nonverbal communicative behaviours, and had difficulties in developing and maintaining relationships, and in adjusting his behaviour to suit social contexts. John also displayed strong interests in a restricted range of topics, had some tactile and visual interests, exhibited a preference for specific routines, and was resistant to change. His language and cognitive development were within the normal range.

Based on the Diagnostic and Statistical Manual of Mental Disorders (5th ed.; DSM–5; American Psychiatric Association, 2013), John was diagnosed to have Autism Spectrum Disorder (ASD) without intellectual impairment or language impairment. Autistic trait severity ranges from Level 1 (requiring support) to Level 3 (requiring very substantial support). The severity levels for both John's Social Communication deficits as well as his Restricted and Repetitive Behaviours were assessed to be Level 1.

Anxiety disorders, phobias, attention deficit hyperactivity disorder (ADHD) and PTSD were considered as possible differential or co-morbid diagnoses. However, clinical assessment (e.g., clinical interviews, school reports, etc.) revealed that John's features of anxiety and hyperactivity did not meet full diagnostic criteria for these disorders. It should also be noted that persons with ASD commonly experience difficulties with anxiety and hyperactivity, which may or may not be severe enough to warrant a diagnosis of co-morbidity.

INTEGRATIVE FORMULATION

Schopler's (1994) iceberg metaphor (Figure 4.1) is helpful in portraying how the underlying characteristics of ASD relate to a child's current presentation. The tip of the iceberg represents overt, observable behaviours (the presenting problem) and the submerged part of the iceberg represents underlying, contributing ASD characteristics. The iceberg metaphor helps us analyse how the triad of impairments in a person with ASD (i.e., social communication, social interaction, as well as restricted and repetitive behaviours and interests) may explain behaviours of concern, and thus aid in intervention planning.

Predisposing Factors

John's underlying ASD characteristics predisposed him to experience difficulties in coping and adapting to change, and resulted in his presentation with a range of anxieties, of which the most recent and pertinent was his fear of the dark. Using the iceberg model, John's presenting behaviour of avoiding dark places and related anxiety symptoms (e.g., crying, needing to use a night light) after his eye operations was motivated by his underlying need to know what to expect, his preference for sameness, difficulties with change, possible sensory issues, and poor emotional regulation.

His other ASD-related difficulties (e.g., inability to read others' facial expression or emotions, poor awareness of social situations, poor perspective taking) made it a challenge for him to understand, take cues from, and react appropriately to unfamiliar social situations. In addition, his passiveness in initiating social contact and avoidance of self-perceived areas of weakness made it hard for John to acknowledge his difficulties and to seek help.

FIGURE 4.1. ILLUSTRATION USING ICEBERG METAPHOR (SCHOPLER, 1994).

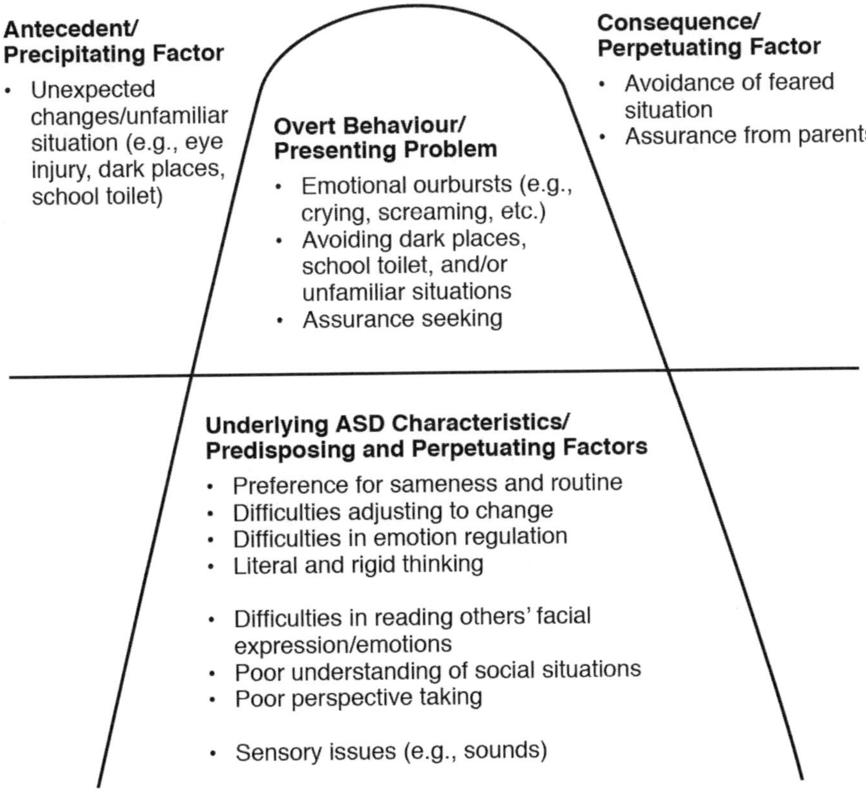

Antecedent/ Precipitating Factor

- Unexpected changes/unfamiliar situation (e.g., eye injury, dark places, school toilet)

Overt Behaviour/ Presenting Problem

- Emotional ourbursts (e.g., crying, screaming, etc.)
- Avoiding dark places, school toilet, and/or unfamiliar situations
- Assurance seeking

Consequence/ Perpetuating Factor

- Avoidance of feared situation
- Assurance from parents

Underlying ASD Characteristics/ Predisposing and Perpetuating Factors

- Preference for sameness and routine
- Difficulties adjusting to change
- Difficulties in emotion regulation
- Literal and rigid thinking

- Difficulties in reading others' facial expression/emotions
- Poor understanding of social situations
- Poor perspective taking

- Sensory issues (e.g., sounds)

Precipitating Factors

John's eye injury had introduced numerous unexpected changes to his routine. He found himself in new and unfamiliar situations—being hospitalised, undergoing an operation, experiencing a temporary loss of vision—which he had difficulties coping with and adapting to. This exacerbated the frequency of his emotional outbursts, triggered his avoidance of uncomfortable situations (e.g., being in dark places, going to the toilet) and reinforced his assurance-seeking behaviour (i.e., needing his parents to accompany him when confronting new situations).

Perpetuating Factors

John's underlying ASD characteristics caused his behaviours of concern to persist. His poor reading of social cues led him to misinterpret others' emotions and intentions. Together with his literal interpretation of situations and rigid pattern of thinking, John's ASD-related deficits perpetuated his perception that unexpected or unfamiliar situations were uncomfortable. Moreover, his poor emotional regulation exacerbated his difficulties in coping with these situations, and led to frequent emotional outbursts and tantrums. His sensitivity to sensory input—certain noises or tastes—further taxed his capacity to cope with his current situation.

Being able to avoid feared situations (e.g., transferring to a different school, having a night light, etc.) and getting constant assurance from parents also reinforced and perpetuated John's avoidant behaviours and emotional outbursts. Being allowed to avoid feared situations deprived him the opportunity to realise that they were not as scary as he believed them to be and reinforced his beliefs that such situations ought to be feared and avoided.

Protective Factors

John's family was accepting of his condition and had actively sought to understand ASD and how it contributed to his difficulties. After his diagnosis, they were very enthusiastic in learning and using ASD-friendly strategies to support him. John himself possessed the cognitive ability to develop new coping strategies and benefitted from his parent's coaching. His close relationship with his family also rendered him receptive to the support they offered.

PROGNOSIS

Given that ASD is a pervasive developmental disorder, as John matures into adulthood he is likely to experience increasing difficulty coping with greater societal demands. However, these difficulties would likely be moderated by his young age, high learning (cognitive) potential, good relationship with his parents, and his parents' dedicated support. These protective factors would facilitate John's acquisition of helpful coping strategies, such as learning about social norms and expectations, conversational skills, and perspective-taking skills. Factors that could reduce his prognosis for treatment included his reluctance to engage in the discussion of topics he perceived to be areas of personal inadequacy or weakness. Thus, rapport between John and his therapist would be an important mediating factor of his prognosis.

INTERVENTION

The therapeutic approach used with persons with ASD varies markedly from a standard therapeutic approach. Prior to John's diagnosis of ASD, his psychiatrist's clinical impression was that he presented with a phobia of darkness with features of PTSD. The initial intervention plan had thus been to deliver Cognitive Behavioural Therapy (CBT) for anxiety, an evidence-based treatment effective in the treatment of anxiety disorders. First, psychoeducation on anxiety was conducted. Relaxation exercises (e.g., deep breathing) were then taught to John and his family. While John was not keen to participate and felt uncomfortable having to close his eyes, he managed to learn deep breathing with his family's prompting and encouragement.

While working with John using CBT, his psychologist began to notice some behaviours that pointed to the need for a comprehensive diagnostic assessment for ASD. For example, it was a challenge working with John to develop his hierarchy of fears. He rated his various fears similarly, and each at the highest level. His psychologist suspected that he had difficulties recognising and understanding his own physiological symptoms and emotions, a common characteristic of ASD. John was unable to articulate his thoughts and fears, which made it hard to for both him and his psychologist to identify his core beliefs. He also exhibited rigid thinking and lack of insight. For example, he did not agree with his treatment plan because he neither like the idea of being exposed to his fears nor saw the need for it. His strong belief that "what I think will definitely happen" also limited his psychologist's attempts at cognitive restructuring work.

While CBT is a well-researched, evidence-based, and commonly used treatment method for anxiety, it is limited in its amenability for persons with ASD. Similar to the challenges faced by John's psychologist, existing research has identified the following issues when CBT was used with the ASD population: clients' difficulty in grasping the concept of cognitive restructuring, therapists' uncertainty about whether gains were sustained, and limited generalisation of CBT techniques to real-life situations (Cardaciotto & Herbert, 2004; Hare, 1997; Weiss & Lunsky, 2010).

While the coping skills and relaxation techniques John learnt helped him manage—and provided him temporary relief from—his physiological symptoms, they were not able to address his poor social understanding, rigid thinking, and difficulty reading social situations. Thus, they were unable to prevent a recurrence of his concerning behaviours. With John's diagnosis of ASD however came the recognition that underlying ASD-related difficulties were what predisposed him to and perpetuated his anxieties. Recurrences of anxiety could now be prevented with ASD-friendly strategies such as visual schedules, social stories^{TM} and comic strip conversation.

In view of the pervasive and lifelong nature of ASD, intervention plans were revised to include psychoeducation with John's parents on ASD. Using the iceberg metaphor, John's psychologist explained to John's parents his underlying need to know what to expect, preference for sameness, and difficulty with change. His parents were then taught to use the iceberg metaphor as a framework that enabled them to analyse John's behaviours of concern, identify his underlying difficulties, and apply appropriate ASD-friendly strategies to prevent their recurrence.

Using the iceberg model, John's parents were able to identify his difficulties in reading others' facial expression, his poor perspective taking, and his misunderstanding of social situations. They were then taught to use comic strip conversations and social stories^{TM} to help John better understand social situations. Comic strip conversations enabled John to become more aware of the thoughts, intentions, and feelings of others.

This caused abstract aspects of social communication to become more concrete and easier to understand (Figure 4.2). Social stories™ are individualised short stories that describe social situations, perspectives, as well as common responses, and are used to help one understand social norms and expected behaviours (Gray, 2010).

FIGURE 4.2 COMIC STRIP CONVERSATION BETWEEN JOHN AND HIS TEACHER

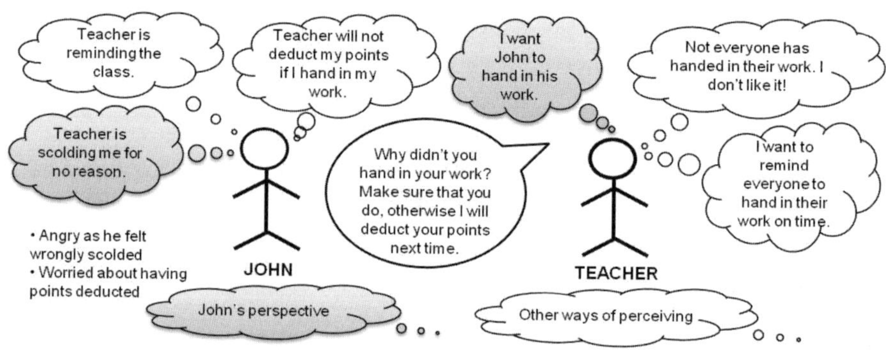

John's parents were also introduced to the use of visual schedules to address his underlying need to know what to expect, preference for sameness, and difficulties with change. Visual schedules present the sequence of one's daily activities with words and pictures. Research has shown that persons with ASD attend better to visual information as compared to verbal information (Garretson, Fein & Waterhouse, 1990). Routine use of visual schedules was aimed at reducing John's anxiety by providing a structure that would allow him to anticipate what would happen next. It was also used to promote flexibility as changes could regularly be introduced to his list of daily activities. This would prevent rigid adherence to a particular routine and would enable him to better cope with unexpected changes. Use of visual schedules could also empower one to become independent of adult prompts and support (Mesibov, Shea & Schopler, 2005).

A number of practical challenges were encountered during the course of John's treatment. Like many other families in Singapore, regular attendance was difficult in view of his family's busy schedule and multiple commitments. His family had little time to practice the strategies taught. Besides issues with attendance, disruptions during therapy session were another challenge. Due to a lack of alternative caregivers, John's parents brought all three children to the clinic. Progress was affected by their having to tend to his baby sister's needs during sessions. His parents' psychoeducation sessions were also occasionally interrupted by John and his brother.

John's reluctance to change, lack of insight, and avoidance of topics perceived to be areas of personal inadequacy and weakness lowered his receptiveness to his psychologist's attempts to engage him. Efforts were thus made to actively involve John's siblings during sessions so he would feel less picked on. Discussion topics and skills were deliberately presented as general life skills rather than skills aimed at countering his "deficits". Furthermore, as John shared a close relationship with his family and was receptive to their attempts to help him, his psychologist worked towards empowering his parents as co-therapists.

Over a period of two years, John's family attended a total of 17 intervention sessions, of which 10 sessions focused on parental psychoeducation. A few months after learning about the iceberg model and the use of visual schedules, his parents reported feeling empowered by understanding John's behaviours in relation to his underlying deficits. They noticed that John no longer avoided the school toilet, nor was he fearful of either dark places or the tree near their home. Although John did not give a reason for this, it was possible that his parents' persistence in practising relaxation strategies as a family had strengthened his coping strategies and the management of his anxieties. Overall, they felt that they understood John better and were more equipped to anticipate and support him in adapting to changes.

Fact Box 4.2. Gender Differences

Consistent with global statistics where boys are about four times more likely to be diagnosed with ASD (Whiteley, Todd, Carr, & Shattock, 2010), in Bernard-Opitz and colleagues' (2001) survey of 176 children with autism in Singapore, 81% were boys and 19% girls. Another local study by Lian and Ho (2012) found that amongst children who were referred in 2003 to the then Child Development Unit at KK Women's and Children's Hospital and received a diagnosis of ASD, the male to female ratio was 4.5:1.

It has been suggested that there are gender differences in the expression of clinical symptoms of ASD. Amongst persons without cognitive impairment, females showed subtler symptoms and less atypical behaviours, which may result in fewer of them being accurately diagnosed with ASD (Tsakanikos, Underwood, Kravariti, Bouras, & McCarthy, 2011). In their 2001 review, Gould and Ashton-Smith found that (compared with boys with ASD) girls with ASD had a better sense of the social world, were more socially inclined, and were better able to observe and follow social action. In addition, the intense special interests girls with ASD held (e.g., cartoons, celebrities, anime) tended to be more mainstream and thus, not deemed "abnormal".

Autism Spectrum Disorders (ASD) are a range of pervasive developmental disorders characterised by difficulties in social communication, and social interaction, and restricted or repetitive pattern of behaviours and interests (American Psychiatric Association, 2000). While prevalence data is not available for Singapore, a recent review of global prevalence estimates that about 1 in every 160 persons has some form of ASD (Elsabbagh et al., 2012), indicating that ASD is not uncommon.

However, it is easy to miss out on an ASD diagnosis or to misdiagnose ASD. For example, John's diagnosis of ASD could have been easily missed if comprehensive and detailed developmental history was not obtained and the underlying reasons for his anxiety symptoms had not been clarified. For persons with mild symptoms of ASD, it may take a period of observation before certain behaviours can be ascertained to be symptoms of ASD. Thereafter, it is common to take more time to gather further information to determine whether ASD diagnostic assessments are warranted.

Bernard-Opitz, Kwook, & Sapuan (2001) surveyed 176 parents of children with autism in Singapore (aged 3 to 12 years) and found that 60% of children were diagnosed before the age of 3 years. Despite having displayed ASD symptoms since young, John fell into the 40% of children whose ASD diagnosis was missed when young. Possibly, his symptoms were mild and did not fully manifest until his eye injury, which imposed demands that exceed his limited coping capacities. In another local study, Lian and Ho (2012) examined the profile of children who were referred in 2003 to the then Child Development Unit at KK Women's and Children's Hospital. Amongst the 170 children who were diagnosed with ASD, 86% were assessed to be in the moderate or severe range. Hence, most children diagnosed at a young age in Singapore displayed moderate to severe levels of symptoms.

With the exception of cases where parents refused or deferred evaluation, clinical observations suggested that persons diagnosed at a later age usually had symptoms that were more ambiguous or difficulties that were not as challenging at a younger age, and thus were not noticed earlier. Other studies have also suggested that many people presenting at clinical or research settings with mild to moderate ASDs are either not identified and diagnosed (Fombonne et al., 2004) or are misdiagnosed (Harpaz- Rotem & Rosenheck 2004). A high prevalence of unrecognised ASDs was also found in children presenting with common developmental psychopathologies (Towbin, Pradella, Gorrindo, Pine, & Leibenluft, 2005). Thus, there needs to be a conscious effort for practitioners to routinely consider the possible diagnosis of ASD.

However, distinguishing between ASD and other psychopathologies can be challenging, especially for those displaying mild to moderate features. This is because the symptoms of ASD often overlap with symptoms of other disorders, for example, anxiety disorder, OCD, depression, and schizophrenia (Helverschou, Bakken, & Martinsen, 2011). A local study by Ooi and colleagues (2011) also found evidence of a high prevalence of behavioural and emotional problems which could result in multiple psychiatric diagnoses among children with high-functioning ASD. This study of 71 children with high-functioning ASD in Singapore found that between 72% and 86% of children had at least one behavioural or emotional problem of clinical concern as indicated by the Child Behavioural Checklist (CBCL) syndromes and DSM-oriented scales. Specifically, the most commonly reported problems were social problems (60.6%), thought problems (50.7%), attention problems (49.3%), and withdrawn/depressed symptoms (40.8%). Using the DSM-oriented scales, the most commonly reported problems were attention deficit/hyperactivity problems (35.2%), anxiety problems (33.8%) and affective problems (31%). John's presentation is illustrative of anxiety actually being a core component of ASD—features of ASD can easily masquerade as and cause anxiety symptoms. Hence, it is critical for practitioners to be able to recognise the characteristics of ASD that underlie presenting behaviours. Thus, there is a need for greater exposure (e.g., clinical attachments and specialised trainings) to enable practitioners to gain expertise in differentiating ASD from other psychopathologies. This is particularly crucial to prevent missed diagnosis and/or misdiagnosis of high functioning individuals with ASD who have milder symptoms.

Finally, parent and caregiver support and dedication play a crucial role in treatment success. Parent training is considered an essential component of successful intervention programs for children with ASD (National Research Council, 2001). A therapist's attempts at intervention would be futile if parents do not accept and understand their child's diagnosis of ASD. Acceptance, as well as a good understanding of ASD and its implications, would place parents and caregivers in a better position to learn ASD-friendly strategies so as to provide a conducive environment for their child. However, it has been found that less than two-thirds of children with ASD in Singapore had parents as their main caregivers. In fact, 28% had foreign domestic helpers as their main caregivers (Bernard-Opitz Kwook, & Sapuan, 2001). In this survey of 176 parents of children with autism in Singapore, it was also found that both parents were working in 39% of the cases. The implication of this finding is that parents in Singapore have competing demands on their time and efforts, as evident in John's case, and this can create serious practical challenges for supporting and treating a child with ASD.

While John's parents quickly accepted his diagnosis of ASD, and were willing to and capable of learning ASD-friendly strategies, a large proportion of parents in Singapore still strongly believe that they can simply engage professionals to "fix" their child. Similar to engaging tutors to improve their child's academic performance, Singaporeans commonly perceive that intervention sessions with therapists alone are sufficient in effecting a significant reduction in symptoms and even an eventual "cure". Many do not realise that ASD-related difficulties persist over the lifespan, although improvements may be demonstrated as their children pick up strategies to help them cope. They may also not realise the impact of continued stress on their family should they not empower themselves to understand and manage their children's difficulties.

Thus, it is important for professionals to engage parents and caregivers in close collaboration in order to meet the needs of a person with ASD. Otherwise, they would likely continue to be dependent on professionals for support, thereby putting unnecessary strain on the healthcare system.

DISCUSSION QUESTIONS

1. While John's family did not practice any religion, they played religious prayer chants on the advice of their elders. Bernard-Opitz, Kwook, & Sapuan (2001) found that 2% of Singaporean parents of children with autism turn to religious healers: consulting temple spirit mediums, fortune tellers, seeking help through the *bomoh* (Malay shaman), and participating in religious healing sessions. How would you respond when families seek advice on these alternative practices?

2. In view of the competing demands from school and work on children and their parents, how would you garner collaboration and commitment from the family to engage in regular therapy and follow through with treatment plans?

3. How can you differentiate between anxiety disorders and anxiety inherently related to impairments associated with ASD, such as difficulties with changes and not knowing what to expect in social situations?

4. ASD is a neurodevelopmental disorder. How do the symptoms of ASD present at different life stages (toddler, child, adolescent, young adult, adult, etc.)? Why is it that some people only get diagnosed with ASD when they are much older?

5. What are pros and cons of having a diagnosis of ASD? Is it okay not to rule out a diagnosis of ASD? Especially when the person's symptoms are mild?

6. Parents and caregivers often ask, "Why should visuals be used when my child can read words?", "Can my child with ASD write his/her own schedule?", "I have been explaining to my child about various social situations, why must I write it out as a social story?" How are you going to respond to them?

7. What are some challenges that you may anticipate in trying to use CBT with a child with ASD? What adaptations may be required?

CHAPTER 5

AKAN DATANG! VOICE COMING SOON

Selective Mutism

KWAN HM CLARE

INTRODUCTION

The psychologist watched as six-year-old Muhriz cautiously and soundlessly moved amongst towards the toys in the consultation room. Muhriz's parents had decided to consult a psychologist at a public tertiary clinic as they were concerned that he only spoke with family members at home, and barely socialized with his peers or extended family members. Over the next three years, Muhriz, his family, and his psychologist began a journey to "help his voice to come out".

BACKGROUND

Muhriz was born and raised in Malaysia. His household comprised his parents, his younger sister and a domestic helper whom they considered part of the family. Being close in age, Muhriz and his younger sister were regular playmates. While his family conversed in both Malay and English, Muhriz had always been more proficient in Malay. Muhriz's immediate family was close-knit and shared a strong relationship with their extended family. When living in Malaysia, Muhriz met his cousins frequently but was generally anxious in their vicinity and tended to communicate with them in a shy and monotonous voice. He would tell his mother, "my voice sounds weird", "voice is only for family" and "I don't like how I sound".

Muhriz's first year at playschool was unremarkable, but in his second year, his parents enrolled him in a new school. This was when he began developing anxieties about school and started becoming increasingly uncommunicative. After a classmate who was a close friend stopped attending his school, Muhriz ceased to speak in class at all. His parents decided to give him a break from school. A year and a half later, Muhriz was enrolled in yet another school. At times he seemed to enjoy going back to school, but at other times, he appeared apprehensive and anxious.

A month after starting school, the family's domestic helper, who had cared for Muhriz since his birth, returned to the Philippines. Upon her departure, Muhriz's parents noticed that, over the next three months, he spoke even less at home and stopped talking in school. To his parents' relief, Muhriz gradually started talking at home. However, he continued to remain completely non-verbal at school. Later, two years into treatment, Muhriz shared another stressful incident that had occurred around this time in Malaysia: a teacher had locked him up in his preschool toilet—he was unsure why but felt scared and was apprehensive about attending school.

When Muhriz was about six, and due to his parents' work commitments, his family relocated to Singapore. Prior to this, Muhriz's parents had consulted clinics and hospitals about his non-verbal behaviour. They were concerned about the discrepancy in his presentation in school and at home—he was shy and withdrawn in the former, but chatty and energetic in the latter. Muhriz had been diagnosed with selective mutism in Malaysia and started psychotherapy sessions a few months prior to his family's relocation. After the move, he was reassessed and began to receive therapy in Singapore.

ASSESSMENT

Comprehensive assessment of a child with selective mutism requires a psychologist to gather information from a variety of sources, including the child himself, his family and teachers. This is on top of the psychologist's own clinical observations during sessions with the child. The assessment should seek to rule out any actual physical problems that prevent speech from occurring, mental disorders or environmental factors. Futhermore, there are considerable challenges in assessing a child who does not speak. For example, Muhriz presented with the hallmark features associated with selective mutism: he was persistently mute across different settings beyond his home environment; he was shy, clingy to his parents, and held little eye contact. He found it difficult to respond verbally to his psychologist and attempted to avoid all interaction. He generally avoided unfamiliar social situations and was behaviourally inhibited when he felt anxious. His psychologist thus had to be prepared to use non-verbal assessments and supplement those with keen observation of his behaviour.

To fully assess Muhriz's selective mutism symptoms and build a stronger understanding of his anxiety and overall psychosocial functioning, his mother was asked to complete three screening measures to supplement the clinical interview: the Selective Mutism Questionnaire (SMQ; Bergman et al., 2008), Screening for Child Anxiety Related Disorders (SCARED; Birmaher, et al., 1995), and the Strengths and Difficulties Questionnaire (SDQ; Goodman, 1997). The SMQ measured Muhriz's frequency of non-speaking behaviour across situations in which he was expected to speak. The scores supported information gained in the clinical interview: Muhriz was not speaking at school, and his mutism was associated with elevated distress and poorer functioning compared to kids his age. The SCARED questionnaire, used to screen for childhood anxiety disorders, pointed to Muhriz having elevated symptoms of separation anxiety and social anxiety. This further supported Muhriz's diagnosis of selective mutism, with anxiety at its core. Lastly, the SDQ is a brief behavioural questionnaire that provides a screening test for emotional symptoms, problems with conduct/hyperactivity-attention/peer relationships, and pro-social behaviour. These three measures provided an overview of Muhriz's current presentation, and the baseline levels that could be reassessed at later stages of treatment.

Aside from Muhriz's diagnosis of selective mutism, it was important that differential diagnoses were taken into consideration. In particular, communication disorder and autism spectrum disorder can both impact on social anxiety and a child's ability to communicate with others verbally and socially. An assessment of Muhriz's speech and language deficits was particularly important as his mother and school teachers had concerns about his language abilities.

A preliminary assessment revealed that while Muhriz had acquired single word and phrase speech within the normal developmental time frame, and was developmentally able to produce speech, he had delayed reading and spelling abilities, having only just learnt to read and spell at the age of six. A comprehensive assessment of his speech and language was postponed so as to provide him with ample opportunities to develop his English language abilities, and such that, through therapy, he could learn to manage his anxiety and develop speaking behaviour for future assessments. It was important that both his expressive and receptive language abilities would be assessed at a later stage.

In order to rule out the differential diagnosis of Autism Spectrum Disorder, a complete diagnostic assessment was administered. This comprised the Leiter International Performance Scale-Revised (Leiter-R; Roid & Miller, 1997), Autism Diagnostic Interview-Revised (ADI-R; Rutter, Couteur, & Lord, 2003), and behavioural observations. The Leiter-R is a nonverbal measure of intelligence that can be administered completely without the use of oral language. It was administered after attempts to get Muhiz to verbalise failed on other assessments requiring verbal responses. It assesses the cognitive domains of Reasoning, Visualisation, Memory and Attention. The ADI-R was conducted with Muhriz's mother. It is a structured interview which assessed Muhriz's developmental history and current abilities in areas affected by autism, including i) reciprocal social interaction, ii) communication and language, and iii) patterns of restricted and repetitive behaviours.

DIAGNOSIS

Muhriz's primary diagnosis was selective mutism. While he presented with some ASD-like symptoms—such as restricted interests in cars and certain songs, which persisted over long periods of time, as well as some degree of inflexibility to routines—and would have met criteria for Pervasive Developmental Disorder Not Otherwise Specified (PDD-NOS) in the DSM-IV (American Psychiatric Association, 2000), he did not meet criteria for ASD using the DSM-5 (American Psychiatric Association, 2013).

Notably, Muhriz was able to develop an intact and meaningful relationship with his sister appropriate to his developmental level. He was able to seek enjoyment and engage in joint attention with his close family members. He also had the ability to communicate with his sister and parents fairly well both verbally and non-verbally. His primary struggle was generalising these social-communicative abilities into unfamiliar situations or social settings. These difficulties were marked by his underlying anxiety. Therefore, the primary target in treatment was jointly discussed with his mother and it was decided that intervention would focus on lowering anxiety symptoms and increasing confidence in social communication.

INTEGRATIVE FORMULATION

Predisposing Factors

Muhriz's shy temperament and hyper-sensitivity to anxiety likely predisposed him to selective mutism, causing him to avoid or withdraw from social interaction due to intense levels of discomfort and anxiety. In terms of familial predisposition, while Muhriz's sister and mother were expressive and natural verbal communicators, his father had a more quiet and introverted nature.

Precipitating Factors

Muhriz's development of selective mutism was likely precipitated by multiple factors. Firstly, Muhriz may have struggled to cope with the unfamiliarity of his new environment. When he entered a new school, he was introduced to a new teaching style and way of relating to his new teacher. Secondly, Muhriz experienced losses of relationships in school and at home. When his friend was enrolled in another school, Muhriz lost a peer who had provided him a sense of comfort and consistency. When his domestic helper returned to the Philippines, the familiarity of his home environment was disrupted. These losses likely triggered a sense of insecurity, precipitated Muhriz's stress reactions and made him feel overwhelmed.

Being locked up in his preschool toilet in Malaysia as punishment could have been the specific incident that triggered Muhriz's selective mutism. As Muhriz was timid by nature and easily frightened by figures of authority, he must have been extremely terrified at being scolded and trapped alone in an enclosed place.

Perpetuating Factors

Muhriz's family's relocation from Malaysia to Singapore brought about significant ongoing changes in his living and schooling environment, which likely perpetuated his selective mutism. For example, while Muhriz's dominant language was Malay, he was enrolled in an international school in Singapore and surrounded largely by peers who were competent and native speakers of English. Muhriz's confidence was affected as his unfamiliarity with the language made responding verbally difficult. More and more frequently, he would communicate by nodding his head or using gestures, rather than speaking in English.

Adding to Muhriz's difficulties in adapting to a new language and environment were his developmental delays in reading and spelling. His struggle to cope with the pace of lessons at school contributed to an increase in his anxiety. Immigration and bilingualism may have put Muhriz at higher risk of developing and maintaining the symptoms of selective mutism (Elizur & Perednik, 2003). From a behavioural theory perspective, his non-verbal responses (i.e., nodding and gesturing) were negatively reinforced when others reciprocated his non-verbal communication. His tendency to ignore others' advances could also have discouraged them from seeking a verbal respond from him. Although remaining silent alleviated his anxieties, it also limited Muhriz's opportunities to practice speaking and expressing himself verbally.

Muhriz believed that his "voice sounded weird". He feared being evaluated by others and described his voice as being only fit "for his family" to hear. These negative perceptions reduced his confidence and increased his anxieties about speaking. When he finally did speak, due to his anxiety, it would generally be in a monotonous voice, thus perpetuating his self-conscious perceptions and his selective mutism.

Protective Factors

Selective mutism is treatable and prognosis is generally favourable. Protective factors that could positively influence the outcome of therapy for a child with selective mutism include the involvement of parents in their child's therapy and the adaptation of therapeutic strategies to provide a personalized and targeted intervention plan for a child. Muhriz's family was supportive and open to recommendations during treatment. His mother, Mdm Siti, possessed insight into his needs and creatively adapted strategies that were discussed during therapy sessions to fit them.

While treatment outcomes for selective mutism may vary, treatment is effective when introduced with consistency. Despite showing improvements over time, many persons with selective mutism continue to experience anxiety in speaking situations, sometimes chronically (Cohan, Price & Stein, 2006). Known predictors of unfavourable outcomes include parents with psychiatric disorders, lower intelligence, and mutistic behaviours within the family (Remschmidt et al., 2001). Fortunately, none of these were applicable to Muhriz.

PROGNOSIS

Muhriz's clinical symptoms of selective mutism co-occurred with a high rate of anxiety symptoms. Current literature has noted high rates of comorbidity with communication disorders (Viana et al., 2009). Children who present with comorbid psychiatric disorders such as anxiety disorders and communication disorders may be at higher risk of underlying psychopathology of a more chronic course. For Muhriz, the impact of his speech and language deficits likely interacted with his anxious predisposition to cumulate in the development and maintenance of selective mutism. For instance, his difficulties in reading and spelling might have caused increased fears in being unable to keep up at school, and likewise, increased levels of anxieties that stifle verbal speech may interfere in his learning at school (e.g., being unable to practise reading out aloud or clarify his doubts with peers and teachers).

In addition, there is much variability in symptomatology among children with comorbid selective mutism and communication disorders (Kristensen & Oerbeck, 2006). Therefore, treatments for these children need to be individualised, and prognosis can vary to a large extent across cases. The effects of such comorbidity can also interfere significantly with the pace of therapy. Due to the lack of longitudinal data on this population, the outcome of treatment for this group of children with comorbidity is still inconclusive.

Furthermore, in view of the changes to Muhriz's country of residence and language use in daily life, the process and length of treatment was expected to be more protracted, as Muhriz needed time to build familiarity in navigating around new surroundings and developing his English. However, if Muhriz received support in terms of anxiety management and intervention to improve his abilities in reading and spelling, the maintaining factors of his comorbid conditions could then be addressed concurrently.

TREATMENT

In accordance with the conceptualisation that Muhriz's selective mutism was being primarily driven by anxiety, evidence-based treatment for childhood anxiety disorder was determined to be an effective treatment plan. Specifically, treatment employed an adaptation of the Meeky Mouse program, a Cognitive Behavioural Therapy–based intervention designed for selectively mute children between ages 8 to 12 years of age (Fung, Kenny & Mendlowitz, 2000). The overall goal of treatment was to teach Muhriz to recognise the signs of anxious arousal associated with speaking and to learn anxiety management strategies in overcoming these feared situations. By reducing his level of anxiety and developing his range of communication, it was hoped that Muhriz would attain increased speech and social confidence.

Using Meeky Mouse, drawn from the work of the Coping Cat workbook (Kendall, 1992) and the Coping Bear workbook (Mendlowitz, et al., 1999), Muhriz was taught the CHAT plan (Check your body's feelings, Having bad thoughts, Attitudes and actions that help, Time for a reward). He was guided in applying these skills to exposure tasks—the major part of treatment—where he would attempt increasingly difficult anxiety-inducing situations. Exposure tasks comprised small activities to help him make incremental progress across three areas: level of verbal communication, varied locations, and varying levels of familiarity with different persons.

The exposure work was based on the Selective Mutism—Stages of Social Communication Comfort Scale framework used in conjunction with the Meeky Mouse program (Shipon-Blum, 2012). In this framework, Muhriz's level of social comfort in speaking was framed in three phrases (*see* Table 5.1). Using segments from the Meeky Mouse program, plans on supporting his mother and the school to help support Muhriz in his exposure tasks were worked out. They included performing Conversational Visits and using Speech Monitoring forms (*see* Table 5.1).

Forming therapeutic alliance with Muhriz was of paramount importance. Careful considerations were made to form a therapeutic relationship that was accepting and validating of him, such that he could experience a positive relationship with a figure of authority. This would set the tone for his future relationships with other unfamiliar adults, such as teachers at school.

Crucially, Mdm Siti was empowered to take on the role of co-therapist as she could provide helpful information about Muhriz's difficulties and strengths. She worked together with his psychologist to draw out a detailed behavioural 'map' of his frequency and volume of speech at different locations and with different persons. This was to obtain an overview of Muhriz's levels of communication across settings and with various people, with the Selective Mutism Severity Rating Form (Figure 5.1) and Selective Mutism Monitoring Form (Figure 5.2).

Mdm Siti's role went beyond just being an informant. She also actively took part in the plans set out for Murhiz. One example was the implementation of the Conversational Visit. The rationale of a Conversational Visit was explained to Mdm Siti and she was encouraged to identify specific times to be present at Muhriz's school grounds. Her role was to practice speaking with him at various locations in school so as to work on desensitising the fear of speaking at these places and to achieve incremental successes in overcoming the anxiety to speak. On top of this, Mdm Siti worked closely with Muhriz's school to provide them with information about selective mutism, as well as to engage teachers in implementing plans that were discussed in therapy to help integrate Muhriz into his school.

Mdm Siti was also encouraged to use positive reinforcement and validation, to build up Muhriz's successes and confidence. These came in the form of verbal praise, encouragement and physical affection. For example, when Murhiz was able to whisper to her at school in front of his schoolmates, she would give him a high five, and whisper back to him, "That was tough but you were so brave!"

FIGURE 5.1. SELECTIVE MUTISM SEVERITY RATING FORM

Instructions: Look at this table outlining 13 Stages in the Emergence of Speech at School Which stage would your child fall into at this point? ______

	Stage	**Description**
1	Complete Mutism at School	Child speaks freely at home but is silent at school. Appears anxious at school. May resist attending school.
2	Relaxed Nonverbal Participation	Child speaks at home but not at school. Child begins participating nonverbally in classroom activities (facial expressions, gestures). May begin to talk positively about school when at home.
3	Speaks to Parent at School	When alone with a parent at school, where students and teachers cannot hear or see, the child speaks at school, often in a whispered voice.
4	Speech Observed by Peers	Child speaks at school, usually to a parent. Peers observe but do not hear the child speaking.
5	Speech Overheard by Peers	Child speaks at school, usually to a parent. Other children observe and hear the child speaking. Child does not speak directly to the other children or teachers.
6	Child Speaks Through Parent to Peers	Child speaks to parent who conveys message to another child sitting nearby. The other child may overhear the child speaking and respond directly.
7	Child Speaks to One Peer-Whisper	Child speaks at school to one peer, often at the playground. Child does not speak to teachers. Tone of speech is low, likely resembles a whisper.
8	Child Speaks to One Peer-Normal Tone	Child speaks at school to one peer, often on the playground. Child does not speak to teachers. Tone of speech is normal (is audible to others).
9	Speech to Several Peers-Whisper	Child speaks to several children at school. Child does not speak to teachers. Tone of speech to peers is low, likely resembles a whisper.
10	Speech to Several Peers-Normal Tone	Child speaks to several children at school. Child does not speak to teachers. Tone of speech is normal (is audible to others).
11	Speech to Teacher-Whisper	Child begins speaking to teacher and speaks to several peers. Tone of speech is low, likely resembles a whisper.
12	Speech to Teacher-Normal Tone	Child begins speaking to teacher and speaks to several peers. Tone of speech is normal (is audible to others).
13	Normal Speaking	Child speaks indiscriminately to most adults (including teachers, other school staff) and peers at school.

FIGURE 5.2. SELECTIVE MUTISM MONITORING FORM

Instructions:

1) List all persons your child speaks to beginning with those he/she talks to most.

2) Next rank those persons at school you believe your child is most comfortable with but does not speak to yet.

3) Mark the situations where your child whispers (W) or has spoken (S) in a voice of normal volume at least once.

4) Finally, using the Anxiety Rating Scale below, rate the degree of your child's distress (from 0 to 1) associated with speaking to the individuals listed on the table.

Note: 0 = no anxiety, the child is able to have a relaxed, friendly conversation with the person; 10 = the child is highly anxious and refuses to speak to the individual.

Anxiety Rating Scale:

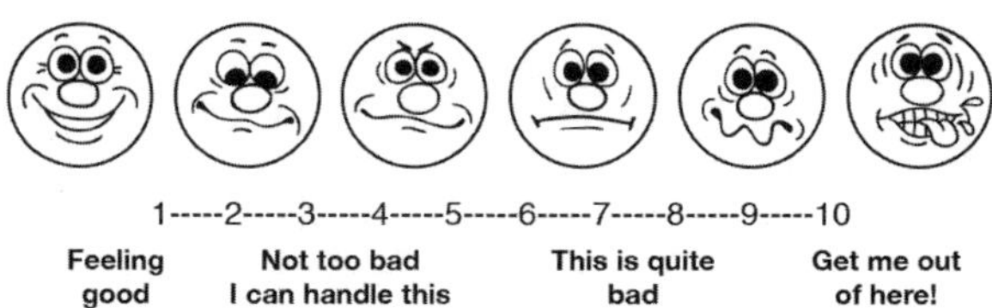

Persons the child speaks or whispers to	Anxiety rating (1–10)	Situations where Child Speaks (S) or Whispers (W)					
		Class	Hall	Play Ground	Other school places: Specify	Home	Other places: Specify
Example: Mother	1					3(S)	
Example: Tommy (Good friend at school)	3		3(W)	3(S)			
Example: teacher	10	N/A	N/A	N/A	N/A		

TABLE 5.1. SUMMARY OF TREATMENT PHASES, GOALS, AND TECHNIQUES

Phases	Goals	Techniques
1 Nonverbal	1. Therapist took non-threatening stance during rapport building. 2. Used non-verbal activities to facilitate social engagement and to enable Muhriz to express wants and needs through non-verbal means. 3. Supported Muhriz to develop self-initiated and self-directed movements.	• Allowed Muhriz to interact and move about therapy room with sister and mother with therapist in the background (e.g., Minimal eye contact, tracked and reflected movements and gestures). • Responses by Muhriz included pointing, nodding, writing, sign language and gesturing • Homework for therapy included sending an email to a friend at school with Mother's help and making personalized cards for teachers, as Muhriz liked drawing. • Requested Muhriz to initiate requests for help, (e.g., to explain what he wanted by gesturing rather than being 'frozen' in movement.) • Mother prepared picture cards for Muhriz to use, e.g., (Cards were creatively bounded up like a newspaper. He could flip them in class and communicate with his teacher.)
2 Transitional	1. Providing alternatives for Muhriz to be involved in verbal activities at school. 2. Used sounds and noises as entry into verbal voice. Used devices as proxy to communicate with others. 3. Psychoeducation on feelings and rating intensity of difficult feelings so that Muhriz was able to inform how manageable tasks were for him.	• Muhriz made video and audio recordings of self. These clips were recorded with Muhriz speaking increasing numbers of words. Played these recordings at therapy sessions and then with identified persons at school. • For show-and-tell and class presentations, Muhriz made audio slides at home, (e.g., PowerPoint slides with audio clip attached.) These were played back at school with Muhriz mouthing words silently in front of class. • Identified favourite friends and teachers in activities in preparation of setting up plans for conversations at school. • Mouthed words and mimicked therapist to voice out letter sounds while reading a book. • Vocalised imaginative play sounds while playing with toys in session, e.g., car moving, aeroplane flying. • Used interactive activities to learn to articulate feeling words and recognise feeling faces; was introduced to the feeling thermometer and voice volume. • Practised rating intensity of feelings through the use of these tools.
3 Verbal	1. Provided positive reinforcement of speaking voice. 2. Activities with increasing difficulty for Muhriz to practise using his voice. 3. Had planned conversations and play dates.	• Used sticker reward for positive reinforcement in game format. Went around the clinic reciting, "Hi, my name is Muhriz." and claimed a sticker from persons that he spoke to as a stamp for his 'speech passport'. • Spoke to therapist and friends over the phone with a script, then with assistance from mother without a script and lastly, without any assistance, using spontaneous speech. • At school, printed out show and tell speech for reference. This was read out in front of class in low whisper, then with increasing volume. Initially, had a friend stand next to him first, till he gradually could do without. • At home, had planned conversations with friends over the phone, then over Skype. • Started with pre-scripted questions and answers and later moved to open ended questions with Mdm Siti who would assist with responses. • Muhriz was expected to speak with increasing volume and for longer duration over these phone conversations as he gained confidence and ability in responding on his own. • Arranged for play dates with friends whom he had previously Skype with. • Mother reminded Muhriz to whisper hello or thank you to all strangers that they met outside home/school environment. • Phrases were adapted from Dr Elisa Shipon-Blum (2012) Social Communication Bridge for Selective Mutism.

Phrases were adapted from Dr Elisa Shipon-Blum (2012) Social Communication Bridge for Selective Mutism.

Last but not least, it was important to help Mdm Siti build her confidence for ongoing therapy. She was validated for her efforts in implementing strategies, and her successes in helping Muhriz complete therapy tasks were identified and celebrated. Therapy also allowed her to process the difficulties that she experienced in parenting a child with selective mutism.

At the end of therapy, his mother filled in a form sharing her experiences. In response to "Please state words of encouragement you would like to share with other parents whose child struggles with Selective Mutism", she wrote, "…it is not your fault that your child has SM. The first step would be to recognise that your child has a problem and plan ways to support your child. Your child need extra love and reassurance—the rest will come. Just know that your child can do it—but don't force it out from them. Support them, and it will happen on its own." In response to "What cultural factors do you think impacted or continues to impact on his communication?", she wrote, "Probably the culture of needing to be right and perfect all the time. I realise that letting kids make mistakes and discovering the 'truth' or 'truths' are important—but I do have to keep reminding myself about this (always in danger of over-correcting)."

Over three years in therapy, Muhriz made steady progress in his social communication abilities. Psychological measures gave an objective indicator of how he responded and progressed through the course of therapy. From the scores on the SMQ and SCARED parent-reported questionnaires, Muhriz presented with a general decrease in symptoms of anxiety and became more verbal communicator across various settings (Table 5.2).

Muhriz's progress in battling mutism was also recognized at school. Here are two excerpts from an email correspondence with the school support teacher, which aptly summarised his progress: "Muhriz is doing really well. He has made such incredible progress this year—I am continually surprised by how far he has come. As a communicator, he speaks regularly in all lessons and is verbalizing his ideas in a much more organized and coherent manner. At times, when speaking he searches for words and relies on his hands to help 'sign' what he is trying to explain. I believe this will decrease as he continues to speak more often…I think in the past, he could be so anxious about trying to take in all of the instructions (as he wasn't asking questions in the past) that he didn't understand or hear everything that was said—as a result of the anxiety. The volume he uses in our classroom is very good, although it can decrease as the group gets larger or when he is in some specialist lessons…".

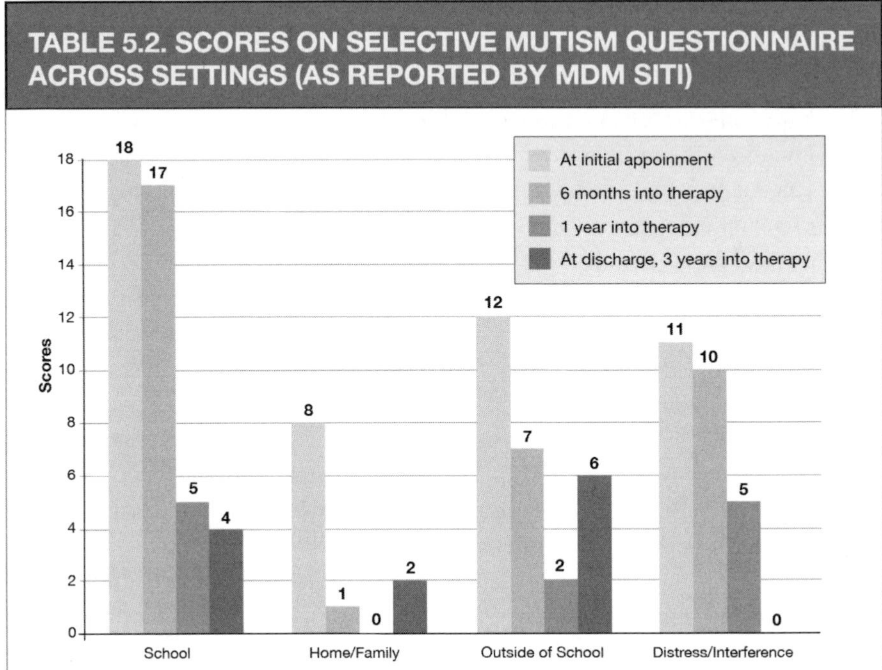

Muhriz had used the tagline used in film publicity, 'Coming Soon' to describe his voice at pre-treatment. Three years on, he could proudly claim that his voice was 'Now Showing'. It will be an ongoing journey for Muhriz, as he encounters various obstacles in life. For instance, apart from ongoing support to tide through academic demands, Muhriz will continuously need to develop his ability in dealing with anxieties associated with setbacks and failures. At times, Mdm Siti had reported that Muhriz would freeze on the spot when he was unable to accomplish a task or if he felt uncertain about how to go about completing it. Recommendations were made for further developing Muhriz's sense of mastery and self-efficacy as he developed and matured, as well as patient guidance and support from his educators to foster his academic development.

DISCUSSION

Locally, treatment approaches for selective mutism differ from practitioner to practitioner. However, commonly used forms of therapy include behavioural therapy and play therapy. Generally, cases with less severe symptomatology are seen within the community or school environment, where students are supported by teachers and school personnel. Cases such as Muhriz's, which are more severe, or present with other psychiatric comorbid disorders, would be surfaced by the community Response

Early Intervention and Assessment in Community Mental Health (REACH) team and be referred to the tertiary hospitals in Singapore.

Literature on selective mutism in Singapore (Carolyn, Fung, & Ang, 2001; Kwan, 2013; Kwan, et al., 2014; Malini, 2011; Ooi, et al., 2012) focuses on intervention methods such as the use of devices in treatment (e.g., audio responses using electronic devices to record voice, computer assisted therapy, and the use of virtual reality systems in exposure tasks) and mother-child characteristics in children.

General guidelines for treatment and resources for selective mutism are mainly sourced from the Western literature. Commonly, support is given to clinic-based clinicians who need guidance on providing therapy through peer supervision or self-learning via online or book resources. A stepped-care model is used in Singapore, in which REACH teams provide regular training to school counsellors and work with more disabling or complex cases. These trainings are usually aimed at providing psychoeducation of the disorder and generally focus on psychotherapy as the first line of treatment for selective mutism in Singapore, medication being less favoured.

Most cases of selective mutism presented at clinics are referred due to a child's non-speaking and inhibited behaviours at school. Teachers and parents are often worried when the child's poor performance in oral exams, class presentations, or group discussions are not a good reflection of their abilities. Likewise, Muhriz's parents were concerned that he was not able to keep up with his schoolwork and would have difficulties making new friends if he was not speaking in his new school.

This is a valid concern as the local education system is shifting from having an emphasis on knowledge-based learning to one that values creativity and innovative learning (Ng & Lee, 2013; Tan & Gopinathan, 2000). A student who is a strong communicator is generally regarded as more competent than a student who aces his written exams alone. This has a significant impact for children who are innately quiet or, like Muhriz, anxious in temperament and less verbally expressive. While this group of children may be identified by teachers as needing support or 'having problems', this form of labeling can potentially exacerbate their anxiety. It is therefore important to carefully consider multiple factors during the assessment of a child presented with symptoms of selective mutism, so as to ascertain the severity as well as the impact on the child's functioning and if it warrants clinical attention.

Teachers and counsellors play crucial roles in the treatment of children with selective mutism, as they may assist in reinforcing behavioural treatment techniques. It is important that teachers understand the behavioural characteristics of the disorder, be aware of their expectations, and are conscious of their reactions when working with a selectively mute child. It is also important that they are taught to understand strategies that can be employed to facilitate a progressive change towards verbal communication, and that they learn to identify the kinds of interactions that may maintain a child's mutism. For example, a teacher who responds with, "Oh, he just never talks!" is inadvertently and negatively reinforcing the child's selective mutism. A psychologist thus plays a dual role in treating a child with selective mutism: as a therapist who works directly with the child, and as a facilitator who integrates intervention plans among the treatment team (e.g., teachers, school counsellor, mother, domestic helper, sister).

Implementing treatment for a child with selective mutism may be taxing because a therapist had to continuously find creative ways to communicate with him or her without overwhelming them with too much speech. As with Muhriz, less emphasis was placed on verbal communication at his initial stages of therapy. Instead, his therapist's goal was to build a trusting, therapeutic relationship with him. During her initial interaction with him, his therapist allowed him to communicate with her in whatever way he found the least anxiety provoking, (e.g., pointing, gesturing). In addition, providing multiple opportunities for a child to choose to respond (e.g., closed factual questions, choice questions) helped to simplify the task of responding.

Activities to encourage speech can be turned into a reward program to positively reinforce a child's progress. One example was Muhriz's speech passport: he was given a sticker each time he introduced himself to a person in the room. It allowed Muhriz to feel in control of his anxiety and to physically record his success at each step. Stickers not only serve as a great confidence booster and provide a natural break to reduce anxiety levels between target goals for the child, it also allows parents to keep track of the little successes their child has made, regardless the extent of their progress.

In conclusion, when working with a child with selective mutism, a psychologist is constantly challenged to develop creative and engaging ways to implement cognitive and behavioural tasks that can keep the child engaged and at the same time, instill hope and a sense of mastery so that the child and family can gradually move their voice from 'Coming Soon' to an eventual 'Now Showing'. It can be trying, but ultimately is a rewarding experience.

DISCUSSION QUESTIONS

1. A child with selective mutism often presents as a very shy and inhibited child. How can you informally assess speech and language abilities if a child is shy or non-verbal in sessions?

2. Both local and international schools in Singapore have a large number of international students. Some of these children may have started schooling at different ages or academic levels. What are some issues to consider when seeing a child and family who have immigrated from a country with a different dominant language and are of a minority race?

3. An important component of therapy for children with selective mutism involves helping them face their fears, a process called exposure. Prior to starting exposure, it is important to create a 'ladder' of feared situations and their associated fear levels, ranked in ascending order from the least to the most anxiety-provoking.

How would your fear ladder look like for Muhriz, if he were working towards giving a verbal presentation at Show and Tell in front of his classmates?

4. For some clinics, there may be limited opportunity for psychologists to work directly with clients in the community setting. Instead, they may be required to carry out their intervention plan in a clinical setting. Thinking creatively, when faced with this challenge, what activities can a therapist carry out during exposure?

5. In local schools, oral exams are one of the main components for assessment of competency in a language subject. How would you respond to a request, by parents of a child with selective mutism for exemption from oral exams or for recommendations for particular test/exams conditions (e.g., having oral exams administered by a teacher their child is familiar with to ease anxiety levels)?

6. Being able to address caregivers' and parents' concerns is a large part of supporting a child with selective mutism. Often, they are unable to decide if their child should be exempted from oral exam. They are often worried that their child may "lose out" in terms of grades as compared to other students. How would you address these concerns?

CHAPTER 6.

OH NO! I NEED A SUPERHERO!

Generalized Anxiety Disorder

ONG GUO XIONG JEFFREY AND EUNICE YAP-WONG

INTRODUCTION

Peter, a nine-year-old, had been a worrier since he was three. "I am scared of everything", he had said. Health concerns gave him significant distress—he was afraid of becoming fat despite his normal weight, he wore full length pants so that "people would not see [his] fat legs", and he avoided sweet foods so as to maintain "healthy sugar levels". Social situations were sources of further anxiety—he avoided talking to strangers and was very self-conscious when he had to "perform" in front of others. Despite having signed himself up for skating and art classes, fear of social evaluation soon resulted in his refusal to participate in group activities, and he soon stopped attending classes altogether.

Threats to his safety preoccupied him. He needed repeated reassurances from his mother that the motor accidents and natural disasters he witnessed on the news were not about to befall him. Furthermore, he was constantly wary of his one-year-old sister and six-year-old brother, who were "tougher and louder" than him. "I cannot overcome my fears", he frequently uttered.

Two months before his referral, Peter had become afraid of sleeping alone and in the dark, believing that "a ghost would kill [him] in the middle of the night" despite neither having seen a ghost nor experienced anything supernatural. Because of nightmares, he had been waking up in the middle of the night. Finding it impossible to get back to sleep, and worrying about oversleeping and being late for class, he would stay up until it was time for school. This made him feel very tired during the day. He had been caught dozing off in class on several different occasions. While his academic performance had always been good, it had now started to deteriorate.

By the time he had turned nine, Peter's worries were so extensive, so disruptive to his sleep and school performance, and so stressful for his family that his mother referred him for psychological treatment.

BACKGROUND

Peter was born full-term. There had been no complications during the pregnancy or birth. He had attained normal developmental milestones and not suffered any major illness or injuries. Observed to be very quiet since young, Peter was slow to warm up to people and did not talk much even to those close to him, such as his mother and his grandmother. He would keep his problems to himself and would not speak out even when he felt uncomfortable. His mother described him as a "reserved" boy who tended to withdraw in unfamiliar situations. He was timid and scared of "everything", including lizards and cartoons.

He was also "stubborn", and often insisted on doing things his way. However, he was sensitive and became easily emotional. For example, he would cry when reading a sad story. This was in stark contrast to his six-year-old brother, who was outgoing and vocal. No other members of his immediate or extended family had seen a psychiatrist or psychologist before. At school, there were no complaints about Peter, except that he seemed too quiet, and that his performance was worsening.

FIGURE 6.1. PETER'S FAMILY GENOGRAM

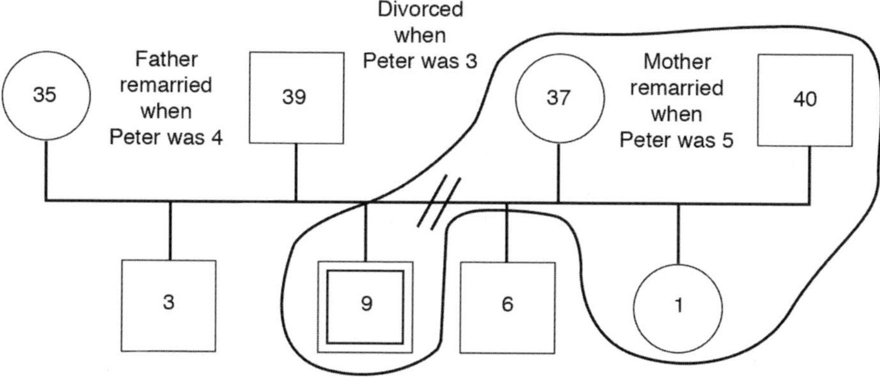

When Peter was three years old, his parents had divorced after the discovery of his father having an affair. While his mother took legal custody of the two boys, their father visited them only once a week. Both his parents had remarried and had children with their new partners (*see* Figure 6.1). Both the events leading up to his parents' divorce and its aftermath left an indelible mark on Peter. He still had vivid memories of the day his mother tried to leave his father. She had tried to walk out on her husband, carrying Peter's baby brother, without Peter. Fearing that his mother would leave him for good, Peter tried to follow, but his father grabbed his arm and refused to let go until he was crying very badly. After his parents' divorce, Peter became very anxious. While finalising their divorce, they had left Peter and his brother in the care of their maternal grandmother and it was from her that Peter sought reassurance. Whenever he awoke from a nightmare, she would pat him on the head, tell him that everything was going to be fine, and sleep beside him.

Peter was soon moved out of his grandmother's house and in with his mother, step-father and step-sister; his mother wanted "all her children to stay under one roof". His younger brother, however, remained with his grandmother. Despite the move, Peter would on some days return to his grandmother's when his mother was too busy with work to care for him. On top of the anxiety arising from his shifts between dwellings, he constantly worried about when his mother would return home from work. Her irregular schedule meant that he seldom saw her and would stay up at night to wait for her. His sense of security was recently shaken again when she told him that their family could be moving overseas in a few years.

ASSESSMENT

The first two sessions, conducted with Peter and his mother, focused on assessing his presenting problems; charting his developmental, medical and family history; documenting significant events in his life; and building rapport with him by talking about his strengths and interests. Peter was quiet and softly-spoken and responded in monosyllables or short phrases. His anxiety was evident in his tense facial expression and rigid body posture. Despite telling his therapist that he felt "okay", he displayed little emotion, even when describing happy moments. Later, he was found outside the therapy room, eavesdropping on a private conversation his therapist was having with his mother. This further highlighted his fear of uncertainty and intense unease about what others had to say about him. In contrast, his mother was forthcoming in talking about his difficulties, her own difficulties, and details of the divorce. She displayed concern about Peter's needs and difficulties and good insight into how the divorce could have affected Peter.

The content of Peter's fears was explored in subsequent sessions and it quickly became apparent that he found it difficult to describe his fears and thoughts. However, as Peter had a keen interest in drawing, his flair for art was used to provide detailed pictures of his fears and nightmares (*see* Figures 6.2 and 6.3) and then used as a therapeutic tool.

Despite his anxiety and difficulties expressing himself, Peter was not depressed. Neither did he have any intention or ideation to harm himself or others. Peter and his mother completed the self-report and the parent-report of the Spence Children's Anxiety Scale (SCAS) (Spence, 1997) respectively. The SCAS is a screening instrument for anxiety symptoms in children. Peter's scores on both versions of the SCAS were in the clinical range, indicating that his level of anxiety was significantly higher than would be expected for boys of his age. These scores served as baseline measures against which his response to treatment was later measured.

FIGURE 6.2. A CLOWN SPIRIT, WHICH PETER FEARED WOULD TRY TO KILL HIM AT NIGHT

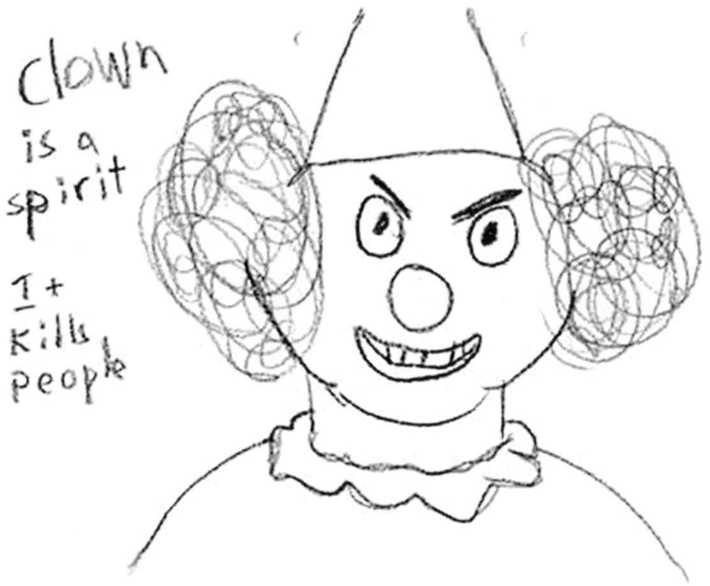

FIGURE 6.3. PETER'S MOTHER LEAVING HIM AND A GHOST APPEARING

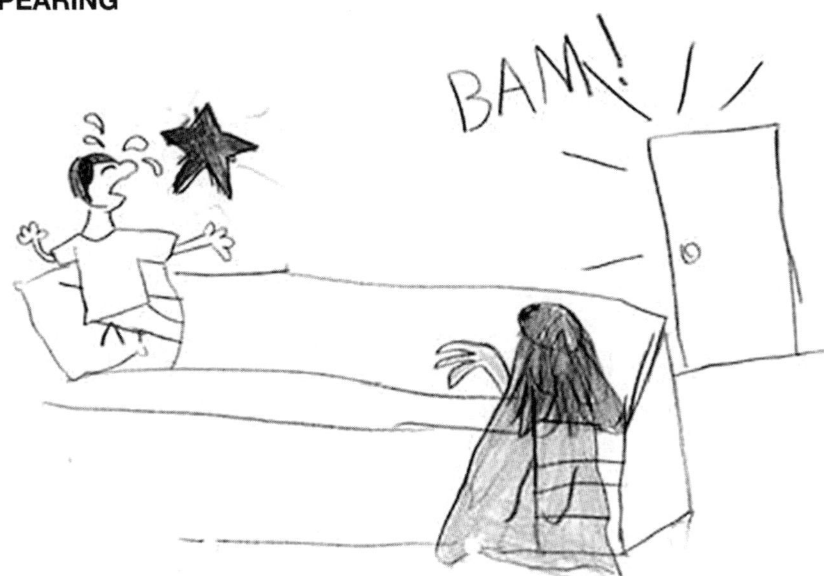

Peter met the criteria for a diagnosis of generalized anxiety disorder (GAD) in the DSM-5: he worried excessively over a variety of concerns, had difficulty controlling the worries, and reported symptoms of muscle tension and restlessness. GAD is characterised by excessive anxiety and worry about a variety of events or activities, over a period of at least six months, causing significant distress or impairment to the person. Someone with GAD has difficulty controlling worry and experiences symptoms such as restlessness, fatigue, poor concentration, irritability, muscle tension and sleep disturbance. While GAD commonly occurs with depression in children (Masi et al., 2004), Peter was not assessed to have depressive symptoms. GAD shares similar features with adjustment, separation anxiety and social anxiety disorders. However, Peter's anxiety symptoms were better accounted for by GAD than an adjustment disorder as his difficulties had been long-standing and did not solely reflect a difficulty in adjusting to stress or change. Furthermore, his anxiety and worries were neither directly attributable to a specific stressor or change as in an adjustment disorder, nor restricted to specific situations such as separation from his mother as in separation anxiety disorder, nor confined to social situations as in social anxiety disorder.

INTEGRATIVE FORMULATION

Predisposing Factors

Peter's temperament was that of behavioural inhibition (BI; *see* Kagan, Reznick, Clarke, Snidman, & Garcia-Coll, 1984). Children with BI often show fearfulness, restraint, reticence and social withdrawal in novel situations (Kagan, Reznick, & Gibbons, 1989). Peter exhibited such behaviour whenever he was in situations involving unfamiliar people and places. There is evidence from literature indicating that children with BI have a lower threshold for limbic and sympathetic nervous system arousal and that BI is a risk factor for anxiety disorders (Hirshfeld-Becker, Biederman & Rosenbaum, 2004; Oosterlaan, 2001).

Peter experienced a number of significant life events in his early childhood. From a tender age, he witnessed his parents' conflictual relationship, was exposed to the shock and horror of his mother trying to leave him behind with his father, and harboured the painful memory of unexpectedly seeing his father with another woman and child. Anxious children experience a significantly greater number of severe life events and chronic adversities prior to the onset of their anxiety disorder (Allen, Rapee & Sandberg, 2008). This highlights the predisposing role of environmental factors in GAD. The traumatic events of Peter's life were likely to have caused him to develop threat and uncertainty-oriented schemas (cognitive models generally developed early in life that influence how a person interprets the world around him). These schemas would be activated whenever the possibility of danger arose, and bias him towards processing information in a way that overestimated the probability of danger, triggering the process of worry that is characteristic of people with GAD.

Precipitating Factors

Peter's parent's divorce was the main precipitating factor of his anxiety—the onset of his symptoms of anxiety was evident following this event. Their divorce was very stressful for him, as it affected many areas of his life, including his living arrangements, the frequency of meeting his parents, the amount of time and attention his parents could give to him and their emotional availability. It threatened his core needs of predictability and stability and contributed to his anxiety. Peter's recent sleep disturbances, which had started to impact on his sleep and schoolwork, was the precipitating factor that prompted the referral to mental health professionals.

Perpetuating Factors

Peter's anxiety was perpetuated by the lack of stability in his life, exemplified by the frequent changes in his sleeping arrangements, his mother's irregular working hours and the looming possibility of moving to another country. These changes and the unpredictability of his life served to reinforce his schemas relating to the uncertainty of the future. Furthermore, he had frequent negative automatic thoughts that tended to overemphasize the probability of death and danger.

When faced with fearful situations such as attending skating lessons and skating in front of others, Peter avoided rather than confronted them. By not dealing with such feared stimuli, he experienced an immediate reduction in anxiety and positive reinforcement for his avoidance. This caused him to be more likely to keep away from subsequent fearful situations, thus reinforcing a pattern of anxiety. Furthermore, while his maternal grandmother's excessive reassurances provided him with immediate relief, they ultimately prevented him from learning how to self-soothe and to problem-solve. This sent an erroneous message to him that his worries were real. His lack of self-confidence, constant undermining of his own abilities, and reliance on others for help, reinforced his belief that he was incapable and perpetuated his anxiety.

Protective Factors

Despite the past adversities, ongoing difficulties and destabilising factors in Peter's life, many factors served to mitigate them. One such factor was his good cognitive ability. He easily understood cognitive behavioural therapy's (CBT) concept of how his thoughts, feelings and behaviour were inter-related and was able to apply the cognitive restructuring skills he was taught. His excellent drawing ability—through which he could readily and clearly express his thoughts and feelings—was another protective factor that could be pivotal in successful therapy.

Both Peter and his mother did not express any prejudice towards either mental health issues or his diagnosis, and were keen to seek treatment. His mother was very motivated to help him and regularly brought him to therapy sessions despite her busy work schedule. Despite the divorce, Peter's parents had remained friends. He thus had positive relationships with both his biological and step-families. With no recent family upheavals and stress that he had to witness and experience, treatment could be set against a more stable family environment.

PROGNOSIS

If untreated, early-onset GAD typically follows a chronic course. Despite the early age of onset of Peter's GAD and the adversities he experienced as a result of his parent's divorce, his prognosis—with evidence-based treatment—was reasonably good. He had no physical or psychological comorbidities and he and his family were actively seeking treatment for his GAD. Furthermore, the presence of several important protective factors such as his current stable family environment and his receptiveness to CBT also made it more likely that treatment would be effective.

TREATMENT

Peter and his mother attended 11 sessions over a nine-month period, with each session lasting just under an hour. Sessions were structured and began with a discussion with Peter's mother about his progress and a review of the behavioural measures that were recorded during the preceding week, followed by a discussion of the following week's plan. The second half of the session was devoted to individual therapy with Peter. His treatment was implemented across the five phases using CBT: (1) psycho-education and rapport building, (2) teaching of behavioural strategies, (3) cognitive restructuring and gradual exposure, (4) generalization of strategies, and (5) relapse prevention.

Phase One—Psycho-education and Rapport Building

In phase one, Peter's case formulation was shared with his mother. Psycho-education about anxiety was also provided; both of them were educated on how fear helps us in dangerous situations by preparing our brain and body to either "freeze", "fight" the danger, or "take flight" from it. They were taught about how the brain and body could be "fooled by false alarms", and result in symptoms of anxiety even when the situation was relatively non-threatening. Peter was taught how to recognize the physiological signs of anxiety in his body. He shared how his heartbeat became louder and faster and his hands and feet felt cold when he was anxious, and related this to his memories of superheroes in movies and comic books experiencing similar symptoms when faced with powerful enemies. Peter and his mother were then introduced to the CBT model of how thoughts affect feelings, which in turn affect behaviour.

Peter loved superheroes. He aspired to be Spiderman and had been training by hanging himself upside-down on monkey-bars and running regularly. Together with his therapist, Peter identified two characteristics common to all superheroes—muscles and fearlessness. As Peter had already been working on his physical strength by exercising, he agreed to begin working on becoming more "fearless". The concept of "fearlessness" was then discussed and introduced into goals of reducing symptoms of anxiety and being able to sleep alone at night.

Phase Two—Teaching of Behavioural Strategies

Following psycho-education, behavioural coping skills were taught to Peter and his mother. For Peter, these skills were likened to the weapons his beloved superheroes used to defeat their enemies. Thinking about superheroes would cue him to utilize those skills. His therapist also explained to him that he would "become stronger" with every successful attempt at defeating "fear" with his weapons.

As his first "weapon", Peter was taught deep breathing. He found it effective in helping him feel less tense. He was then instructed to teach deep breathing to his mother. This served to reinforce his learning, to promote self-efficacy, and to give his mother the opportunity to practice with him daily. As a cue to practice deep breathing when he felt anxious, he created a poster and hung it in front of his bed. Visualization was the second "weapon" Peter was "equipped" with to fight his fear. He was first asked to imagine himself in a place where he felt safe and untroubled. He drew and described a scene in New York City, in which he was surrounded by skyscrapers and felt happy and carefree (Figure 6.4). He was then asked to use his five senses to describe what he saw, heard, smelled, touched and tasted in his imaginary New York City. At the end of this exercise, he said that he felt more relaxed.

Peter's mother was introduced to parenting strategies to help him. Firstly, she was taught to reduce the reinforcement of Peter's anxiety by using "planned ignoring" and by rewarding his brave behaviour by giving him attention and using specific praises. To address the lack of stability in Peter's life, his therapist also discussed strategies with her for improving predictability. These included having a fixed day and time every week during which she and her son could spend an hour on an enjoyable joint activity; preparing a timetable of her work schedule for Peter, and preparing Peter for changes by discussing them with him in advance.

Phase Three—Cognitive Restructuring and Gradual Exposure

Cognitive restructuring was the third "weapon" Peter was taught to use. Through the use of comic strips of two scenarios (Figure 6.5), Peter identified the thoughts of a superhero who succumbed to his enemy in one scenario, and the thoughts of a superhero who stood up to his enemy in the other scenario.

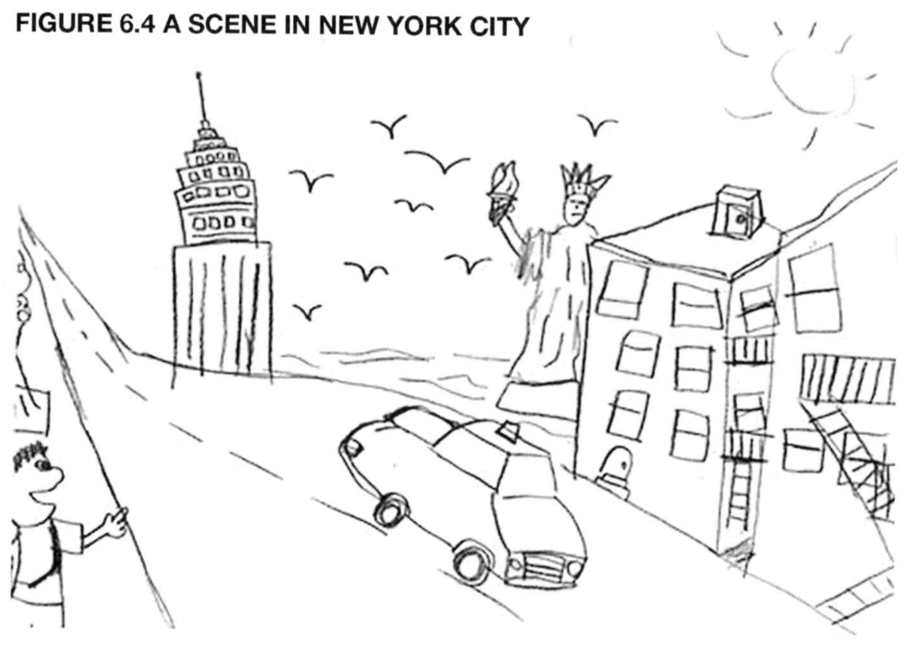

FIGURE 6.5 COMIC STRIPS HELPED ILLUSTRATE HOW THOUGHTS, FEELINGS AND BEHAVIOUR ARE INTER-RELATED

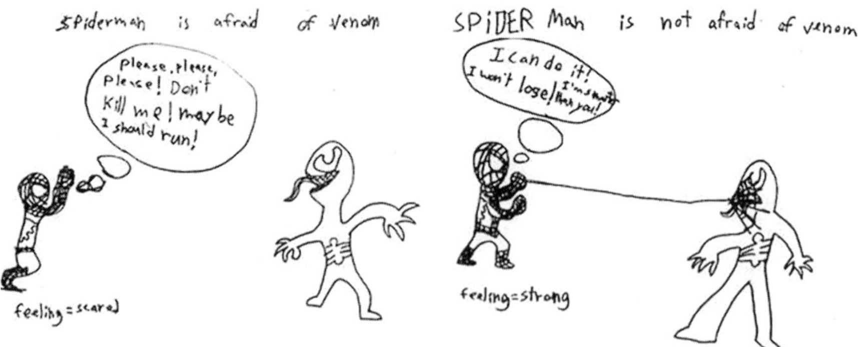

This gave Peter insight into how his feelings and behaviour were very much influenced by his thoughts or interpretation of situations. Using specific examples of his recent fears and accompanying negative thoughts, his therapist taught him to challenge his negative thoughts. For example, Peter had been worrying that snakes and poisonous spiders would harm him at night when he was asleep. To counter these thoughts, Peter was guided in creating a list of counter-evidence (Figure 6.6).

Peter's therapist explained that this cognitive restructuring was not simply a process of replacing negative thoughts with positive ones but was about challenging the basis of his negative thoughts in order to evaluate their validity. Eventually, Peter was able to come up with coping statements that targeted his common negative thoughts (e.g., the creatures are not real; they are just my imagination; I am safe), and which he could articulate whenever he felt anxious.

To address Peter's avoidance of feared situations, exposure therapy was conducted. He had to learn to use extinction and to put his earlier taught coping skills into practice. Peter and his mother's goal for exposure therapy was for him to be able to sleep alone at night for increasingly longer periods of time. An exposure ladder was jointly created in which one-hour increments of "sleeping alone time" were rewarded with points that could be exchanged for presents. These presents were also accompanied by specific praise from his mother and the therapist. This reward system was based on the operant conditioning principle that desirable behaviour can be facilitated and increased through appropriate reward and reinforcement. By the time this phase of the treatment drew to a close, Peter was able to sleep unaccompanied in his own room. A month later, this was still maintained. His improvements coincided with his mother staying at home full-time as the family's helper had gone on leave.

FIGURE 6.6. THOUGHT CHALLENGING BY PETER

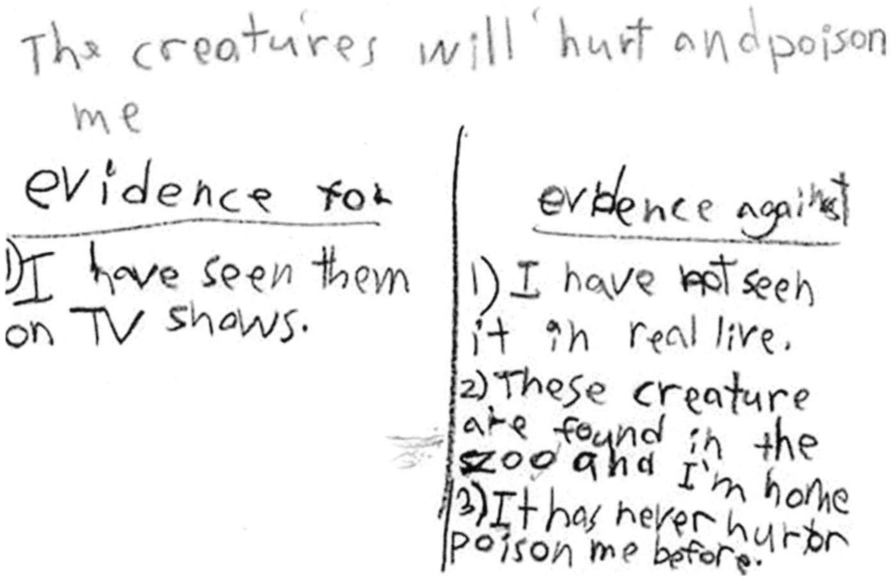

Phase Four—Generalization of Strategies

It was at this stage that Peter's mother noticed new unusual behaviours. For example, Peter would communicate with his teachers only in short sentences and was afraid of playing football for fear that the ball would hit his face and affect his teeth. His therapist realised that his underlying anxiety was still prevalent and pervasive, and increased treatment intensity to include repeated exposure to the various new events and situations he feared. Together with Peter and his mother, another list was constructed and ordered in terms of degree of fear.

However, Peter's therapist also noticed that he had not kept up with the practice and usage of previously taught strategies to manage his anxiety. The reasons for his difficulties were explored and strategies were devised to help him to overcome these challenges. For example, as Peter found it tiring to constantly examine the reality of his negative thoughts, he was taught to write several coping statements on pocket cards and to carry them around as reminders to refer to whenever he got anxious. To ensure that this was followed through, his mother was also taught about cognitive restructuring and how she could help Peter create coping statements. Peter's mother was also asked to keep a diary and to make note of three incidents per week during which she observed Peter using what he had been taught in therapy. At the end of the week, she would discuss these with Peter. This gave her an opportunity to reinforce his behaviour through praise, and increase the amount of positive interaction with her son.

Phase Five—Relapse Prevention

During this phase, two more strategies were introduced to Peter—problem solving and distracting himself from his fears and worries. He was taught to solve problems using the simple steps of defining the problem and goal, generating solutions, making decisions, and evaluating their effectiveness (D'Zurilla, & Goldfried, 1971). The concept of a toolbox from which Peter could pick different strategies to tackle problems was introduced to help him organise the strategies he had learnt. A behaviour chart was also put in place to measure his progress and achievements. Because he enjoyed drawing, each achievement was rewarded with the opportunity to add to a drawing on the jungle-themed chart. His achievements also allowed him to redeem tangible rewards, such as an Avengers comic book.

Over the sessions, Peter grew more confident in expressing himself. He finally revealed that he was very fearful that his mother would leave him for good. This exposed a strong need for assurance and security in his life, particularly from his mother. His therapist discussed this issue with her, and she acknowledged his better behaviour and more settled manner when she remained at home to care for her children. Subsequently, she decided to aim at resigning and becoming a full-time homemaker.

Towards the end of treatment, Peter's mother reported that he had overcome his fear of crowds and his avoidance of strangers. He had also shown unusual perseverance in not giving in to fear and nervousness. His mother had exposed him to different scenarios such as bringing him to attend big events and signing him up for a kid's running event. She encouraged him to carry out his own purchases and transactions. He was eventually able to approach a salesperson for assistance with his mother providing a script for him, or prompting him.

By his final therapy session, Peter had drawn eight achievements on his jungle-themed behaviour chart in one month and received several rewards. He continued to be able to sleep alone and was observed to be less anxious. This was congruent with his improved scores on the parent and self-report SCAS, both of which were no longer in the clinical range. Both Peter and his mother felt confident of the strategies learnt and were sure of how to proceed. Together with his therapist, it was jointly agreed that sessions would conclude. Peter shared, "I, Spiderman, have finished my training … I am ready to take on the villains".

DISCUSSION

GAD in children impacts multiple areas of life, and engenders different worries at different developmental stages. In children and adolescents with GAD, these worries often revolve around performance in school, punctuality and catastrophic events (American Psychiatric Association, 2000). These were characteristic of the content of Peter's worries.

To address the wide-ranging worries and issues of GAD, various psychological treatment approaches have been used, ranging from cognitive-behavioural based treatments to psychodynamic therapy (Moore & Carr, 2000). Across treatments, CBT has the most evidence supporting its efficacy and has been found to be "probably efficacious" in the treatment of anxiety in children and adolescents (Ollendick, & King, 2000; Silverman, Pina, & Viswesvaran, 2008). Silverman and colleagues (2008) found

Fact Box 6.1. Use of Anti-Anxiety Medication for Children with GAD

There are a variety of anti-anxiety medication commonly prescribed to those with GAD such as Fluoxetine (Birmaher, et al., 2003), Setraline (Rynn, Siqueland, & Rickels, 2001), Diazepam and Lorazepam (Hidalgo, Tupler, & Davidson, 2007). However, these medications may produce side effects such as headaches, stomach upset and confusion. Furthermore, the person taking these medications may build up tolerance if they are taken over a long period of time, and may need increasingly higher doses to get the same effect. These issues are pertinent for the clinician to consider, especially when treating a child. Hence, CBT is often used as the first-line treatment for GAD and medication is indicated only if other measures such as CBT have not been found to be effective (Patel, & Fancher, 2013).

that 62% of children and adolescents treated with CBT for anxiety no longer met DSM criteria at post-treatment. Treatment gains achieved with CBT have also been shown to be maintained for as long as three to six years after treatment is completed (Barrett, Duffy, Dadds, & Rapee, 2001; Kendall & Southam-Gerow, 1996). Hence, CBT was the primary treatment used to help Peter with his GAD.

CBT treatment for children with GAD includes a wide gamut of methods such as gradual exposure, cognitive restructuring, problem solving and practical modifications to the child's environment. Peter's quantifiable progress from the exposure ladder and his improvements in SCAS scores demonstrate that CBT can be an effective treatment for children with GAD. Using an exposure ladder for gradual exposure was chosen over flooding because it has been shown to be more effective with children (Silverman, & Kurtines, 2005), and can help the child develop a sense of mastery by gradually building upon his success (Kendall, 2006). This has been shown to be successful in a variety of anxiety-related behaviour (Kendall, 2006), including avoidance of the dark (Leitenberg & Callahan, 1973).

A contingency management program has been found to be more effective than one without reinforcement procedures (Sheslow, Bondy, & Nelson, 1982). Hence, behaviour charts and rewards system were set in place to motivate Peter effectively to confront feared situations. Equipping children with good problem-solving skills reduces post-treatment relapses in anxiety disorders (Kleiner, Marshall, & Spevack, 1987) and behavioural problems (Dubow, Tisak, Causey, Hryshko, & Reid, 1991; Kazdin, Siegel, & Bass, 1992; Webster-Stratton, Reid, & Hammond, 2001). He was therefore taught to use them in school and at home. For example, Peter had been worrying over his upcoming Math test. He did not understand a particular topic and had been procrastinating over revising for the test. After going through the steps of problem solving, Peter had approached his teacher and requested extra help on the topic. He also implemented his own revision schedule.

Peter's mother's involvement in his treatment was crucial because parents have been identified as the ideal change agents in the lives of children of divorced families (Wolchik et al., 1993). Grych and Fincham (1992) have highlighted that a stable environment is necessary to decrease disruption and reduce the levels of stress a child is subject to after a divorce. Hence, a major goal of Peter's treatment was to increase the stability in his life by targeting environmental factors such as his mother's work.

As can be seen in this case, working with children with GAD requires creativity on the part of the therapist because their worries vary and they have different levels of insight and understanding. The importance of creativity and of adapting therapy for children through the use of art work, simple metaphors and game-like exercises (Whitton, Luiselli, & Donaldson, 2006) has been well-documented in published case studies. Tailoring treatment to the unique needs of clients is particularly important for children with anxiety as they may have difficulty feeling safe in a novel environment such as the therapy room or clinic.

Given Peter's reserved temperament, together with the consideration that children from Asian cultures may be less verbally and emotionally expressive than children from Western cultures, it was a struggle for him to verbally express his thoughts and feelings. Without the use of art work, it would have been very difficult to understand what his difficulties were. Without the use of alternative mediums to express himself, his sessions in therapy would have been one-directional and the rapport with his therapist minimal. Instead, building on Peter's strength and interest in art gave him a sense of accomplishment and made sessions enjoyable. Having him play the role of a detective who gathers evidence to challenge his negative thoughts proved both engaging and effective in helping him to master cognitive concepts.

Michael and colleagues (2012) used the character of Batman, described to be "strong and relaxed" as a cue for a six-year-old boy with GAD to utilize his adaptive coping skills. Similarly, when faced with anxiety, Peter was taught to use superheroes like Spiderman as a cue to put his coping skills into practice. This proved to be an effective move, as his strong interest in superheroes and his aspiration to become one motivated him to learn skills to manage his anxiety and gave him the willpower to go through with exposure tasks during therapy. Rubin (2006) explained that children are likely to identify with superheroes because superheroes are seen as being in the same situation as them, having to overcome obstacles and being transformed by the experience in the process. Challenges faced on certain steps of Peter's exposure hierarchy (e.g., feeling like giving up when he was too afraid to sleep alone after watching a horror movie) were equated to obstacles faced by superheroes in their quests. Because he saw himself as a superhero, Peter's surmounting of each obstacle raised his confidence. He felt "stronger and braver" as he progressed through on exposure hierarchy.

Balancing time and focus can become a challenge during therapy, especially when working with a child and their parents, and particularly when a child has GAD. GAD is associated with many worries, which can change over the course of therapy. Some of Peter's behavioural problems that were of concern to his mother included stealing money, lying, and loitering in the neighbourhood without permission. However, addressing these issues often left the therapist with little or no time to review Peter's progress in managing his anxiety, or to go through his CBT homework tasks. Furthermore, his therapist had to make it clear to his mother that his behavioural problem should be addressed separately from his anxiety treatment. This issue came to light when his progress on the exposure ladder was affected due to his mother punishing him for lying by making him forfeit his points for one week.

As it has been found that GAD in childhood was a risk factor for adolescent conduct disorder (Bittner et al., 2007), much time was dedicated to equipping his mother with parenting skills from Triple P—Positive Parenting Program (Sanders, 1999) in order to ensure that Peter's behavioural problems did not escalate. Peter's lack of supervision after school was consistent with findings in the literature linking childhood GAD with inadequate supervision and control (Nordahl, Wells, Olsson, & Bjerkeset, 2010). This prompted a recommendation that Peter be enrolled into an after-school care facility.

Another challenge encountered was the difficulty in engaging Peter's grandmother in his intervention. Given cultural expectations for respect for elders and the notion that elders are more knowledgeable due to their greater life experiences, Peter's therapist recognized his grandmother's expertise and positioned ourselves as requiring her help in helping Peter. However, she felt that there was "nothing wrong with him" and that he would naturally "outgrow" his difficulties with anxiety. Furthermore, her permissive caregiving was believed to be perpetuating his behavioural problems. Hence, a fair amount of time was spent discussing with Peter's mother on how she could persuade his grandmother to attend a meeting. However plans for her involvement in his therapy fell through, despite much planning and a phone call to her. This was a pity but it was also a learning point for the therapist—sometimes in therapy, despite our best intentions and efforts, human behaviour and thinking is not something that we have complete control over.

DISCUSSION QUESTIONS

1. The lifetime prevalence rate for GAD in the United States has been found to be 5.7% (Kessler et al., 2005) while the lifetime prevalence rate for GAD in Singapore was found to be only 0.9% (Chong et al., 2012). What factors might account for this difference?

2. Given that Peter's mother has plans for the family to move overseas and that Peter's GAD causes him to worry excessively about the future, how would you help mother prepare Peter for this significant life event? What factors would be important to consider?

3. Based on the case formulation, Peter's parents' divorce seemed to be the precipitating factor for his anxiety. Do you think it is necessary to discuss or process the divorce with Peter? What would drive your decision? If yes, how would you as a psychologist, go about doing so?

4. Would you have involved Peter's other family members or even his school in the intervention? What would affect your decision? If yes, who should be involved and what would their roles be?

5. Exposure can either be done in a graduated manner (i.e., systematic desensitization) such as with Peter, or it can be done in a way where the client is immediately exposed to the stimulus that is most aversive to him/her (i.e., flooding exposure). What are the pros and cons of flooding exposure? In what situations would you consider using it?

CHAPTER 7.

LAZY, NAUGHTY AND IRRESPONSIBLE

Frontal Lobe Epilepsy
CATHERINE ANNE COX

INTRODUCTION

Tim was a nine-year-old boy who had a diagnosis of Frontal Lobe Epilepsy (FLE) since the age of three. His neurologist was concerned about his current behavioural issues and suspected a diagnosis of ADHD over and above his FLE. He was also worried about the family's compliance with anti-epileptic medications: Tim's parents preferred Traditional Chinese Medicine (TCM) and as a result Tim's seizures had not been well controlled. A neuropsychological assessment was requested to develop a clearer picture and diagnosis of his behaviours and cognitive abilities, and to determine the effect of poorly controlled seizures on his well-being.

Tim's parents, Mr and Mrs Lim, complained that he was lazy, naughty, and irresponsible. At home, they clashed with Tim over his homework and computer time. If they did not sit with Tim and "scold" him, he would refuse to do his homework. These difficulties had become more pronounced in Primary 3, when his homework load increased. He would only get started on his assignments when his parents returned home from work at 8:30 pm. Keeping him focused then required another two hours of family energy. As Tim had managed to negotiate for computer time before bedtime, he was not sleeping until well after 11pm. To discipline Tim, his mother shouted at him and threatened to ban computer games. Both parents resorted to caning him, at least once a week, as this was the only effective means of directing him.

Tim also had a temper. He fought frequently with his younger sister whom he always envied. He defied his domestic helper, particularly when she was caring for him alone, and had hit her on several occasions. He rarely complied when his grandparents asked him to do homework.

Tim lived with his working parents, two younger siblings and an Indonesian domestic helper. Developmentally, Tim was born at full term, following an uneventful pregnancy. He began walking at ten months of age, and his mother described him as "very busy" and "into everything". Although he only spoke his first words at 18 months, his parents attributed this to his high level of activity, and were not particularly concerned. By three, he was just beginning to put words together (e.g., "my car").

It was at this time that Tim presented to the hospital. His parents had noticed that he would sometimes cry out in his sleep, grunt, smack his lips and that his left leg and arm would stiffen. These episodes had been happening for about six months, but it was not until his parents witnessed an episode during which his whole body jerked uncontrollably for 10–15 minutes, that they brought him to A&E. During inpatient admission, a video electro-encephalogram (EEG) showed seizures originating from his right frontal lobe. Further monitoring revealed not only visible seizures of 3–4 per night but an additional 3–4 very short seizures. Consequently, management of his seizures required anti-epileptic medication (AEDs) His MRI brain scan was normal, indicating that his seizures were unlikely to either have been caused by an underlying brain malformation such as a tumour, or a disorder of brain development (i.e., 'cortical dysplasia'), both of which could potentially be treated by surgery.

At the same time, Tim's neurologist had observed that he was not speaking at an age-appropriate level and thus referred him for speech and language therapy (SLT). He was found to have moderate expressive and receptive language delay, as well as poor attention. Ongoing therapy was therefore recommended to help Tim develop pre-reading skills like narrative skills (the ability to tell a story well) and phonological awareness (rhyming, letter-sound recognition). However, Tim only attended speech therapy until he was about five. When asked why they did not continue with SLT, Tim's parents explained that it was inconvenient to bring him to therapy during the week. Furthermore, they felt that he was progressing adequately.

One year after the admission to A&E, at four years of age, Tim's seizures were well-controlled with two AEDs. His parents also brought him for acupuncture sessions and had him use Traditional Chinese Medicine (TCM). When he was six, his parents no longer observed him to have any seizures. Being concerned about the potential side effects of his prescribed Western medication, they ceased his AED usage. Six months later, Tim had a seizure, was readmitted to hospital and restarted on another course of AEDs. This became a repeating pattern: his parents would stop his AEDs whenever he had a period of freedom from seizures, but continue with TCM, till his seizures began again. When Tim was eight he experienced another long seizure. By this time his seizures had become much harder to control.

At the age of six, concerns about his concentration and school readiness led to a neuropsychological assessment. While his verbal skills, literacy and numeracy were significantly lower than expected for his age, his visuo-spatial skills were average. His attention was below age expectations—he was distractible, did not persist with difficult tasks and needed frequent prompts and cues. These corroborated his kindergarten teacher's and parents' reports of clinically significant attention problems. These problems were considered consistent with his poorly controlled seizures, language delay, and his slower progress in English than his first language Mandarin. However a possible diagnosis of ADHD was also raised. It was thus recommended that he repeat K2 as well as be put on a trial of a stimulant. Tim repeated K2, but his parents rejected the use of a stimulant. Support from his neuropsychologist and speech therapist was also suggested, but his parents cancelled subsequent appointments.

When Tim was again seen in Primary 3, his form teacher reported that his class performance had been below average and that he had failed most subjects. Although he had been in his school's Learning Support Programme (LSP) for Maths and English, his gains had been hampered by poor attention. His teachers reported a range of concerns about his lack of attention ("fidgety", "cannot sit still", "needs reminders to complete work in class", "does not persist"), poor social functioning ("has few friends", "can be quarrelsome"), and language ("is very quiet", "rarely contributes"). He had come to the school counsellor's attention six months before his referral, for getting into a physical fight with a boy who had called him "stupid". Tim's teachers were not aware of his nightly seizures, and parents had never informed them: they preferred to keep details about his condition within the family.

ASSESSMENT

Tim's clinical neuropsychologist conducted a comprehensive neuropsychological assessment over three sessions. The first involved history taking with his parents and an evaluation of their concerns; sessions two and three focused on Tim's cognitive and emotional assessment. A hypothesis-testing approach was used to direct the assessment. Following a review of his medical and developmental history, a number of diagnostic hypotheses for his condition were suggested, either alone or in combination: ADHD, FLE, uncontrolled seizures, and language delay with perhaps dyslexia. Despite their overlapping symptoms, seizures and language difficulties were accounted for independently of ADHD because treatment for each condition is different.

An important aspect of neuropsychological assessments with children is to determine whether their performance and behaviours are age-appropriate or not (Jones-Gotman et al., 2010). For this reason, Tim's results on the standardised psychometric tools were adjusted for age, and where possible, gender.

Parent and teacher reports of behaviour can vary as a function of their different perspectives and across different situations. For example, parents of children with epilepsy have been found to report more ADHD behaviours than teachers, whereas the reverse has been found in community samples (Sherman, Brooks, Akday, Connolly & Wiebe, 2010). Differences in reporting may also be of diagnostic relevance. For this reason, a range of questionnaires was given to both Tim's parents and teachers so as to assess his attention, executive skills and emotional and behavioural functioning across different settings.

To make direct comparison with his previous assessment at six years of age, the same tests were used. However, this was not always possible. For example, he was administered the Wechsler Intelligence Scale for Children—Fourth Edition (WISC-IV; Wechsler, 2004) for children aged six to sixteen years old, rather than the Wechsler Preschool and Primary Scale of Intelligence—4th Edition (WPPSI-IV; Wechsler, 2012), which was used in his previous assessment.

Tim's assessment was carried out in the absence of his parents. He was quiet and did not initiate conversation, except to ask when the session would be over. When he did reply to questions, his speech, although clear and easily understood, consisted only of short phrases and single word responses; he had to be encouraged to elaborate on his answers. Longer questions that were asked had to be repeated, and he was slow in responding. However, when doing tasks that did not require a verbal response he was quick, but also careless and prone to making errors. Tim needed repeated prompts to stay on task, as he would look around the room, get distracted easily and fiddle with items on the desk, such as his water bottle, pencils and the stopwatch. These items had to be removed from his reach.

Intellectual Ability

A comprehensive neuropsychological assessment was conducted starting with general intellectual skills (IQ), to allow for an understanding of Tim's general functioning and to determine whether low IQ or poor verbal skills were factors in his current difficulties. His intellectual abilities were significantly varied. His visually based skills remained strong and fell in the high average range, whilst his verbal skills were in the borderline range and fell below age expectations, consistent with his prior assessment.

Attention and Processing Speed

Tim had a range of moderate to severe difficulties with attention when he had to focus on a boring task, or hold and manipulate information in his mind (working memory). When he had to do two things at once (divided attention), he would end up focusing on one task while almost completely neglecting the other. From questionnaires completed by his teacher and parents, it was clear that, compared to other boys his age, he had more difficulties with working memory, attention and hyperactivity. They reported that he struggled to stay on task, could not maintain a sustained effort, was easily distracted and more "on the go" than others his age.

Executive Skills

Executive skills include planning, volition, and purposive action (Lezak et al., 2004), which are basic to good problem-solving, and the ability to work towards a goal (e.g., a school project). Tim's executive skills were assessed through both cognitive tests and by observation of his approach to tasks. His reasoning and problem-solving skills were age-appropriate for tasks that had visual support, such as picture puzzles, but below age expectations for tasks that used language, such as verbal reasoning questions. He was not well organised, tended to rush through tasks, and did not use his earlier errors to correct his later performance. On questionnaires that examined executive skills in daily life, his parents and teachers indicated impairments in his ability to inhibit his responses ("blurts out answers"), and in organisation and self-monitoring.

Memory

Tim's attention and executive difficulties impacted on his memory: when given information to learn and remember, he was easily overwhelmed. Although he exhibited better recall when information was repeated, his haphazard and disorganised approach to learning resulted in his poorer performance than others his age. Once he was able to learn new information however, he did not forget it.

Academic Functioning

Tim's academic skills were assessed to rule out any underlying learning difficulty like dyslexia, and to monitor how much knowledge he was acquiring at school. His academic skills—reading, spelling and numerical skills—were all age-appropriate when compared against overseas norms for some tests. However, they were in line with his teacher's report that his performance was below average in class. For example, children who are failing maths at school in Singapore often obtain high-average to superior scores in standardised maths tests developed overseas.

Emotional and Behavioural functioning

Rating scales completed by Tim's teacher and parents indicated that he tended to be more withdrawn and shy than was typical for boys his age. At home however, he was more oppositional than other boys. This was consistent with his parents' reported difficulties with discipline.

DIAGNOSIS

Tim met the criteria for ADHD Combined Presentation, with inattention and impulsivity, over and above his current diagnosis of FLE. His pattern of cognitive performance was consistent with his poorly controlled seizure disorder, early age of seizure onset, language delay, multiple AEDs, and Mandarin-speaking background.

Determining which of these factors resulted in him meeting diagnostic criteria for ADHD was difficult. Children with epilepsy can appear to have ADHD due to underlying seizures, language impairments, or even anxiety. In Tim's case, attention and executive functioning were the most severely impaired components of his profile. This lent support to the hypothesis that his ADHD arose from a combination of seizures and poor attention. His language impairment was less pronounced than previously assessed and there was no suggestion of any mood disorder (e.g., anxiety) that could account for his poor attention. Pragmatically, a diagnosis of ADHD is easily understood by educators and allows parents to apprehend why medication would be of use.

INTEGRATIVE FORMULATION

Predisposing Factors

Early age of seizure onset is known to lead to greater levels of cognitive and behavioural impairment, and seizures that originate in the right frontal lobe are known to impact on social functioning, executive and behavioural functioning, and attention (Braakman, Vaessen, Hofman, Debij-van Hall, Backes, Vles and Aldenkamp, 2011). Tim's language delay also placed him at risk of developing a language-based learning difficulty (Stoeckel, Colligan, Barbaresi, Weaver, Killian, Katusic, 2013), and his Mandarin-speaking background predisposed him to poorer English, which would compromise his performance on tests normed in Western countries (Dixon, 2011).

Fact Box 7.1. Medicating ADHD

Methylphenidate (Ritalin, Biphentin, Concerta) is a stimulant, and most commonly used in the treatment for ADHD. It has been found to improve the attention span, short term memory and academic performance of a child with ADHD (Bedard et al., 2007; Evans et al., 2001). However, side effects of this drug include appetite loss, growth retardation, sleep disturbances, anxiety and depression (NIMH, 2012; Fung & Lee, 2009). A major contention is that the effects of its long-term use have not been quantified. A recently released longitudinal study, which set out to measure the medium- to long-term effects of stimulant use among children with ADHD, found a deterioration in academic performance over time and increases in mood disturbances (Currie, Stabile & Jones, 2014). A more recently discovered selective norepinephrine reuptake inhibitor, Atomoxetine, has been found to be associated with fewer harmful side effects, and a potential alternative to methylphenidate (Garnock-Jones & Keating, 2009).

Precipitating Factors

Tim's referral to psychological services was precipitated by him failing at school. This was due to a combination of the academic rigours of the Singaporean education system and the more demanding schoolwork he was assigned as he got older. The severity of his academic difficulties, together with his parents' frustration over his 'laziness' and lack of progress, finally led his parents to seek help.

Perpetuating Factors

Perpetuating Tim's problems were his epilepsy, cognitive weaknesses and his family's variable compliance with his neuropsychologist's recommendations. His poorly controlled epilepsy would have impacted on his brain development and compromised his cognitive and academic functioning (Westerveld, 2010). His EEG showed ongoing abnormal discharges that may have further reduced his attention in daily life. Further, seizures during sleep are known to alter sleep architecture and to result in poor sleep quality; this potentially reduced the consolidation of his memories during sleep, resulting in reduced learning and memory (Van Bogaert, Urbain, Galer, Ligot, Peigneus & Tiege, 2011).

Tim's cognitive weaknesses in language and reading made it hard for him to keep up at school. His weak attention and executive functioning kept him from benefitting from traditional classroom teaching. They undermined his ability to manage his homework independently and in a developmentally appropriate manner. His lack of success and positive experiences at school led to a downward spiral of reduced motivation and effort.

Tim's difficulties in school were compounded by poor compliance with other therapies and interventions. His parents' choice to discontinue speech therapy when he commenced primary school deprived him of support to manage his language disorder in a school setting. And while he had been given the chance to repeat K2, his parents had decided against following up on recommendations for medications targeted at the control of his seizures and attentional deficits. Lack of structure and supervision at home, coupled with his parents' expectation that he should be completely independent in completing his homework, meant that he had no opportunity to acquire relevant skills to support his poor executive functioning (e.g., planning and organisational strategies). Finally, the absence of good sleep patterns resulted in fatigue, which impacted both his attention and seizure frequency.

Protective Factors

Tim had a close and intact family unit. They were sincere in their efforts to seek help for him. Their difficulties in compliance with western medications resulted from their cultural beliefs and a general mistrust of western medicine, rather than a lack of willingness to see their son improve.

PROGNOSIS

As seizures are a symptom of disordered brain development (Westerveld, 2010; Hermann, Jones, Dabbs, Allen, Sheth, Fine, McMillan & Seidenberg 2007), it is likely that Tim would always display an uneven pattern of cognitive strengths and weakness. It is possible that he will be increasingly unable to keep pace with his peers cognitively and academically, especially when demands for better language skills and more advanced executive skills (such as inferencing, problem-solving, planning and analytical thinking) come to the fore in higher grades at school. Furthermore, it is difficult to project how a child's developing brain will respond to seizures and treatment. Because one cannot assume that a child has deficits in a particular skill (such as reading or problem solving) until they reach the point of having to learn that skill, a definitive prognosis is seldom possible (Jones-Gotman et al., 2010).

Tim's prognosis was dependent on his family's ability to treat his epilepsy and ADHD consistently, his regular attendance at speech and language therapy sessions, and increased structure and support at home. Without such support and intervention, his future is likely to be clouded by academic failure, more extreme oppositional behaviour, and even more restricted social opportunities. A review by Harpin (2005) noted that children with ADHD are more likely to display conduct issues and fail to complete school. A recent, large, longitudinal study by Wei, Yu & Shaver (2014) found that "ADHD has a long-term deleterious effect on academic, social, and behaviour outcomes for students" with learning and emotional difficulties. Furthermore, students with both ADHD and learning difficulties had more reading, social and behavioural difficulties than those with only a learning difficulty. These problems did not lessen with age.

Whilst Tim did not have an emotional disorder during the period of his assessment, people with epilepsy have much higher rates of depression. The development of a mood disorder also indicates a poorer outcome for seizures (Kanner, 2011). However, treatment of ADHD has been shown to moderate the condition's long-term impact (Shaw et al., 2012) and an evidence base is building for a range of interventions targeting learning difficulties and reducing poor outcome.

TREATMENT

Feedback and psycho-education are crucial components of intervention, and one of the first few steps to engaging parents. Feedback on Tim's assessment was shared first with him, and then with his parents. Tim's therapist assured him that it was not his fault that he experienced more difficulty concentrating than other kids his age and highlighted his strengths in visuo-spatial skills, like drawing and creating toys from Lego. While

Tim did not say much during this session, he acknowledged his decided preference for subjects like art and sports. His shy smile reflected his pleasure at being recognised for what he was good at.

Tim was also told that a report would be written to provide his parents and teachers with ideas of how they could "help him to think better". The therapist then held a separate session with Tim's parents and his grandparents, during which they could freely ask questions about his formal report. During this session, they discussed three main recommendations: medication compliance, home-based strategies and school support.

Compliance with Tim's anti-epileptic medication was reinforced as it played a critical role in managing his condition. Because his parents did not understand how attentional deficits and academic problems could arise in the absence of visible seizures, his therapist explained that small, unnoticeable seizures or abnormal brain waves—for example, an unusual inter-ictal (between seizure) EEG—could lead to transient problems in cognitive functioning (Van Bogaert, et al., 2011). This modified their tendency to blame Tim for his reduced attention. The therapist also emphasised that even if his EEG were normal, the high incidence of ADHD and epilepsy (MacAllister Vasserman, Vekarla, Miles-Mason, Hochsztein, & Bender, 2012), particularly for children with FLE (Zhang, Li, Zhu and Sun, 2014), warranted the use of a stimulant medication.

Fact Box 7.2. Supporting Parents of Children with Epilepsy

Programs which address parent education for epilepsy are rare in the Asian context. In 2013, KKH implemented its Epilepsy Action Plan, an instuctional guide for caregivers of children with epilepsy, across all of its paediatric disciplines. These plans, presented in brochure format, are customised for each patient. They include pictures and instructions on medicine dosage, frequency and administration, seizure management and documentation, resources for emergency treatment, and answers to frequently answered questions about the side effects of medication. Tim and his family subsequently attended sessions with his neuropsychologist every three months. These sessions involved psycho-education about the long-term impact of uncontrolled seizures on the brain, and the evaluation and adjustment of behavioural strategies. Tim's parents were also repeatedly reassured by various members of the epilepsy team, including the epilepsy nurse, epilepsy pharmacist and the neurologist, that any "toxic" side effects of AEDs were preferable to uncontrolled seizures. His EEGs improved and were repeatedly normal; this was explained to be the result of their compliance with medication.

The therapist outlined practical guidelines for managing behaviour at home, such as the implementation of home-based schedules and routines. In order to support Tim's weak executive skills, he could be trained to follow a schedule with prompts, rather than being directly supervised step-by-step. A list of acceptable behaviour within the family was also drawn up (e.g., no hitting or name calling, no hand-held devices or computer games near bedtime). To help his parents enforce computer guidelines, the therapist suggested that the whole family stop using their computers at bed time so that light from these electronic devices would not disrupt the onset of sleep.

Lastly, the therapist highlighted academic recommendations, including special accommodations for exams: extra time, a separate room for examinations, and prompts to stay on task. She proposed exemption from his mother tongue, Mandarin, if he continued to struggle with it after receiving learning support. Specialist interventions were also proposed. Rather than regular tuition, which could be expensive and yield few results for children with difficulties like Tim's, attendance at classes run by organisations with educational psychologists on staff was suggested. A strong focus was placed on addressing and improving on significant areas of weakness like executive skills (e.g., planning, problem-solving and organisation). This was crucial as his school syllabus had started placing more demands on the use of executive skills to tackle mathematics problem sums.

Effectively engaging Tim's parents in his intervention required his therapist to understand their key concerns. Local data has revealed that parents in Singapore are primarily concerned about cognition and academic functioning, followed by social and emotional problems (Yap et. al., unpublished data). Parents from Western societies, however, are more concerned about seizure and medication management, and dependency in adulthood (VanStraten & Ng, 2012). While Tim's parents were clearly concerned about his academic performance, his father was initially sceptical that his cognitive problems arose from epilepsy. He repeatedly claimed that Tim was "lazy" and could do better "if only he tried". Research findings that difficulties in cognition and behaviour often pre-date seizure onset (Taylor et al., 2010; Herrman, et al., 2007) were thus shared with his parents to illustrate that his cognitive problems could not be blamed on either seizures, AEDs, or poor effort alone. The potential consequences of not adhering with recommendations to manage his seizures and ADHD were outlined: he would lose any motivation to excel at school, fail academically, develop a range of behavioural problems, fall in with the "wrong crowd", and even end up being suspended or expelled (Wei et al., 2014). Furthermore, Asian cultural values of the importance of academic success and of not losing face were emphasised to motivate treatment.

Caring for children with special needs is challenging for parents, and Tim's parent's wanted to relate to him in a more positive manner. They were thus encouraged to praise him for each attempt he made to improve, and to spend time with him on enjoyable activities apart from academic work. As caning did not affect his behaviour much, alternative disciplinary methods were explored. A combination of rewards for appropriate behaviour (computer time, choice of dinner cuisine on the weekend, a computer game with his dad) and withdrawal of privileges (less computer time) for less appropriate behaviour was suggested.

Tim's parents wanted to test the efficacy of behavioural intervention in the absence of medication. However, when six months saw little change in his behaviour they finally agreed to put him on a slow release stimulant prescribed by his psychiatrist, and he was monitored for any increase in seizure frequency (Fosi et al., 2013). At their next session they reported that behavioural strategies had become much easier to implement. Tim had also begun to proactively complete his homework instead of avoiding it. At school, recommendations from his assessment were implemented with the assistance of an Allied Educator and school counsellor. His teachers also noted an improvement in his behaviour, and in the grades he attained upon commencement of taking the stimulant.

A few months later, Tim's social skills were observed to have improved in school. Whereas he had initially shied away from interaction with other children, he was beginning to demonstrate more enthusiasm during play with his peers. He was also participating more actively in co-curricular activities, such as his school's Audio-Visual Club, taking more care of the equipment under his charge and interacting more appropriately with other club members.

Tim's initial prognosis had been complicated by non-compliance with treatment and support. However, once his parents and teachers understood his diagnosis, his needs, and the complexity of his condition, their willingness to engage with his therapist and epilepsy team gave him the appropriate treatment and support needed to turn the outcome of his condition around.

DISCUSSION

Many children, teenagers and parents with epilepsy who are seen for neuropsychological assessment present with considerable distress. For children and teenagers, when seizures occur just before major exams, they are faced with the disappointment of poorer grades, the daunting prospect of not qualifying for the same school or stream as their friends, and the fear of their grades being compared with those of their extended family members at events such as Chinese New Year or Hari Raya. Some teenagers report that their parents discourage them from talking to others about their epilepsy to avoid bringing shame to the family.

Children with epilepsy have been found to be more concerned about the social stigma associated with their condition than with the seizures themselves (VanStraten & Ng, 2012). Even cognitively intact children with epilepsy experience significant social rejection from their peers (Westerfeld, 2010). When teachers and parents exclude them from activities such as physical education, it further highlights their differences from their peers and increases their social isolation.

Epilepsy is a heterogeneous disorder and a neuropsychological assessment is a key method of understanding its impact and the impact of its treatment on everyday life (Jones-Gotman, et al., 2010). Assessment provides crucial information for an accurate diagnosis and helps in guiding treatment. Neuropsychologists who work within epilepsy teams play a role in helping children and their families to manage the psychosocial impact of this condition (Jones-Gotman et al., 2010). Tim's case illustrates how establishing a good therapeutic relationship is critical to treatment compliance and a positive outcome.

Within an epilepsy team, a neuropsychologist possesses the expertise to bring together all the elements that impact on a client's cognition, academic performance, and psychosocial functioning. Tim's case illustrates how neuropsychological comorbidities can vary widely. This is common in paediatric epilepsy because a range of problems that present in childhood—brain malformations, tumours, insults, and genetic disorders—can give rise to seizures and alter brain development, leading to more global difficulties with brain anatomy and function (Westerveld, 2010). Such disordered brain development means that the typical lateralising and localising signs found in adults are not always present in children (Jones-Gotman et al., 2010), and the occurrence of a wide range of cognitive and behavioural outcomes can lead to significant challenges for the pediatric neuropsychologist (Westerveld, 2010). As well as being a clinical challenge, symptoms associated with childhood epilepsy can also be confusing for parents, who see an otherwise normal child but cannot understand why he or she is experiencing so many problems.

Tim's parents exemplify how little the average person knows about epilepsy, despite it being a fairly common neurological disorder with a lifetime risk of 2–5% (Rugg-Gunn & Sander, 2012). Some of the main challenges to be overcome when working with parents of children with epilepsy include improving their understanding of epilepsy, explaining its complex set of comorbidities, dealing with stigma, and implementing an appropriately tailored treatment plan. A key part of engaging Tim's parents was helping them understand that a child with epilepsy will underachieve even with a normal IQ, and explaining how Tim's other deficits in attention, executive skills, memory and specific language and learning difficulties contributed to his overall presentation (Westerveld, 2010).

Parents often want to know the cause of their child's cognitive challenges. Making parents aware of Hermann and colleagues' (2007) findings of deficits in cognition occurring soon after seizures start—which suggest that neurodevelopmental brain abnormalities are likely to be responsible for the multiple cognitive and academic difficulties found in children with epilepsy—is critical so that they do not solely lay the blame for their child's condition on either seizures or medication, as they are wont to do. Tim had frontal lobe epilepsy (FLE), the second most common localization-related epilepsy in childhood (Braakman et al., 2011). It is often related to a structural or functional (a seizure focus) lesion and can be difficult to control. This was seen in Tim's case, with his seizures recurring after medication was ceased. In Braakman and colleagues' 2011 review of the literature on FLE in children, they concluded that attention difficulties, including ADHD, executive deficits and behavioural impairments, are common and occur at very high rates. Thus any psychologist working with children with epilepsy should consider ADHD a comorbidity (MacAllister et al., 2012), assess both parents and teachers, and use objective testing to confirm their observed symptoms (Sherman et al., 2010).

Finally, understanding that children with epilepsy are much more likely to have ADHD, (MacAllister et al., 2012; Hermann et al., 2007; Westerveld, 2010), helps parents to realise that they should not blame their child for being naughty or for not trying hard enough. This in turn opens up an avenue for treatment, as was the case for Tim. In fact, improvements in Tim's overall behaviour and progress were largely related to higher rates of compliance to his AEDs and stimulant medication, which was facilitated by his parents' better understanding of his comorbid ADHD.

The need for both behavioural and pharmacological approaches to help these children highlights the utility of a multi-disciplinary team and the importance of good communication among its members. When all professionals on the team are able to be on the same page with regards to their client's treatment, families are not only reassured, but receive reinforcement for their adherence to treatment. However, for some families like Tim's, it can take several years to build a trusting relationship with a client's family, particularly if they are sceptical of western medicine and hospitals.

In conclusion, this case illustrates the range of common coexistent problems that surface in children with epilepsy, and emphasises the need for neuropsychological involvement to provide the best care for a child. The neuropsychologist plays a valuable role, integrating findings from current literature into clinical practice to provide evidence-based care. Of equal importance is possessing a sound grasp of cultural norms and values for working with families and engaging them in the treatment process.

DISCUSSION QUESTIONS

1. This case study involves parents who have chosen not to proceed with traditional western medicine to treat their child's seizure disorder. This presents ethical questions for medical professionals. At best, the parent's decision would result in some form of cognitive problems for their child; at worst, it could end in severe disability from status epilepticus, or even death. How do you think that you would work with such a family and preserve rapport and a good working relationship whilst advocating medical treatment for the child?
2. How do you think multiple comorbidities found in children with epilepsy impact on diagnosis and treatment? Do you think it is helpful to diagnose a child with "everything?" Under which circumstances would such a diagnosis be beneficial?
3. Children with epilepsy in overseas research reported being most concerned about stigma (VanStraten & Ng, 2012). What kinds of discrimination or psychosocial

issues do you think children in Singapore may face that may be different from children in western countries?

4. What do you think were the advantages of Tim being seen by a neuropsychologist who understands epilepsy as opposed to other psychologists (e.g., clinical or educational)? How is the neuropsychologist's input different from the rest of the epilepsy team?

CHAPTER 8.

FROM OSTRICH TO EAGLE

Physical Abuse and Post-Traumatic Stress Disorder

TAN LI JEN AND CHEW QIAN RU CHARIS

BACKGROUND

Daniel Tan was an eight-year-old Singaporean boy referred to the Clinical and Forensic Psychology Branch, Ministry of Social and Family Development (MSF) for assessment and treatment in response to severe physical abuse by his biological father. Spotted with bruises and burn marks on his arms and legs in school one day, Daniel was questioned by his form teacher who found out that he was frequently hit by his father. The school immediately alerted Child Protection Service (CPS). Following investigations by the police, Daniel's father, Mr Tan, was charged in court and sentenced to prison. Mrs Tan was the sole breadwinner of her family, had a full-time job, and struggled to be available at home for Daniel, so CPS placed him in his relatives' care. Within a few months, however, family conflict, coupled with practical and financial limitations, brought an end to Daniel's stay with his extended family. Having exhausted other care options, Daniel was subsequently placed in a voluntary children's home.

Daniel was referred to a psychologist after living in the children's home for three weeks. During his assessment, he presented as a thin boy who looked downcast and guarded. He exhibited significant symptoms of post-traumatic stress, including nightmares, poor appetite, and hypervigilance (e.g., he was afraid of people running towards him during physical education lessons). He was also extremely fearful of loud noises because they reminded him of his father's shouting. He avoided talking about his family problems and was reluctant to disclose details of his abuse, as he was worried about getting his parents into more trouble. Daniel also presented with depressed mood and low esteem, and blamed himself for causing his father's imprisonment and his family to be broken apart. Daniel was also disappointed that his mother had been unable to protect him. However, he rationalised that she "[could not] stop Daddy [from hitting him] because she is too small and he is too big."

Daniel could not concentrate in school and his grades dropped while he was adjusting to his stay at the children's home. Despite having been described by his father as an active boy who required frequent punishment, staff at the children's home did not report any significant behaviour problems during his stay. Instead they were concerned that he might be a target of bullies, as he tended to be shy and unassertive.

Daniel was an only child. His parents had met in school and his mother had become pregnant with Daniel when she was 17. Both parents received little caregiving and financial support from their families. As a young mother, Mrs Tan struggled to balance managing the household and caring for her child. Mr Tan recalled seeing the home in disarray and Daniel in soiled diapers. When Daniel turned five, Mr Tan quit his regular job for a daily rated job so that he could assume the role of his son's main caregiver, while Mrs Tan started full-time work. Unfortunately, this arrangement also led to the start of Mr Tan's own parenting struggles and his harsh discipline of Daniel.

Mr Tan's own childhood was marked by harsh physical punishment by his father. He had suffered from clinical depression since adolescence, but had stopped taking his medication after a few years. While both Mr and Mrs Tan reported a generally good marital relationship and positive moments with Daniel (e.g., outings, playing with toys), Mr Tan had a violent temper. The couple argued frequently about their finances and Daniel's care. These confrontations would often escalate to spousal violence, which included scolding and pushing, and the throwing of both punches and objects. Daniel witnessed this and would hide under the table in fear.

In addition to witnessing violence between his parents, Daniel had experienced multiple forms of violence and trauma. His father meted out harsh discipline on him, and had used various implements such as a ladle, cane and chopping board to hit Daniel's arms, legs and backside. He would also kick Daniel when he was angry with him. Other forms of punishment included tying Daniel to a water pipe in the toilet for hours, and making him do push-ups. For Daniel, being punished was a weekly affair, triggered when his father felt that he had misbehaved or messed the house up during play time. Daniel's mother was usually unaware of those harsh punishments as Daniel never told her about them for fear of triggering an argument between his parents. Even when Mrs Tan saw her son being hit, Daniel said that she was unable to restrain her husband because of his strength and his position of power at home.

During his clinical interviews, Daniel revealed that he was also a victim of repeated bullying in school. He described how he was locked in the toilet by his classmates during recess, and had his school bag thrown off the school bus by another group of older boys. As a result of the stress faced both at home and in school, Daniel's grades suffered. While teachers regarded him as a polite child who did not exhibit any significant behavioural problems, Daniel had low assertiveness and seldom told his teachers about being bullied for fear of causing more trouble.

ASSESSMENT

Clinical assessment of child abuse and trauma involves extensive interviews with multiple informants and caregivers. Several interviews were conducted with Daniel individually, and his psychologist also interviewed Mr and Mrs Tan separately to gain information on his presenting problems and background. Corroborative information from the school, the children's home and CPS were also considered to ensure a holistic assessment of Daniel's functioning and needs. Interviewing a child also requires knowledge of trauma-sensitive and child-friendly interviewing skills, and the active use of engagement and rapport building throughout the sessions. Expressive arts techniques such as drawing were used to encourage Daniel to share his thoughts and feelings, and games and role-playing were weaved into the sessions so as to make therapy more fun and engaging for Daniel.

Several psychological questionnaires were administered to Daniel, including UCLA PTSD Index for DSM-IV (Pynoos et al, 1998), a measure that assesses a child's exposure to traumatic events and assesses DSM-IV PTSD diagnostic criteria (fn. 3); Child Depression Inventory—2 (CDI-2; Kovacs, 1992), a self-report instrument designed to measure depressive symptoms in school-aged children and adolescents; Pier-Harris Children's Self-Concept Scale, 2nd Edition (PH-2; Piers, Harris & Herzberg, 2002), a self-report questionnaire for assessing self-concept in children and adolescents; and the Family Relations Test (Bene & Anthony, 1957), a projective test that assesses a child's perception of family members. Mrs Tan also completed the Parent's Version of the Strengths & Difficulties Questionnaire (SDQ) (Goodman, 1997), a brief behavioural screening questionnaire for 3 to 16 year olds.

DIAGNOSIS

Based on Daniel's clinical presentation and corroborative reports from his mother, his school and the children's home, Daniel was assessed to meet the criteria for a diagnosis of post-traumatic stress disorder (PTSD). His responses on the UCLA PTSD Index indicated that he had reported significant concerns related to post-traumatic stress, and had elevated severity scores for the primary PTSD symptoms of intrusion and hyperarousal. Although his avoidance and total scale scores were slightly lower than the clinical cutoff, the psychologist's clinical impression was that Daniel could have minimized some of his symptoms during the assessment, due to avoidance or caution about whether his statements would reflect negatively on his parents.

Daniel was also assessed as having a secondary diagnosis of depression. He presented with low mood associated with his abuse experiences and separation from his parents. During his initial stay at the children's home, staff reported that Daniel was often tearful and showed poor sleep and low appetite. These symptoms lasted for more than a month. Daniel blamed himself for "separating the family" and missed his parents. His total depression score on the CDI-2 fell within the very elevated range and his PH-2 scores were indicative of significantly low self-esteem. His mother perceived him as having high levels of difficulties in terms of overall stress and peer relationships.

Differential diagnoses considered included either depressive disorder or adjustment disorder. However, Daniel had a clear history of multiple traumatic abuse experiences, and was assessed by the clinical interviews and his scores on the trauma assessment measure to have experienced significant symptoms of trauma. These symptoms also had an impact on his daily functioning at school and at home. Hence, PTSD emerged as the primary disorder for Daniel.

INTEGRATIVE FORMULATION

Daniel presented with symptoms of traumatic stress, including nightmares, hypervigilance and fear of loud noises and perceived danger. He avoided talking about his abuse and had depressed mood, poor concentration and low self-esteem.

Predisposing Factors

Daniel's exposure to violence between his parents from a young age, and a lack of positive attention and nurturing from his parents due to their personal psychological issues and family conflict, were the predisposing factors.

Precipitating factors

Daniel's emotional problems were precipitated by the chronic physical abuse by his father and poor protective action from his mother and other family members. In addition to the trauma and violence at home, Daniel also experienced trauma in school as a victim of bullying. While he was removed from his family home for safety and protection, having to adjust to a new environment also added to his emotional stress.

Perpetuating Factors

Daniel's negative beliefs and inappropriate self-blame about his abuse perpetuated his anxiety and depression symptoms. His perception that people could not be trusted and caused harm also maintained his hypervigilance and fears. In turn, his avoidance of thinking or talking about his abuse experiences maintained trauma symptoms such as his nightmares. His heightened anxiety and perceived vulnerability also made it difficult for him to be more assertive or to protect himself when faced with school bullying. His physical separation from his parents and lack of attachment figures in his new care environment also contributed to his depression and anxiety about the future.

Protective Factors

In spite of the multiple risk factors in Daniel's situation, some protective factors existed. Firstly, the disclosure of physical abuse to CPS resulted in concrete safety measures to prevent Daniel from being further abused by his father. While his mother had been unable to intervene and stop the abuse, she still cared for Daniel and expressed her wish to support him and to be involved in his care. Daniel's school teachers were also concerned about his well-being and were motivated in putting measures in place to address school bullying. Prompt police and legal intervention was also effective in ensuring that firm consequences were meted out to Daniel's father, which would also help deter future recurrences of abuse.

PROGNOSIS

In view of the multiple levels of support and intervention provided to the family and Daniel's own willingness to engage in therapy, there was a good prognosis for recovery. Daniel was assessed to have a range of trauma symptoms, and while his total PTSD severity score fell below clinical cutoffs, the TF-CBT consultant opined that he would still benefit from trauma-focused treatment. This is consistent with research indicating that even children with subclinical levels of post traumatic stress symptoms benefit from treatment as they may be at risk for future mental health problems (Dorsey et al., 2011). Moreover, some of Daniel's symptoms could have been minimized or suppressed due to his anxiety and avoidance.

TREATMENT

Trauma-focused psychotherapies have been recommended as "first-line treatments for children and adolescents with PTSD" (AACAP, 2010, 421). In contrast to general non-directive counselling approaches, which may not have a specific focus on past traumas, this type of treatment directly addresses the child's traumatic experiences and symptoms. TF-CBT was selected for Daniel's intervention as it has received the most empirical support from multiple randomized controlled studies (AACAP, 2010; Cary & McMillen, 2012; Foa, et al., 2009), and has been used with child and adolescent victims of abuse, including children with multiple trauma histories and complex trauma (Cohen, 2012; Ford & Courtois, 2013). Intensive clinical supervision was provided by senior psychologists within the department and was augmented by monthly case consultation sessions by the TF-CBT consultant.

Therapy was aimed at reducing Daniel's post-traumatic stress symptoms, increasing his sense of safety and emotional stabilization, processing the trauma associated with his physical abuse, and enhancing his self-protection skills. It was also targeted at improving the protective abilities of his adult caregivers. Therapy was provided over the course of 15 months. A total of 26 individual therapy sessions were conducted every three weeks, with each session lasting 1.5 hours. Weekly sessions were conducted during the trauma narrative phase of treatment. As Daniel's mother worked long hours and his father was in prison, additional effort was made to engage them in therapy. Three individual therapy sessions were conducted with Mrs Tan, and several joint sessions were conducted between Daniel and his mother. Additionally, Mr Tan joined in a restorative session conducted in the prison.

The following core TF-CBT treatment components were provided (Cohen, Mannarino, & Deblinger, 2006; Cohen & Mannarino, 2008). They can be easily remembered by using the acronym "PRACTICE": P: Psychoeducation/Enhancing Safety, P: Parenting Skills, R: Relaxation Skills, A: Affect Modulation Skills, C: Cognitive Coping Skills, T: Trauma Narration and Processing, I: In Vivo Mastery of Trauma Reminders, C: Conjoint Child-Parent Sessions, and E: Enhancing safety.

Phase I: Stabilisation Phase

The first phase of treatment focused on helping Daniel to stabilise and learn basic coping skills and information about trauma. Of utmost importance in the first session was engaging Daniel in therapy by helping him to understand why he was seeing a psychologist, and why his psychologist was asking him to describe his previous abuse experiences, even though it was difficult for him. By using a practical analogy, this therapy rationale (Fact Box 8.1*)* was shared with Daniel and revisited at different points throughout the course of therapy. Given Daniel's avoidance about sharing his feelings, which is very common in trauma victims, the initial phase of therapy also focused

Fact Box 8.1. Introduction to Therapy Rationale

Therapist: Let's imagine that you were walking home from school one day, and you accidentally fell on hard ground and had a really bad cut on your knee, with blood coming out. What will you do?

Daniel: Go home and clean it, then apply ointment. But it will hurt.

Therapist: What happens if I just decide to put a plaster over the wound and tried to forget about it? What will happen to the wound?

Daniel: It will grow worse because of infection.

Therapist: Yes! Sometimes when bad things happen to kids, they are like wounds and injuries in their hearts. If we simply put a plaster and try to forget about it, the hurt just grows bigger and you will have an infection or a bad scar. If we clean the wound and apply ointment, it may hurt initially, but it will become better and the wound in the heart will heal. Therapy is like the medication. Healing happens when they apply medicine and ointment, by sharing their bad experiences with a doctor or a trusted adult.

on making him comfortable and developing a therapeutic alliance through games and stories.

Because Daniel was experiencing difficulties in adjusting to staying at the children's home and handling the bullies at school, his therapist also spent the initial sessions working with the social worker and school staff to increase Daniel's physical and emotional safety in these environments. Steps were taken to have his teachers and peers to look out for him at school and a routine was established for him to increase his sense of control in the children's home. Through worksheets on assertiveness skills and role-play, Daniel was taught strategies for responding to potential bullies (Figure 8.1). He was also taught to identify situations in which he would face a high risk of being bullied, and practised a combination of assertive thoughts and actions in response.

FIGURE 8.1 LEARNING ASSERTIVENESS SKILLS THROUGH EXAMINING BODY LANGUAGE

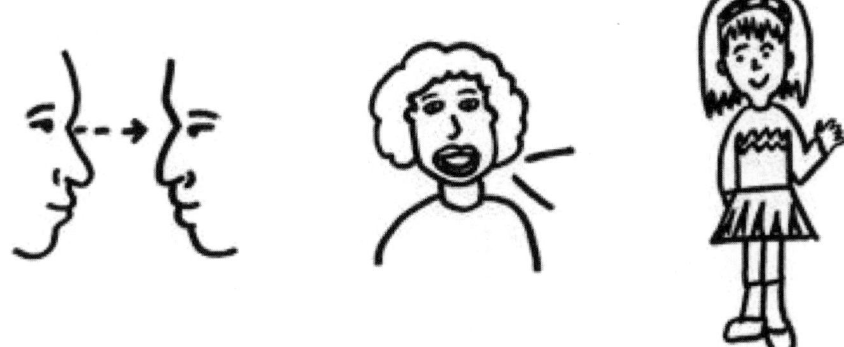

Once a measure of safety was established, subsequent sessions progressed to psychoeducation about trauma and post-traumatic stress reactions, with the goal of normalising and helping Daniel to understand his own trauma reactions. Relaxation and coping skills (e.g., progressive muscular relaxation, controlled breathing, grounding; Fact Box 8.2) were also taught to help Daniel manage and regulate his feelings associated with his experiences of being bullied and physically abused. Daniel also learnt to use positive imagery techniques such as going to his imaginary safe place (i.e., a quiet room) to cope whenever he missed his parents, and was encouraged to play the piano or soccer to relieve negative feelings.

Concurrently, his therapist also had sessions with Daniel's mother to provide psychoeducation about the effects of abuse and trauma on Daniel, to help her to understand her child's feelings and thoughts, as well as to discuss parenting strategies such as validating his feelings and spending quality time with him to support his recovery. During the Affect Modulation component of therapy, Daniel learned to identify and express different feelings. He was introduced to the Subjective Units of Distress Scale (SUD), using a scale of 0 (no anxiety or distress) to 10 (most anxiety and distress imaginable) to communicate the intensity of his feelings about different situations. Daniel was able to utilize the SUD to communicate that the physical abuse was the most distressing experience he had ever had (10 out of 10).

Cognitive coping involved teaching Daniel about the interrelationships between his thoughts, feelings and actions, and how he could reduce his negative feelings by developing more helpful thoughts, which would in turn lead to more positive outcomes. Although he initially held very negative self-beliefs and tended to self-blame ("I am a bad child for sending Dad to jail"), Daniel was gradually able to develop a more helpful self-belief ("I am a brave boy"). Throughout therapy, Daniel was empowered to identify and share his thoughts and feelings, and to engage in practical strategies to regulate his negative affect.

Fact Box 8.2. What is Grounding?

Grounding is a set of simple strategies to allow individuals to anchor on the present by focusing on the external world, rather than the past or future. Individuals who benefit from grounding are those who suffer from PTSD and have overwhelming emotions and memories or tend to feel numb with dissociation.

Staying grounded: A trauma self-help exercise (adapted from www.helpguide.org)

If you are feeling disoriented, confused, or upset, you can do the following exercise:

- Sit on a chair. Feel your feet on the ground. Press on your thighs. Feel your behind on the seat and your back against the chair.

- Look around you and pick six objects that are red or blue. This should allow you to feel in the present, more grounded, and in your body. Notice how your breath gets deeper and calmer.

- You may want to go outdoors and find a peaceful place to sit on the grass. As you do, feel how your body can be held and supported by the ground.

- Eat something, describing the flavours in detail to yourself.

- Focus on your breathing, notice each inhale and exhale.

Phase II: Trauma Narrative Phase

As Daniel began to display improvements in his mood and adjustment, and with ongoing checks to ensure his continued safety at school, his therapist progressed to the trauma narrative phase of therapy, and emotional processing of Daniel's physical abuse experiences. The development of a trauma narrative functions as a means of therapeutic gradual exposure to fearful memories and thoughts. In this phase, a good therapeutic rapport within a safe and caring environment was critical in helping Daniel to feel comfortable about sharing upsetting thoughts and painful memories associated with the abuse he had experienced. His therapist had to constantly be attuned to Daniel's behaviour and emotional reactions while developing the trauma narrative, so that she could pace his introduction to various trauma narrative tasks, which would facilitate his recovery and mastery over his traumatic memories.

Daniel was first encouraged to create a baseline narrative in session, to help him gradually ease into sharing his trauma narrative. During this session he typed out and described a neutral family event (i.e., family outing). Over the next few sessions, he typed out his trauma narrative, choosing to share the most distressing memory of being beaten by a fishing rod. His drawing and an extract from his trauma narrative is shown below in Figure 8.2.

FIGURE 8.2 DANIEL'S ABUSE SCENE

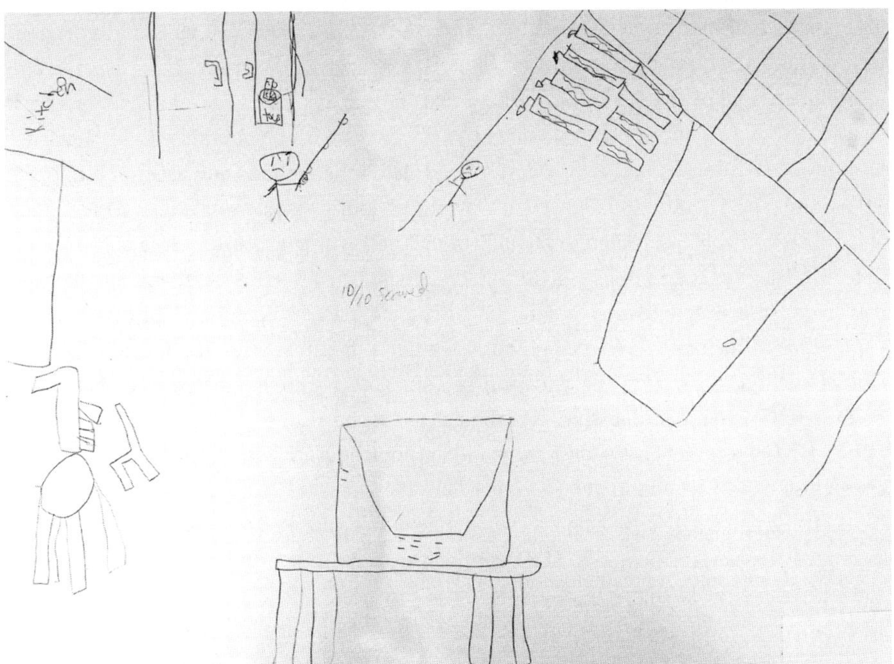

To accompany his drawing, Daniel wrote: "At night I put my things at the corner of the cupboard that belongs to my dad. I was in my daddy's room alone. Some of the family went shopping and my dad was in the toilet. Suddenly my dad asked me, "Why are your toys at my room?" He was very angry, and his eyebrows were going up. I said nothing because I was very scared. I thought, "Uh-oh my daddy is going to beat me" and he beat me with his fishing rod. He beat me until I cry and all the blood came out. He beat me at my legs and my hands. I was sad and also crying. I did not stop because I was very scared. He asked me to stop crying. He stopped and he kicked my toys away. I felt very, very sad. I washed my blood away at the toilet."

With support from the therapist, Daniel elaborated on his thoughts, feelings and behaviours during the abuse incident. As he recalled and wrote about his abuse experience, his therapist would periodically check on his levels of distress by asking him for his SUD ratings, which Daniel identified as a 7 out of 10. Daniel's therapist validated his fears, encouraged him to use controlled breathing and imagery techniques to regulate his feelings, and affirmed his efforts to talk about what had happened. She also challenged his inappropriate self-blame (e.g., he was naughty, which was why his father hit him; it was his fault his father was imprisoned), encouraged his development of more positive beliefs, and helped him to feel less guilty and depressed.

A joint parent-child session was arranged where Daniel read out his trauma narrative to his mother. Prior to this, Daniel's therapist held discussions with his mother on how to provide supportive and caring responses, and how to cope with her own emotions when listening to Daniel's trauma story. While Daniel was initially hesitant to read his narrative aloud, rating his anxiety as 8 out of 10 on the SUD, he was able to use deep breathing to calm himself. He was noticeably relieved to have been able to share his thoughts and feelings about his experiences with his mother and his SUD fell to 4 out of 10 after his narrative. Mrs Tan validated his feelings and assured him of his safety, and specifically told Daniel that "it [the abuse] was not your fault". Much praise and validation was also given to Daniel for accomplishing this difficult task.

Mr Tan was living in prison during the course of Daniel's assessment and therapy. As he expressed repentance about the abuse he had inflicted on Daniel and was supportive of his son's recovery process, Daniel's therapist arranged for and prepared Daniel for a session with his father in prison. Safety and support was given to him by having his therapist and Mrs Tan present when he read his trauma narrative to his father. Daniel's father listened intently and apologised for hurting him, "I wounded you physically. And I wounded you in your heart."

Mr Tan also affirmed Daniel's resilience and assured Daniel that he was learning to control his anger. Daniel's SUD rating dropped from a 9 to 3 after the session, and he was relieved that he could share his thoughts and fears with his father. This session served both as a form of in-vivo exposure for Daniel, as well as a positive initial restorative session between father and son. Through his positive trauma narrative experience, Daniel was more comfortable with sharing his thoughts, and his self-esteem and skills increased significantly.

Phase III: Integration and Consolidation Phase

The final treatment phase focuses on helping the child and his family to integrate the skills and insights they have learnt, in order to build safety and support for the future. With significant progress in Daniel's mood and esteem, his final therapy sessions focused on establishing his goals and enhancing his safety. A personal safety plan (*see* Figure 8.3) was developed to boost Daniel's level of protectiveness. Steps included walking away when he sensed danger, and talking to trusted adults (e.g., his mother, caseworker, form teacher in school, psychologist) about his problems.

FIGURE 8.3 DANIEL'S SAFETY PLAN

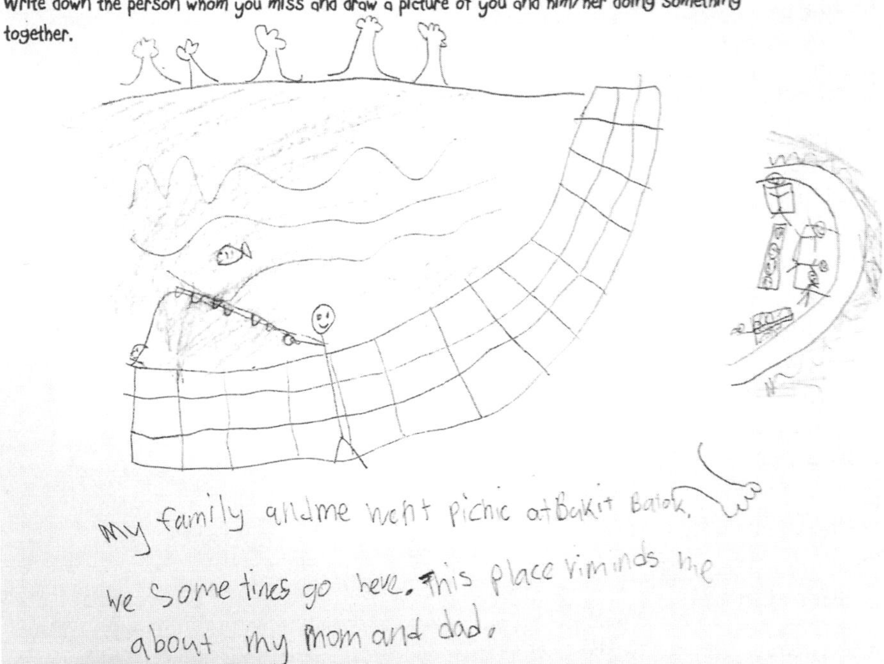

By the end of therapy, Daniel's post-traumatic stress symptoms had been significantly reduced and his self-esteem improved. Based on his clinical presentation, self-report on psychological measures (*see* Table 8.1) and feedback from his mother, Daniel no longer met the criteria for post-traumatic stress disorder and adjustment disorder. Many of his symptoms had fallen to normal levels when measured post-treatment. These improvements were maintained; at his three-month follow-up assessment, his functioning across all measures was within the average ranges for a child of his age.

Daniel's academic work also improved and he received a school award. In the children's home, he started to develop friendships with peers and was given responsibilities to help the staff. Mrs Tan expressed the desire to work on her protectiveness and relationship with her child, and was regular in visiting Daniel in the children's home. Mr Tan was eventually released from prison after a jail term of two years, and returned to live with his family. Daniel then began to have regular outings and home leave with his parents as part of his family reintegration process. Job opportunities were provided to the father to support his reintegration into the community. Mr and Mrs Tan were also referred to a family service centre in the community so that they could continue to obtain support and guidance on their parenting and protective abilities.

TABLE 8.1. DANIEL'S IMPROVEMENT THROUGHOUT THE COURSE OF THERAPY			
Treatment phase (T-score) / Questionnaire	Pre-treatment	Post-treatment (after 25 sessions)	Three-month follow up
UCLA PTSD Index for DSM-IV	29 *	13 (Normal range)	9 (Normal range)
Child's Depression Inventory—II	70T **	61T *	47T
Piers Harris 2	30T **	44T	56T
Strengths and Difficulties Questionnaire (SDQ)	18 (High)	9 (Average)	5 (Average)

** indicates scores in the subclinical range, ** indicates scores in the clinical range*

Daniel wrote this reflection at the end of therapy: "I cried a lot at first. I learnt how to do tummy breathing and relaxation. I also learnt how to stop thinking sad and bad thoughts—I learnt how say "no" and protect myself from danger. My mummy helps me and she reads story to me because she cares for me. I know there are other people who believe in me and can help me. They are my social worker, psychologist and teacher. I feel better. There is no beating now. I hope the wound in my heart recovers as the body wound gets better. I am brave to tell people what happened to me. I am happy now and my crying is getting lesser. I am more like an eagle [carefree and happy] and less an ostrich [timid]."

FIGURE 8.4. DANIEL'S PREPARATION FOR HIS FATHER'S RELEASE

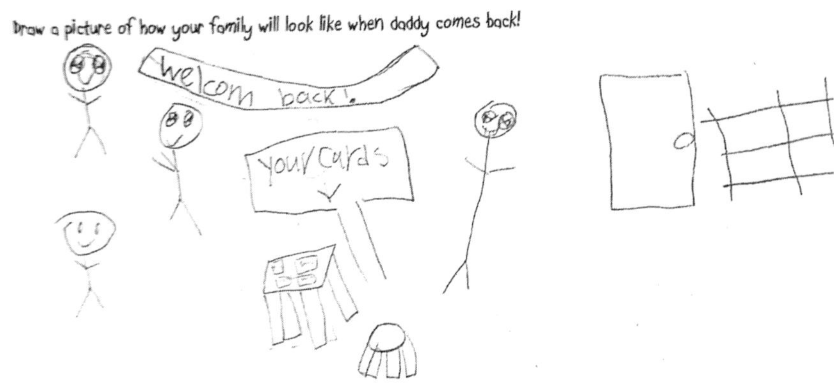

DISCUSSION

Childhood is often seen as a happy, innocent and carefree season of life. While children in Singapore may be less likely to be exposed to certain types of trauma such as natural disasters or gun violence, they are not spared from "man-made" or interpersonal trauma such as traffic accidents or violence in the family, community, or among peers. This case study describes evidence-based trauma treatment provided in a "real world" setting, for a child with a complex and severe history of physical abuse, who came from a family of a lower socioeconomic status, beset with multiple social and legal problems.

In the psychological treatment of children who are in Singapore's child welfare system, therapists are often required to work in multidisciplinary teams of professionals, including Child Protection Officers, professionals from the judicial system, substitute care providers, support service providers (e.g., Family Service Centres), educators (e.g., teachers and school counsellors), and concerned community members (e.g., immediate family members, relatives who are providing care for the child, members of a church or temple). All relevant parties must be aware of both their role in protecting the child, and the unique knowledge and skills they bring to their community's prevention and intervention efforts. Effective communication between professions helps in the child's recovery from abuse. Therapists also can act as an advocate for trauma-informed care, and help to build a psychological net of safety around the child and his or her relationships with significant persons.

This multi-disciplinary collaborative approach was undertaken in Daniel's intervention. Apart from direct therapy sessions with him, his therapist also worked closely with his mother, his teachers, and the children's home staff to expand his support system. This even included arranging for a prison visit to engage Daniel's father in understanding Daniel's needs. His therapist ventured out of the office "clinic" to conduct these community-based sessions.

When a vulnerable child experiences abuse, the resultant emotional hurt and scars are deep. It is thus essential to make the child's physical and emotional safety and stability a treatment priority, before moving on to trauma processing. Therapists need to assess a child's immediate risk for repeated abuse or trauma exposure through ongoing monitoring of safety needs within his or her immediate care environment. Safety planning depends on several factors such as the nature and severity of danger involved in the trauma, the child's developmental level and ability to carry out concrete safety plans, the non-offending parent's availability and ability to serve as a source of safety, and the availability of other support figures (Cohen, Mannarino & Murray, 2011).

In Daniel's case, Child Protection Service's safety assessments indicated that letting him stay in his home with active domestic violence and a history of physical abuse posed a high risk to his safety. Hence, temporary removal to a children's home was effected. During the initial phase of Daniel's therapy, the bullying he experienced in school, his new living arrangement in the children's home, and his low self-esteem and poor assertiveness made him vulnerable to re-victimization. Hence it was imperative that initial sessions focused on ensuring his physical and emotional safety and stabilizing his adjustment to the children's home, before the trauma narrative phase of therapy commenced. Staff at the children's home regularly monitored his needs and safety, and Daniel was taught to build his safety figures and learnt coping strategies. Discussions were also held with his mother, teachers, and caseworkers to help identify safe places and people he could turn to for support in coping.

Therapists should also be sensitive when working with non-offending carers, and take note of their emotional state. Mrs Tan was tearful on several occasions and shared her feelings of guilt about failing to protect Daniel from abuse. However, as she herself was a victim of domestic violence, her own emotional and safety fears made it challenging for her to be attentive and protective to Daniel's needs. Mr Tan also displayed remorse for his actions. The guilt Daniel's parents expressed was suggestive of their hope of restoring their relationship with him and was helpful in his therapist's facilitation of a restorative family session in time. However, as his family had multiple needs, they continued to require ongoing follow-up support from community agencies even after the conclusion of Daniel's therapy.

The engagement of caregivers is a critical part of TF-CBT since betrayal of trust is a core issue for abused children. Therapists aim to restore children's trust in their non-offending caregiver by teaching the latter how to communicate both their assurances of future protection and their acknowledgement that the abuse was not the child's fault. While it is important to involve non-offending caregivers in therapy, therapists should first assess these caregivers' levels of emotional functioning, commitment and priorities. This is because non-offending caregivers often experience a tension between protecting their children and maintaining their own relationship with the perpetrator of abuse. This tension may be further intensified by the non-offending caregiver's own trauma history as a past victim of abuse. In this case, Mrs Tan was referred to a Family Service Centre to help her to process her experience of domestic violence.

Various research has shown that caregivers who prioritise their children's well-being and show insight and commitment in protecting and supporting them aid in their children's recovery (Cohen & Mannarino, 1997; Cohen, et al, 2004; Deblinger et al., 1996). Psychoeducation and training about trauma and abuse provides insight to the caregivers and help them to understand how their children might feel, what their children's symptoms mean, and how they can best respond to their children's needs. Through updating parents about their children's therapy progress and involving parents in therapy sessions, therapists empower caregivers to show their support and play an active role in their child's recovery.

In Daniel's case, Mr Tan was imprisoned and unable to participate in regular therapy sessions to address his parenting methods. Nonetheless Mr Tan received intervention for his depression and supportive counselling in prison. The lack of support from Mrs Tan's extended family and her long working hours also limited her ability to attend every therapy session with Daniel. Nonetheless, she was committed to keeping herself updated about his progress and tried her best to attend sessions when available. When working with clients from lower socioeconomic strata, practical barriers to treatment engagement are often present. These include their inability to take time off work to attend sessions as it would directly impact on their income. Mrs Tan's willingness to be involved and appraised of Daniel's treatment was actually uncommon for child welfare cases, as parent resistance, denial, or hostility is more often encountered. Mrs Tan's responsiveness to feedback on Daniel's progress and her efforts to attend sessions were key positive factors in Daniel's treatment progress.

This case study illustrates the provision of TF-CBT for a local child abuse victim. Core TF-CBT components, such as the trauma narrative, were relevant and easily understood by Daniel and his parents, and minimal localizations or adaptations to the model and components were required. Consistent with other TF-CBT implementation in low-resource countries such as Zambia, any adaptations that were made involved the alteration of techniques rather than changes in TF-CBT core elements (Murray, et al., 2013). For example, using local stories and analogies to illustrate therapeutic messages helped to increase children's engagement and understanding. Key components such as the cognitive triangle have been shown to be relevant and easily understood by Zambians, Singaporeans and Americans alike.

More sessions than usual were required because of the complexity of Daniel's case. Some sessions also had to focus on dealing with current crises (e.g., bullying incidents), before continuing on with trauma processing work. As Daniel had been placed in out-of-home care, extra effort had to be made to arrange for his parents to be involved in joint sessions. Daniel's case is a promising example of how an evidence-based treatment developed in a Western society can be used effectively in the local context with a complex family with high needs.

DISCUSSION QUESTIONS

1. What are some key considerations in treating a traumatized child or adolescent in order to ensure that their social-environmental system is able to support their recovery? In Daniel's case, was individual child therapy sufficient, or were additional interventions needed?

2. What were the challenges and the benefits of addressing Daniel's system of care (e.g. school, family, other caregivers or settings) in his treatment?

3. Is trauma and PTSD uncommon in Singapore compared to other countries in Asia? What kinds of traumatic events could children and adolescents in Singapore experience? How can Singaporean children and adolescents who are exposed to trauma be more effectively identified and provided with help in our local context?

4. PTSD is a common condition, but the diagnosis of PTSD has long had its controversies. With the recent major changes in the DSM-5 for PTSD criteria, such as the inclusion of some depressive symptoms, how might PTSD overlap with other disorders? What is the clinical utility of the new DSM-5 criteria, and what are some of the limitations or disadvantages?

CHAPTER 9.

CHILDREN SEE, CHILDREN DO

Oppositional Defiant Disorder

DESIREE CHOO AND RANJANI UTPALA

INTRODUCTION

Jason was a 14-year-old boy of Thai ethnicity who was suspended from school for getting into a physical fight with a classmate. Following suspension, Jason's school mandated that he see a psychologist before he could return to school. He attended the outpatient psychology clinic with his mother, Julie. He was a tanned, well-groomed teenager of athletic build, but he was sullen and indifferent, avoiding eye contact with his mother and only speaking when prompted. When seen alone, he remained guarded, but was more forthcoming with the psychologist. He was well-spoken and seldom used slang or colloquialisms.

Jason's fight was precipitated by a classmate writing a remark which was "offensive to a large group of people" on the whiteboard. He felt furious, shouted at his classmate and demanded it be erased. His classmate had not complied and tried to lay the blame on someone else instead. Jason got angrier, "lost control" and hit the classmate once on the neck with a "scout's branch" that was lying nearby. His parents were called and a decision was made to suspend him from school. This was Jason's first instance of suspension.

Jason spent a lot of time after this incident thinking about his anger. He was concerned about missing school and worried that his rash act would have serious consequences. His father had threatened to send him back to Thailand if he were expelled from school and he dreaded that possibility. However, Jason did not feel guilty about the actual assault on his classmate because he claimed he had "been taught that a liar deserves to be beaten". Despite this, he said that he would not hit a person in the future in order to avoid negative consequences.

Jason's mother, Julie, described Jason as a well-mannered boy who did not have any behavioural difficulties until the age of 12. Upon entering secondary school however, Jason had become increasingly moody and reserved. Around this time, Julie had noticed racist remarks written on his school exercise books by his classmates. Julie had advised him to ignore those classmates, and informed his form teacher of the comments, but she was uncertain as to whether the teacher had ever confronted the students. Jason revealed that he had continued to experience verbal bullying, often during heated or tense situations such as soccer games.

During Jason's Secondary One and Two years, Julie began receiving calls from Jason's teachers about his "difficult and aggressive" behaviour. Jason "behaved as if the world hated him", was frequently defiant in his remarks toward teachers and had outbursts of anger that were clearly out of proportion to their triggers. For example, if he received a poor grade on his tests and assignments which he felt was "unfairly" given, he would hit his table or flip it over. Such incidents escalated in intensity and frequency over time until the latest incident with his classmate.

In response to his mother's disappointment over his behaviour, Jason insisted that he had been unfairly treated by teachers. He felt that he was "the only one in class who dares to talk back as I do not believe in sitting quietly and not saying anything". He believed that he was frequently punished because most teachers did not like that he often voiced his opinions about their "unfair treatment". He held an intense dislike for their "do as I say because I am superior" attitude. He much preferred his English teacher over the others because he felt that she was willing to listen to his views and was not dismissive of him.

Despite these challenging behaviours at school, Julie described him as a sensitive and artistic person. He had taught himself to make large origami structures at a young age and loved to draw, especially intricate sketches of dragons. Jason also reported that he enjoyed listening to and playing multiple musical instruments and aspired to be either a turntablist or a hip-hop artist.

BACKGROUND

Jason was born in Thailand and lived there with his parents until his family migrated to Singapore when he was eight years old. Until then, his main caregiver had been a hired nanny as both his parents worked full-time in administrative positions. According to Julie, there were no complications with her pregnancy and Jason's birth, and he had attained all developmental milestones as expected.

The family seemed to adjust well following the move to Singapore. They were all fluent in English, and Jason had no major problems, academically or socially, despite enrolling halfway through the year. The only observation made by teachers was that he tended to appear distracted and fidgety during lessons. In subsequent years, however, Jason had been assigned to different classes and found it increasingly difficult to cope. More and more, teachers began to report that he was "naughty" and unable to sit still in class. Nevertheless, Jason had qualified for the Express stream after his Primary School

Leaving Examinations (PSLE), in spite of not having received any extra tuition other than a short-term PSLE preparation program.

FIGURE 9.1. GENOGRAM OF JASON'S FAMILY

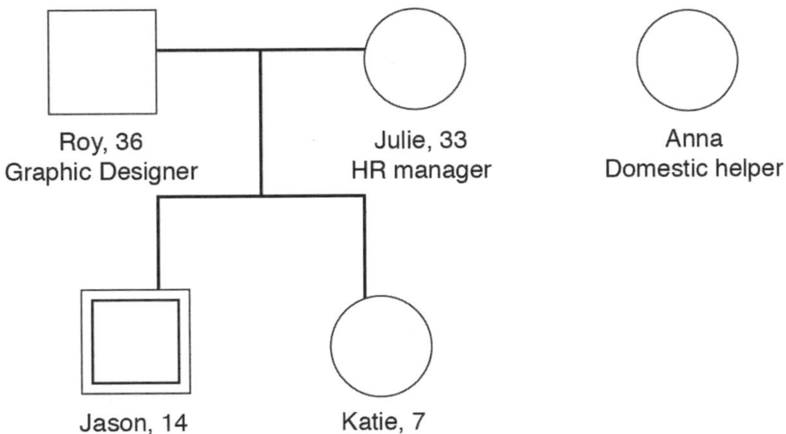

Jason described his relationship with both his parents as distant; he had little to say to them and only spoke with them about practical matters. Julie described her and Roy's parenting style as "stern, strict and disciplined" and admitted to pressuring Jason about his studies till it "sucked the life out of him", especially for his PSLE. In terms of discipline, she shared that she would usually talk to Jason first, but that his father would beat him with a belt for lying or doing badly in exams, although she reported that these were not frequent occurrences. Julie shared that Roy had begun to distance himself from his son after he had "beaten him very badly" for having failed a PSLE trial examination. And while Roy had regretted his actions, he had not spoken to Jason about it subsequently.

After two to three sessions, Jason revealed a more detailed history of domestic violence in the family. He reported numerous occasions when his father had hit him with a belt and punched him. However, Jason quickly tried to minimize the impact of his father's violence, saying, "There was no blood; it wasn't very serious." His father would frequently damage furniture at home out of anger, at times in a drunken state; the police were called in by neighbours during one of the instances. The most recent incident of violence had occurred just a week before the intake assessment. Roy had punched a hole in the wall because Julie had refused his demands to know what had transpired during her individual session with the psychologist.

Julie corroborated Jason's views that the family violence she was experiencing had not been serious and assured the psychologist that she and Roy were engaged in couples counselling at a Family Service Centre (FSC) for marital and parenting issues. Julie gave permission for the psychologist to liaise with the FSC counsellor, who shared that Roy was aware that his own difficulty in anger management likely had an influence on Jason, and seemed open to seeking help for his own difficulties during couples counselling.

Socially, Jason reported being closest to members of his church's youth group, which he had been a part of since the age of 12. He spent every weekend in church and was involved in ministry preparation work and Sunday worship. He also had some friends in school with whom he played computer games with, but reported being not as close to them as compared to his youth group peers. At the time of assessment, Jason was not in a romantic relationship or sexually active, and denied having experimented with drugs or alcohol.

ASSESSMENT

When working with children and adolescents, a systemic approach to assessment and intervention is recommended as it allows us to understand how various family members may contribute and respond to the presenting problem. Furthermore, the therapist can assess which family members can be used to help out in treatment. Although it would have been ideal for both parents to be involved in the intake assessment, Roy refused to attend, citing heavy work commitments. As a result, two 90-minute intake interviews were conducted with Jason and his mother. In order to assess Jason's behaviour across different settings, telephone interviews were conducted with Jason's school principal and form teacher. The psychologist also liaised with the FSC counsellor to better understand the intervention his parents were receiving.

Although the main reason for Jason's referral was his aggression, a more comprehensive assessment, the Achenbach System of Empirically Based Assessment (ASEBA; Achenbach & Rescorla, 2001) was used to screen for other common difficulties in childhood and adolescence. Eight 'syndromes' are assessed: anxiety, depression, somatic complaints, social problems, cognitive problems, attention difficulties, rule-breaking behaviour and aggressive behaviour. The ASEBA includes a caregiver report (the Child Behaviour Checklist, CBCL), which was completed by Julie, and a Youth Self-Report (YSR) completed by Jason.

On the YSR problem scales, Jason's score on the Aggressive Behaviour syndrome was in the clinical range while his scores on the Anxious/Depressed syndrome was in the borderline clinical range. He reported experiencing occasional bouts of low mood and irritability. These results indicated that Jason reported more problems than are typical of boys his age. On the DSM-oriented scales, Jason's scores on the Oppositional Defiant Problems and Conduct Problems scales were in the clinical range, indicating that diagnoses of Oppositional Defiant Disorder (ODD) and Conduct Disorder (CD) should be considered.

Julie's responses on the CBCL, surprisingly, did not highlight any clinically significant problems on the syndrome scales. Possible reasons for this response are explored in the *Discussion* section. Her score of Jason's behaviour on the DSM-oriented Attention Deficit/Hyperactivity Problems scale, however, was in the borderline clinical range. Qualitatively, Julie indicated that her main concern was Jason's aggression in school and his withdrawal from family members.

As school aggression was what precipitated his referral to the psychologist, information from Jason's schoolteachers was an important part of the assessment. Unfortunately, the Teacher Report Form (TRF) was not completed, but the psychologist spoke with Jason's school principal and form teacher over the telephone to obtain qualitative information about his functioning in school. They provided a vivid depiction of Jason's defiant behaviours toward certain teachers (e.g., rude comebacks, lying on the floor for the entire class period when a teacher upset him) and expressed exasperation at the lack of respect he displayed for these teachers.

Jason's risk of harm to others was assessed as moderately high. Whist he denied ongoing thoughts of wanting to hurt anyone, he was struggling to manage his anger and frustration and this had recently caused his classmate harm. At home, Jason denied recent incidences of physical abuse, maintaining that physical punishments had tapered off about two years ago. Although his father continued to have frequent angry outbursts, Jason explained that the abuse was mostly verbal and that the violence was directed at the furniture. Although Jason was confident of keeping himself safe, he was given information on services he could contact in an emergency and was encouraged to tell other adults if he felt unsafe at home.

Jason reported having fleeting thoughts of suicide but denied any intention to harm or kill himself as it was against his religious beliefs and he did not want to hurt his mother by hurting himself. Jason also denied engaging in self-harm behaviours in the past. His risk of self-harm was assessed to be low.

DIAGNOSIS

Jason's presentation was consistent with the diagnostic criteria of Oppositional Defiant Disorder (DSM-5; American Psychiatric Association, 2013). He met criteria displaying a "pattern of negativistic, hostile and defiant behaviour lasting at least 6 months", comprising of the symptoms of "angry/irritable mood" and "argumentative/defiant behaviours" but not "vindictiveness". As these behaviours resulted in his suspension from school and were distressing to Jason, they were assessed as causing significant impairment and distress. Although there was no evidence of current child physical abuse, given the information provided, it was evident he had previously been abused. This information was integral in the conceptualization and formulation of the treatment.

A differential diagnosis of Conduct Disorder (CD) was considered but not substantiated due to an absence of clinically significant deceitfulness and theft. Further, Jason was neither a recurrent rule breaker nor repeatedly aggressive toward people.

Research on conduct-related problems suggests that anger management problems are developed and maintained by interactions between biological, psychological and social vulnerabilities. These patterns are evident with Jason, a young person from a foreign country who was transitioning into adolescence in the context of a volatile family environment and school bullying.

Predisposing Factors

Biologically, heritability coefficients of up to 0.8 in young people with conduct-related problems suggest a strong genetic component in the development of anti-social behaviour (Simonoff, 2001). Possible influences with a genetic basis include difficult temperament, neurotransmitter dysregulation, and lower levels of autonomic arousal/responsiveness. Roy's own impulsive temperament and difficulties with anger management suggest a possible biological influence on the development of Jason's current emotional and behavioural difficulties.

According to social learning theory (Bandura, Walters & Sears, 1959), aggression is learned through the process of modeling (e.g., a child's imitation of parental aggressive behaviour). This is supported by a substantial body of research evincing transmission of aggression within the family (Hill, 2002). Jason's witnessing of domestic violence at home likely modelled dysfunctional methods of coping with negative emotion, which predisposed him to adopt a similar coping style in his interactions with others. Moreover, the increased psychological pressure and physical punishment from his parents concerning his PSLE performance seemed to increase the emotional rift between him and his parents. The difficulties with his parents might have made it more difficult for Jason to respond to bullying at school and increased the likelihood of social difficulties at school.

Cognitive theories highlight social information processing difficulties and social skills deficits as key etiological factors of conduct-related problems. Specifically, research has shown that young people with conduct-related problems tend to exhibit a hostile attribution bias in their cognition in the context of socially ambiguous situations (Crick & Dodge, 1994). These young people also show a lack of skills to generate and implement alternative, non-aggressive solutions to difficult social situations (Spivack & Shure, 1982).

Precipitating Factors

Jason's outbursts of anger were commonly triggered by instances of peer bullying (e.g., racist remarks), perceived injustice or unfairness, and others imposing authority on him that he perceived as unreasonable.

Perpetuating Factors

His self-perception of being "the only one in class who dares to talk back" as "I do not believe in sitting quietly and not saying anything" reinforced his propensity to react aggressively in class when he suspected his teachers or classmates of picking on him. Furthermore, rebelling against his teachers and responding aggressively to peers gave Jason a sense of control, which was a feeling that he had lacked at home. Notably, his lack of opportunity to learn adaptive methods to cope with negative emotion was a key perpetuating factor in his difficulties in regulating his emotions. The rapid changes in physiology that accompany the period of adolescence was also likely both an important risk and perpetuating factor for Jason's emotion regulation difficulties.

These biological, social and cognitive predisposing, precipitating and perpetuating factors are encompassed by the multi-systemic ecological theory based on Bronfenbrenner's (1986) ecological model of child development. This model posits the importance of multiple systems (the individual, family, peers, school and broader social/societal networks) in the development and maintenance of conduct-related problems, thus necessitating that each of these systems are addressed during treatment planning. Jason was exposed to violence from a young age. Furthermore, he lived in a society where corporal punishment is still widely used in schools and in the judicial setting. Being exposed to physical acts of violence as a form of discipline may have led Jason to develop beliefs about the use of physical aggression when he felt wronged by others. Such beliefs were likely maintained by witnessing continued violence within the family.

Protective Factors

A number of factors surfaced as protective elements that boded well for Cognitive Behavioural Therapy (CBT) based intervention. Jason was an insightful, articulate individual able to express his thoughts and emotions clearly. The presence of social support in the form of his peers in church as well as his strong interests in artistic pursuits were also sources of strength that could be drawn on during the process of change. The willingness of his parents to seek counselling as a family and his father's reported openness to seeking help for his own anger management issues provided a strong basis for a systemic approach to intervention. These factors, together with Jason's keenness to remain in school, provided valuable motivation and support for him to stay engaged in and benefit from therapy.

TREATMENT

In accordance with the formulation based on the multi-systemic ecological theory, the treatment plan included individual sessions with Jason, then with his parents only, and later, with both Jason and his parents. As Jason's parents were concurrently engaged in counselling at a Family Service Centre, the initial focus for intervention was on individual work with Jason to improve his emotion regulation skills.

Treatment material was adapted from a skills-based group program manual for adolescents by French (2001), which was based on Novaco's (1975) cognitive behavioural model of anger and aggression. Treatment components for the first eight individual sessions included psychoeducation about anger and aggression, identifying his personal triggers and early signs of anger, as well as learning assertive ways to manage triggers and adaptive ways to reduce physical tension and regulate negative emotions (*see* Table 9.1). Jason's primary goal was to return to school and learn anger management skills to avoid further negative consequences. Specifically, he wanted to learn to be able to calm himself down when provoked without reacting either physically or verbally. Since the school mandated he attend therapy before he could go back to school, this was the key motivation behind his continued engagement in therapy.

Over the course of therapy, Jason, like many adolescents, experienced significant difficulty in challenging his thoughts and struggled to take the perspective of other persons. Specifically, his belief that people who lie or treat others unfairly should be punished, and his self-perception of being the 'only one in class' who dared to stand up for this belief remained intact.

Additional psychoeducation included normalizing the emotion of Jason's anger, distinguishing different stages of anger in his own words on the anger thermometer (e.g., annoyed/irritated, pissed off, angry, furious etc.), distinguishing anger from aggression, and discussing the costs and benefits of aggression from an evolutionary "fight or flight" perspective. Log sheets were used as therapy assignments to help Jason identify common triggers by recording daily hassles. When Jason reviewed his weekly logs, he was able to identify situations that involved perceived injustice, unfairness and/ or physical or verbal abuse as common triggers to his angry outbursts. These occurred across settings with parents, teachers and peers. Some examples he gave were of his teacher singling him out to reprimand him in front of his classmates when he was not the only one talking during a lesson, and of a schoolmate cheating on the soccer field. In all these instances, Jason reported experiencing the same quick and intense surge of anger that had led him to hit his classmate.

Alternative, adaptive coping methods that were explored include relaxation techniques (e.g., deep abdominal breathing), distraction techniques (e.g., listening to music on his headphones or walking away), cognitive reappraisal strategies (e.g., challenging his thoughts, "letting it go", thinking through potential consequences, and weighing the costs and benefits of aggression), as well as responding assertively instead of aggressively or passively. When Jason became irritated at school, he substituted listening to music or walking away with deep breathing. However, as he usually had his headphones around his neck at all other times (even during therapy sessions), he found listening to music very helpful as a distraction in most other settings.

TABLE 9.1. OVERVIEW OF INTERVENTION SESSIONS	
Session	**Session content**
Session 1	Goal-setting Psychoeducation Orientation to treatment
Session 2	Recognizing triggers Recognizing signs of anger Introduction to self-monitoring
Session 3	Learning behavioural emotion regulation strategies
Session 4	Exploring cost and benefits of aggression
Session 5	Learning assertiveness skills
Session 6	Reinforcing assertiveness skills Introduction to cognitive reappraisal technique
Session 7	Effective communication and cognitive reappraisal (cont.)
Session 8	Review of skills learnt Reflection Preparation for lapses

Despite this, he was able to make behavioural changes due to his main motivation of avoiding punishment. Recognising the strength of these beliefs, the initial goal of treatment was to work towards behavioural change while the secondary goal was to work on his more deeply rooted beliefs.

The therapist strived to maintain a collaborative, client-centred approach in sessions with Jason so as to build and sustain trust and rapport that was essential to his engagement in therapy. Interestingly, unlike what had been observed and reported in the classroom by his schoolteachers, Jason's 'defiance' was not particularly evident during sessions. He responded respectfully to the therapist's attempts to understand his worldview and her suggestions of ways to manage his difficulties with anger. The only issue that arose was his repeatedly not completing his therapy assignments. When this was brought up, Jason explained that he had either forgotten to fill out his log sheet or that there had been no hassle or disturbance during that week. He was, however, cooperative and willing to complete the assignments in session whenever he had not done them prior.

Jason's progress for this treatment phase was assessed after the completion of eight weekly sessions via an adaptation of the pre- and post-group self-report form (French, 2001), which assesses clients' perceptions of the nature, intensity and disruptiveness of their anger problems, as well as their perception of progress toward the therapy goals they had set prior to intervention (Table 9.2).

TABLE 9.2. JASON'S RESPONSES TO TREATMENT

	Pre-intervention	Post-intervention
Aggression problems	6*	4
Level of worry about aggression problems	6	5
Goal 1: Ability to manage triggers effectively	4	7
Goal 2: Reaction to anger	6	5
Goal 3: Ability to calm down when provoked	3	7

1 = least, 10 = greatest

Jason also rated his perception of how effective individual techniques used in therapy were for him. Of note, he indicated that relaxation/breathing and assertive communication techniques were "extremely helpful", but that "thinking differently about situations which make you angry" had not been very helpful. During these initial therapy sessions, Jason struggled to generate or even accept suggestions of alternative thoughts or perspectives and maintained a rigid view that people who disrespect others deserve to be punished. He shared that he had been "brought up to believe this". While he found it difficult to accept different ways of thinking, he was motivated to avoid getting into trouble; he found that considering the consequences and the pros and cons of aggression were more helpful than directly challenging his own cognitions.

In sessions one and two, Jason's thoughts and feelings about his experience of domestic violence and its influence on his own beliefs about violence were explored and processed using cognitive reappraisal techniques. Cognitive reappraisal involved changing the way Jason thought about his experiences in order to change its affective impact on him. This process was enabled by Jason's well-developed metacognitive skills and ability to articulate his worldview. Jason demonstrated notable maturity for his age and was able to acknowledge the influence of his father's own violent childhood and family upbringing on his own challenges with frustration and anger. However, Jason was sceptical about the likelihood of his parents, especially his father, making changes in their interaction with him through receiving counselling at the FSC. Despite the belief that his father was unlikely to change, it was interesting to see a shift in Jason's rigid beliefs about people by this stage in therapy. He was now more open to both talking about and considering the perspective of others and seemed to hold less rigid ideas about "being disrespected".

Jason's parents had been able to attend only one parents' session with the therapist, which occurred after nine individual sessions with Jason. The main aim of the parents' session was to discuss ways they could support Jason in his application of newly learnt skills. During this meeting, both Roy and Julie reported noticing marked improvement in their relationship with Jason, the most significant of which was his willingness to open up to them about the difficulties he had been experiencing (e.g., relating to the recent development of a romantic relationship with a girl from church), in contrast to his previous reticence and isolation at home. They attributed this change to a combination of an improvement in Jason's overall mood, and their efforts to rebuild their relationships with him through introducing weekly family dinners and Roy adopting a more patient stance toward Jason.

Roy recognised the negative effects of using physical punishment on Jason and acknowledged his need to continue working on his own anger management issues. He wished to provide a safe and supportive environment for Jason to learn respect, honesty and industry on his own rather than by "telling" him what to do, but also acknowledged that this was not always easy. Roy and Julie agreed to attend a joint session with Jason toward the end of therapy in which they would share with him what they had learnt from attending counselling at the FSC and their commitment to applying those skills to further improve their relationship.

In subsequent individual sessions with Jason, consistent with his parents' reports, he presented as more cheerful and described a change in the way his parents related to him. For example, he recounted an incident in which he had been practising on his drum set in his room late at night, and shared that his father had surprised him by knocking on his door and asking him calmly to stop practising for the night. He shared that this was a significant positive change from how his father would have reacted in the past and seemed heartened by the change.

When the idea of the joint session with his parents was proposed to Jason, however, he seemed uneasy and unwilling to engage in it. He balked at the idea of writing or sharing his observations of his parents' efforts to change and how it made him feel, retorting, "That's not me; I wouldn't do that". He was, however, more willing to tell his parents about some of the anger management strategies he had learnt over the course of therapy and how they had helped him cope with his emotions more effectively. When the majority of the individual work with Jason and his mother was completed, the therapist tried to arrange a family session with his parents. However, despite their initial promising level of commitment and engagement, Julie stated that both she and her husband were very busy with work, and she felt that Jason should be "responsible enough to go for therapy himself". She also admitted that they had only attended two sessions altogether with the counsellor at the FSC, which focused on Roy's anger management issues. Julie eventually agreed to attend a family session but only at much later date due to work commitments.

At this point, Jason's therapy was ongoing. The focus of therapy was shifted toward working with both Jason and his parents in reinforcing Jason's therapy gains, as well as increasing his parents' motivation to support Jason in the process of change.

DISCUSSION

Based on a study in Hong Kong, rates of externalising disorders among Asian children and adolescents appears to be comparable to or even slightly higher than among American children (Leung, Hung, Ho, Lee, Liu, Tang & Kwong, 2008). Within clinical settings, conduct-related problems comprise up to half of all referrals and most commonly occur in individuals with profiles like Jason's—men between middle childhood and adolescence (Carr, 2006). In Singapore, a similar trend was reflected in data from an outpatient child psychiatric centre, which showed that 31% of all referrals from 2001–03 were for children and adolescents with disruptive behaviour disorders (Fung & Cai, 2005). Research on malleability of disruptive behavioural disorders has identified early age of onset, hostile parenting, deviant peer association, and poor scholastic performance as predictors of poorer treatment prognosis (Fergusson, Lynskey, & Horwood, 1996; Pevalin, Wade, & Brannigan, 2003).

In Jason's case, problems with parenting and the home environment were the main predictors of poor treatment prognosis. Despite this, Jason's protective factors improved his prognosis. These included the late onset of his behavioural problems, having a support network of friends in church, and his inherent motivation to stay out of trouble at school. Though his home environment was far from ideal, Jason's parents had taken some steps to address their levels of conflict at home by seeking counselling. Furthermore, they initially expressed an apparent commitment to adopting a more effective parenting style, which was also indicative of a positive prognosis of present intervention efforts. However, as therapy progressed, their initial engagement and motivation dwindled.

One explanation could be that this initial engagement was influenced by social desirability. Significant amounts of research have highlighted systematic cross-cultural differences in social desirability, with individuals from collectivistic societies tending to have higher social desirability scores (Johnson & Van de Vijver, 2003). In Singapore's multicultural, yet largely collectivistic culture, this is an important factor to consider in the formulation and treatment of disruptive behaviours in our youth. Jason's parents may have presented false positive responses toward therapy in order to maintain a courteous and harmonious relationship with the therapist. In fact, they may have initially acquiesced to the therapist's recommendation to attend family sessions without having an actual intention to follow through with them.

Further evidence of possible social desirability was seen in Julie's minimization of Jason's behavioural and emotional difficulties on the CBCL. However, a more plausible explanation for Julie reporting fewer externalising problems and her and Roy's resistance to engaging in treatment could be poor mental health literacy and help-seeking behaviour among Asian parents. There is some evidence that parents from ethnic minority groups report significantly fewer externalising symptoms on the Achenbach scales than their offspring when compared to European American parents (Lau, Garland, Yeh, McCabe, Wood, & Hough, 2004).

Lau et al. (2004) suggested two possible reasons for this discrepancy. Firstly, ethnic minority parents may be more prone to acculturative stress (i.e., stress surrounding immigration/discrimination etc.) and consequently less sensitive to their children's distress and less likely to notice symptoms. Secondly, lower levels of mental health literacy when compared to their Caucasian counterparts may cause ethnic minority, Asian parents to be more oblivious to specific symptoms of emotional and developmental problems. In addition to possible acculturation stress, Julie was coping with violence within her marriage. These two significant factors may have led to her lowered awareness of the extent of Jason's difficulties. This may explain also why Julie did not realise that Jason was having difficulties until his suspension from school and why she only brought him to therapy upon being mandated by the school.

Although Julie had referred Jason for therapy, poor parental understanding of the extent of his problems combined with a lack of appreciation of the importance of parental involvement in the therapeutic process may have hampered the outcome of the planned systemic intervention. Poor engagement from his parents made it challenging to employ a multi-systemic approach and eventually decreased Jason's motivation to participate in family sessions. The psychologist tried to address this by meeting with the parents to discuss the pros and cons of family sessions. Though both parents engaged well during this session, identifying several pros and cons of engagement and disengagement, the work done was insufficient to increase their motivation to attend. The psychologist was required to shift the focus to individual work with Jason.

Other culturally related factors that likely influenced the progress of therapy with Jason and his family is the common cultural expectation in Asian societies of obedience toward one's elders, and the relative social acceptance of caning and other forms of physical punishment of children in the local setting (Tong, Elliot & Tan, 1996). In Singapore, even different professionals have differing definitions and views about what constitutes physical abuse of a child. Chan, Chow and Elliott (2000) found that professionals from different disciplines hold different opinions about what constitutes child abuse and neglect. This in turn has an impact on both reporting and intervention. Chan et al (2000) warned that "a lack of strong consensus among the professions regarding the acceptability of actions may pose a problem for effective efforts to combat physical child abuse and neglect in Singapore" (p. 44). In the Phillipines, Maxwell (2001) found that the effect of parent-to-child aggression on delinquency may be attenuated by such cultural perspectives. These widely held public and even professional beliefs about the use of physical punishment as a form of discipline present a unique challenge for the implementation of interventions that are based on western societal values. Such differences in cultural values and beliefs underscore the need to carefully consider the context of the client's cultural background in distinguishing physical abuse from other forms of socially acceptable physical punishments.

If Jason's parents had engaged in therapy as planned, the psychologist would have worked on exploring Julie and Roy's own beliefs and attitudes towards physical punishment and the effectiveness of these measures on Jason. In such an instance, it would have been imperative that the psychologist did not blame his parents or insinuate that they had practiced poor parenting as this could lead to a rupture in the therapeutic alliance and eventual parental disengagement. Rather, it would have been important for the psychologist to work together with parents to identify and reinforce effective self-regulatory and parenting strategies while simultaneously identifying and replacing ineffective or harmful disciplinary practices with more effective ones.

Working with parents who use physical punishment can be challenging for various reasons. In Jason's case, the therapist personally disapproved of corporal punishment and her beliefs may have inadvertently manifested during her session with the parents and negatively impacted her therapeutic alliance with them, thus contributing to the challenge of engaging them in the therapeutic process. When working with client populations that challenge a therapist's personal values, it is important to identify these through reflective practice and the use of supervision.

Jason's case also highlighted the importance of acknowledging the prevalence of racist attitudes and racially discriminatory behaviours among youth in schools, as well as the impact this may have on the emotional well-being of foreign youth or those of minority ethnic groups. Although Julie had reported the racist remarks made by Jason's classmates to his teacher, no apparent appropriate follow-up action was taken by the school to correct Jason's classmates' negative behaviours. This lack of action taken by authorities was processed with Jason in therapy. Jason was then taught to be assertive without resorting to the use of physical or verbal aggression.

Due to the transgenerational nature of conduct-related problems and relative unresponsiveness to treatment, a majority of referred individuals show poor prognosis, thus making conduct-related problems the most costly disorder of childhood and adolescence (Carr, 2006). Considering the magnitude of the problem and potential long-term consequences of disruptive behaviour disorders on the young person, his family and community, public awareness of the importance of early intervention and the crucial role of parents and teachers in the effective intervention of such problems remain important areas for development.

Jason's case clearly illustrates the multitude of factors that influence an adolescent boy's oppositional behaviour, and the consequent prognosis of psychological therapy. The positive impacts of therapy are evident—but must be considered within the context of challenging individual, systemic and therapeutic dynamics and challenges.

DISCUSSION QUESTIONS

1. In Singapore, caning is widely accepted as a method of physical discipline (Tong et al., 1996). What are your personal views on corporal punishment of children/ adolescents and how might they influence a therapist's approach to therapy with young persons and their parents?

2. How would you distinguish between corporal punishment that is aimed to discipline and physical abuse of a child?

3. Poor parental engagement is often the norm when working with cases of conduct problems. What strategies do you think would be useful in engaging parents?

4. It is widely accepted that unconditional positive regard for the client is an essential component of a therapeutic relationship. What are some challenges with achieving this when working with oppositional or aggressive clients or parents who have different beliefs or values from you? How can a therapist manage their personal beliefs to ensure that they do not interfere with the therapeutic process?

5. In the present case study, Jason had multiple personal protective factors. How can a therapist approach assessment and therapy with an adolescent who lacked insight, motivation and the ability to effectively articulate his thoughts and emotions?

PART 2.

ADULTS

CHAPTER 10.

PLAYING WITH FIRE

Pyromania

HO WEI TSHEN AND CHU CHI MENG

INTRODUCTION

Wally was a 20-year-old man charged with ten counts of mischief (Section 426 [Cap 224] of the Penal Code) for fire setting. He had been caught burning cardboard boxes and bicycle tyres at the void deck of apartment blocks in his neighbourhood. Pending his presentence court hearing, Wally had been referred for an assessment of the psychological dynamics underlying his fire setting behaviour, as well his risk of reoffending. He was subsequently ordered to serve two years of probation, as well as to attend regular therapy sessions to address his fire setting behaviour.

Wally's interest in fire began about two years before his sentence, when he stumbled upon a pile of burning paper at the base of a residential block. He recalled being mesmerised by the way the fire consumed the paper and described its "colour, shape, and movement" as "magical". Since then, he had been preoccupied with fire. After his first arrest, Wally had desisted from setting more fires for fear of being sent to jail. However, his obsession with fire continued to be fuelled by his regular viewing of videos depicting explosions and major fire events, such as war reports, forest fires and riots during which property and combustible materials were burnt.

The sight of discarded cardboard and combustible material at refuse collection points of apartment blocks was a key trigger for Wally's thoughts of fire setting. This typically occurred when he was alone, had nothing to do and was taking a stroll around his neighbourhood. His modus operandi was consistent and fairly unsophisticated. After making sure that no one was watching, he would set fire to the pile of discarded material before retreating a safe distance away to watch it burn to ash. Reminiscing his successful fire-setting incidents gave Wally a feeling of pleasure. He denied the intention to harm anyone.

While Wally evinced regret for his actions, he did not appear to be fully able to fathom the impact of his actions on his family and those who lived in his vicinity. He was initially unaware of the severity of his actions and thought that it was legitimate to set small fires to discarded paper material after watching others burn incense paper. Nevertheless, he expressed a willingness to engage in psychotherapy because he was afraid of going to prison should he reoffend.

His parents initially minimised his fire setting behaviour, and tried to defend his actions—"It was just a small fire"—but eventually understood the severity of his offences through the course of the interview. Furthermore, they expressed disappointment and blame toward Wally for committing the offences. However, they concurred that they would provide the necessary support to assist Wally with his rehabilitation.

BACKGROUND

Wally was the younger of two children in his family; he had an elder brother aged 26. He had an unremarkable childhood and reportedly met his developmental milestones. At the point of assessment, he was living with his family and serving National Service (NS). Wally shared close relationships with his parents and brother, but usually would not confide in them with personal issues. Apart from his offences, no familial history of criminality or mental illness was uncovered.

With regard to his education, Wally was emplaced in the Normal Technical stream and subsequently in a vocational institution. However, after losing interest in the subjects he had chosen and frequently skipping classes, he had dropped out of the institution and, with the support of his parents, opted for early enlistment. Wally had planned to continue his studies after completing NS.

Wally had few friends while growing up and subsequently lost touch with them after he left school. In camp, he interacted mainly with four fellow National Servicemen, but did not mingle with them outside of camp. Wally recalled being teased in school. Despite being angered by his schoolmates' verbal taunts, he reportedly ignored his provocateurs. He had never been involved in a romantic relationship.

In general, he appeared to have limited ability to develop peer relationships that required him to be sensitive to the needs of his peers and to respond to them appropriately. In his free time, Wally engaged in mostly indoor hobbies, such as reading comics, playing chess and computer games (by himself as well as with friends). Aside from his fire setting, there was no evidence of other deviant behaviours.

ASSESSMENT

Six sessions—totalling seven hours—of interviews and psychometric testing were conducted with Wally. These interviews were administered with the purpose of obtaining relevant information about his family and personal history in order to evaluate his psychological, emotional and social functioning. They also aimed to assess the psychological dynamics underlying his fire setting behaviour, including the function, extent, severity and modus operandi of his behaviour, as well as the way in which it was reinforced. In order to verify the information obtained, Wally's mother was also interviewed, and his secondary school, NS, and Institute of Mental Health (IMH) reports were perused.

During the assessment, Wally presented with restricted affect and somewhat rigid thinking (e.g., he minimised his difficulties, and disliked altering his daily schedule to accommodate the interviews or any last-minute changes). He also did not speak or offer any kind of information unless spoken to; even then, his responses were brief and usually expressionless. Nonetheless, Wally was compliant and polite during the entire process.

Research suggests that fire setting tends to be associated with multiple forms of antisocial behaviour and psychiatric comorbidity (e.g., Gannon & Pina, 2010; Grant & Kim, 2007; Vaughn et al., 2010). Hence, it was important to screen for other types of antisocial behaviour in different social domains during the assessment process. Wally's collateral reports and mother's account indicated that he did not have a history of prior antisocial behaviour or any significant behavioural difficulties, and took his NS duties seriously. However, two areas of concern were his lack of organised leisure or recreational activities and his lack of prosocial peer support.

Fact Box 10.1. Making Yourself Look Better Than You Actually Are

Socially desirable responding (SDR) is a well-documented form of response distortion, especially on self-reports of personality. SDR is exhibited on a continuum in any population; in fact, people may be inclined to respond more negatively if they have poor self-evaluation, low self-esteem, high humility, or are attempting to malinger. Paunonen & LeBel (2012) explained that one way of dealing with desirability bias is to design psychometric assessments with neutrally worded items. However, this is not always possible when attempting to measure traits deemed to be positive (e.g., hardworking), or negative (e.g., impatience). A second method is to appeal either directly or indirectly to a respondent's integrity. For example, the MMPI-2 has a set of validity scales to detect the 'faking' of responses. However, a person's motivation to present themselves in a positive light may override their motivation for integrity. Various studies have found SDR to have a small to large effect on the criterion validity of different measures.

See Paunonen and LeBel (2012) for a comprehensive overview of SDR and an example of research that suggests that SDR only minimally affects criterion validity.

Wally did not appear to be exhibiting any post-traumatic stress or depressive symptomatology, nor any mood or psychotic phenomena. To determine if he had anger expression and management difficulties that compromised his psychological functioning of physical health, Wally completed the Novaco Anger Scale and Provocation Inventory (NAS-PI; Novaco, 2003). His NAS profile suggested that he had a tightly controlled emotional life and was not likely to exhibit clinically significant anger-engendering cognitions, anger arousal, or aggressive behaviour in the presence of provocation. Notwithstanding this, his PI subscales suggested that he could be easily annoyed and provoked, in particular by disrespectful treatment, unfairness, frustration, and annoying traits of others.

With regard to his personality functioning, Wally was assessed using the Minnesota Multiphasic Personality Inventory—2nd Edition (MMPI-2; Butcher, Dahlstrom, Graham, Tellegen, & Kreammer, 1989), a reliable and well-validated instrument that is widely used to assess possible psychopathology and personality characteristics for persons aged 18 years and above. As the MMPI-2's validity scales indicated that Wally responded to items in a defensive manner, his results were not considered an accurate representation of his psychological status. His MMPI-2 validity scales results were further corroborated by his responses on the Paulhus Deception Scale (PDS; Paulhus, 1984), a 40-item self-report instrument that measures one's tendency to give socially desirable responses. His responses indicated that he was trying to present himself in a positive light, not surprising given he was awaiting his sentencing outcome (*see* Fact Box 10.1).

As Wally's fire setting behaviour had the potential for serious property damage and loss of human life, it was necessary to assess his risk for future reoffending. This was carried out using the Level of Service/Case Management Inventory (LS/CMI; Andrews, Bonta, & Wormith, 2004), a structured risk assessment guide that makes recommendations relevant to the offenders' supervision and treatment based on an examination of his needs. A violence risk assessment was not carried out as Wally was not deemed to have either currently or previously harboured the intention to physically or psychologically harm others. Had there been concerns about his propensity to hurt others through fire setting, a violence risk assessment tool (e.g., Historical, Clinical, Risk Management—20 Factors; HCR-20) could have been used. In such a case, fire setting would be considered part of a wider array of antisocial or violent behaviour.

Wally did not have significant antisocial antecedents or an extensive criminal history. His behaviour appeared to be neither an expression of socio-political ideology, anger or vengeance nor intended to conceal criminal activity or improve his living circumstances. Moreover, he did not experience any psychotic phenomena or intoxication during the commission of his offences. Although he did not condone an offending lifestyle, he held fire-supportive attitudes such as, "The fires were not harmful to anyone" and "I was in control of the fires as they quickly burned out". These ideas were consistent with his responses on measures that assess attitudes toward fire and fire interest (i.e., the Fire Attitude Scale [Muckley, 1997] and Fire Interest Scale [Murphy & Clare, 1996]).

Furthermore, he had difficulties controlling his urges to engage in fire setting. Relative to other adults who have committed criminal offences, Wally's risk of general reoffending was assessed as being low, while his risk of future fire setting behaviour was deemed moderate to high. His fire-setting risk was based on clinical judgement with the aid of other proxy measures as there were no psychometrically valid and localised risk assessment measures of risk for fire setting or arson. Effective intervention was expected to lower his risk of reoffending.

DIAGNOSIS

Following his arrest, Wally had consulted an IMH psychiatrist, who had diagnosed him with pyromania (DSM-IV-TR 312.33). His intellectual functioning, as assessed on the Wechsler Adult Intelligence Scale—4th Edition, was within the "Low Average" range, indicating that he scored above approximately 22% of his peers. His current psychological assessment had yielded a similar diagnostic finding of pyromania. However, it should be noted that DSM-5 does not include pyromania as a distinct diagnosis as there is insufficient evidence to retain it as distinct disorder. Pyromania is now classified as an "Impulse-control Disorder Not Otherwise Specified".

INTEGRATIVE FORMULATION

Case conceptualisation (and subsequent treatment targets) were based on the Risk-Need-Responsivity model (RNR; Andrews & Bonta, 2010) and the Good Lives Model (GLM; Ward, 2002). According to the RNR concept, the risk, needs and responsivity of the offender, after identification, should inform the level and kind of treatment that he receives. The GLM postulates that every individual has a set of primary goods—experiences and states of being—that, if attained, would increase their sense of fulfilment and happiness (Ward, 2002; *see* Fact Box 10.2). Offending behaviour might thus arise when the individual is unable to attain his primary goods in a prosocial manner (Emmons, 1999; Ward & Stewart, 2003; Yates & Ward, 2008).

Predisposing

Wally's self-regulation deficits in the form of impulsivity were likely to have predisposed him to his fire-setting offences. In particular, although his cognitive functioning was assessed to be in the *Low Average* range, Wally appeared to be relatively naïve and claimed not to know that it was wrong to set fires. More importantly, Wally's significant interest in fire and pyrotechnic paraphernalia was a key factor that predisposed him to fire setting.

Precipitating

Wally's urges to set fires were initially triggered by his setting fire to combustible materials in his surroundings, and subsequently generalised to television and internet videos depicting fires and explosions. Over time, he developed a habit of setting fire to alleviate his negative affect (e.g., boredom). Hence, high-risk situations for fire setting

Fact Box 10.2 Primary Goods and Criminogenic Needs

In the Good Lives Model (Ward, 2002), offending behaviours relate either directly or indirectly to the pursuit of one of a combination of 11 primary goods and are flawed attempts at gaining fulfilment in individuals' lives. Criminogenic needs are dynamic risk factors linked to the perpetuation of offending behaviour and are internal and external obstacles that hinder or prevent the acquisition of primary goods in prosocial ways. More information on the Good Lives Model can be found at www.goodlivesmodel.com.

Primary Goods	Criminogenic Needs
Community	Antisocial Associates
Creativity	Unemployment and/or Offence-Supportive Beliefs and Attitudes
Excellence in Agency	Impulsivity
Excellence in Play	Criminal and/or Deviant Sexual Preferences
Excellence in Work	Unemployment
Inner Peace	Emotional Dysregulation, Adjustment Difficulties, and/or Dysfunctional Coping Through Criminal Offending
Knowledge	Offence-supportive Beliefs and Attitudes
Life	Substance Abuse and/or Lack of Stable Living Environment
Pleasure	Addictive Behaviours, Sexual Preoccupation, and/or Deviant Sexual Preferences
Relatedness	Intimacy Deficits and/or Lack of Perceived Social Support
Spirituality	Offence-supportive Beliefs and Attitudes

included situations during which he was not constructively occupied, when he was constantly exposed to videos and sights of fires and explosions, as well as when he had access to combustible and pyrotechnic material.

Perpetuating

Wally's fire setting behaviour was maintained by his fire-supportive cognitions, the reinforcement that he obtained from successful fire setting, as well as limited coping mechanisms. Specifically, he was reinforced by the intense sensory stimulation, pleasure, and soothing feelings that arose from fire setting. He neither sought support from his parents regarding personal problems, nor did he have readily available prosocial peer support because of his limited social skills and inability to build and maintain peer relationships. This could have led Wally to develop deeply entrenched coping scripts involving fire, which helped him to calm himself during times of high stress.

Protective

Wally did not have significant antisocial cognitions and behaviour, and crucially, had not engaged in substance use that could exacerbate his fire setting behaviour. He appeared to be regretful of his actions and motivated to attend treatment to prevent future trouble with the law. He was also suitably engaged in NS duties, which he fulfilled responsibly. His primary goods were autonomy, relatedness, excellence in play, and inner peace. It was important to him to exercise responsibility and autonomy over his life, to engage in fulfilling relationships with others, and to feel a sense of accomplishment and enjoyment in his hobbies.

PROGNOSIS

The prognosis of individuals with pyromania is often linked to severe consequences both personally and financially when treatment is not given; specifically, it can lead to serious injuries, death, and property destruction. Wally had a number of risk factors for future fire setting behaviour—his interest in fire, fire-supportive attitudes, lack of readily accessible prosocial support, an inability to maintain prosocial peer relationships, and poor stress coping. While there are very few treatment programs for adult fire setters (Gannon & Pina, 2010)—stemming from a rather limited knowledge of effective interventions with this population (Palmer, Hollin, Hatcher, & Ayres, 2010)—his therapist believed that he would benefit from cognitive behavioural therapy guided by principles of the Good Lives Model (GLM; Ward, 2002) and the Risk-Need-Responsivity model (RNR; Andrews & Bonta, 2010). Factors that could potentially improve his prognosis included regular attendance and compliance with therapy, and the addressing of his risk factors.

Wally attended a total of 16 therapy sessions over the course of a year. Although weekly therapy was recommended, he was only willing to attend therapy once every three weeks so as to cause minimum disruption to his NS duties. Nevertheless Wally was highly motivated to refrain from reoffending. He was compliant throughout the course of therapy, attended all sessions punctually and completed all his therapy homework. After his sentence, and without the need to engage in impression management, he had dropped his initially defensive stance.

Some challenges arising from Wally's lack of responsiveness were apparent from the onset of treatment. Firstly, his rigid thinking affected his willingness and ability to effect change in his life. For example, he refused to alter the frequency of his therapy, even though his NS schedule permitted it. He also found it difficult to respond during activities that did not interest him. Secondly, Wally's lack of emotional expressiveness made it hard to engage him. He would nod in response to requests or statements by the therapist, even when he was confused or did not understand them. He did not initiate conversation or volunteer information unless first spoken to; even then, his responses were brief and expressionless. Thirdly, while Wally had an adequate grasp of language and vocabulary, he was fairly inflexible in his thinking due to his lower level of cognitive functioning. This combination of factors caused therapy to be a very slow and frustrating process for his therapist, who had to frequently check on his understanding.

To address Wally's issues with responsiveness, initial sessions focused almost exclusively on rapport building and engagement. The use of humour and discussion about his interests (e.g., comics) made him more relaxed and engaged. To help him to feel more at ease, sessions and homework tasks were highly structured, and concrete analogies were used to help him understand concepts better. Motivated to change, Wally responded seriously when he understood that therapeutic progress was dependent on his participation. He was receptive when his therapist shared her difficulties in reading his social cues, and earnest in working on her feedback to indicate whenever he did not understand or disagreed with what was being communicated.

Wally soon became more engaged during sessions. He smiled more readily and was more vocal when he had doubts or queries. In order to increase insight into his risk factors, his assessment findings were shared with him. However, he continued to minimise some of them; he denied having engaged in fire-supportive cognitions or experiencing negative mood states prior to his offences. While not ready to process and address his offending behaviour just then, he was motivated to work on other risk factors and primary goods such as his peer relationships. His therapist thus used this as a springboard for setting other goals. For instance, the question "What behaviours or skills are needed to develop and maintain friendships?" was processed repeatedly with him. Over time he was able to generate a list of skills such as "being able to put myself in their shoes", "being able to know and feel more emotions (so I can put myself in their shoes)" and "being able to start a conversation with people I don't know". Acquiring these skills was subsequently incorporated into his therapy goals, as they were consistent with his risk factors and primary goods (i.e., inner peace and relatedness) (see Chu, Ward, & Willis, 2014).

Wally's rather restricted affect impinged on his emotional awareness, as well as his ability to regulate his affect and to build the friendships he desired. In order to expand his emotional range, Wally was taught to identify and differentiate his daily emotions more accurately. For instance, Wally's reports of being "tired" were processed and differentiated into similar but distinct emotions like "boredom", "fatigue," and "lack of motivation". He was also asked to keep daily logs of his activities and affective states. For example, whilst engaging in an activity, he would rate his affect on a 10-point scale, with 1 being most negative affect and 10 being most positive affect. This allowed him to monitor his daily behavioural and emotional patterns. Through such practices, Wally came to the realisation that he had a narrow emotional range; while he seldom experienced significant negative emotions in his daily life, he experienced few positive feelings as well. He was thus determined to increase his sources of pleasure, such as his hobbies and interests, in order to expand his emotional range and reduce his dependence on fire setting for positive affect.

As Wally became more emotionally aware, more perspective-taking and empathy exercises were employed during sessions to increase his capacity for victim empathy. Therapeutic goals were addressed through small, structured homework tasks that were expanded incrementally until a goal was reached. For example, in a bid to increase his repertoire of pleasurable and constructive activities, Wally set incremental goals to increase his fitness, go to the library more often, and to resume drawing and online chess. Being able to experience success in achieving these goals also put him on the right track to attaining his primary goods of excellence in play and autonomy. He finally felt that he was "living [his] own life instead of waiting for time to pass". By the end of therapy, Wally had started to work on his education and vocational goals, including exploring taking courses to become an interactive media designer.

To meet his need for relatedness, Wally set goals to socialise more and to build deeper friendships. These included initiating outings with his friends, carving out time to spend with them every weekend, reconnecting with those whom he had lost contact with, and getting to know new people that he met at the gym. He also became more open in sharing his problems with friends and more proactive in approaching them for advice. These goals gave Wally the opportunity to work on his social competence by practising skills of self-introduction and small talk in real-life situations.

Wally's progress in the attainment of his primary goods was matched by an increased sense of well-being and personal efficacy. This was corroborated by his mother's account of his progress. She confirmed that he socialised and exercised more, and shared more about his life with her on a daily basis. His presentation during sessions also changed—he smiled more often, was slightly more vocal, and readily indicated displeasure, disagreement or confusion. By this stage, Wally "[didn't] have to set fire to get the happy feeling". He was assessed to have sufficient alternative sources of pleasure and enjoyment, such that desensitisation to fire-related stimuli could be carried out without significant loss of pleasure in his life. Wally was also able to process his offending behaviour and anticipate the negative outcomes of fire setting without minimising them. He eventually gained insight that even though his fire setting had been minor, when he focused on the fire, he could not think clearly, so he might put people's lives in danger.

Covert sensitisation was subsequently employed to address Wally's sensitivity, positive emotional and physiological response to fire-related stimuli. Covert sensitisation is a form of behaviour therapy in which an undesirable behaviour is paired with an unpleasant image in order to eliminate that behaviour (see Plaud & Gaither, 1997). Sometimes it is unethical and even dangerous to elicit certain behaviours in session—fire setting, in this case—in order to extinguish it. The major advantage of covert sensitisation is therefore that it allows for the targetting of such behaviour without actually eliciting it.

Firstly, a hierarchy of fire-related stimulus was generated based on the amount of positive affect and thoughts of fire setting they engendered. Wally's sources of stimuli were first and foremost watching people burn things, and secondly, watching the daily news depicting wars, bombings, and major fires—he would do the latter every day. Baseline ratings were also taken of the positive affect or excitement induced by internet videos depicting fire-related events (typically 7 out of 10), and Wally noted the physiological arousal he would experience, such as sweaty palms and an increased pulse rate. Secondly, his therapist explained how his "substitute behaviours" for fire setting—watching videos involving fires and bombings—though seemingly harmless, reinforced his interest in fire and constituted a risk in the long run. Thirdly, Wally identified aversive stimuli that could be used in the reconditioning process: his negative experience in the police lock-up after being arrested. Recalling the experience evoked hopelessness, failure, and intense disgust. He then wrote a detailed and immersive recollection of it that included aversive input from all five senses. Fourthly, Wally was given the daily task of pairing a targeted number of relevant internet videos with a brief visualisation of his aversive imagery.

After a few weeks, Wally reported lower ratings of positive affect and excitement (about 3 to 4 out of 10) in response to videos depicting fire-related events. He had started to find such videos "neutral" and television watching had become a less pleasurable. In order to maintain the conditioned effect, but to prevent habituation to aversive imagery, covert sensitisation continued for a few more weeks.

Lastly, to ensure generalisation of effects for covert sensitisation, Wally monitored his affective and physiological responses to stimuli that were previously evocative, such as discarded cardboard boxes. He reported a lack of evocative response in his bodily sensations, thoughts and emotions, which suggested that his fire setting impulses had been sufficiently reduced. Furthermore, his responses on subsequent administrations of the Fire Interest Scale and Fire Attitude Scale revealed a gradual decrease in his interest toward fires and pyrotechnic material. To pre-empt future situations where Wally might encounter evocative fire-related stimuli, he was taught basic mindfulness skills (e.g., as selective attention) and self-soothing (e.g., controlled breathing and progressive muscle relaxation) to strengthen his emotional regulation. Mindfulness involves the focusing of attention and awareness on the present experience, and is used in therapy to improve self-regulation of attention and emotion.

Wally kept his parents updated on his therapy activities, homework, and learning points throughout the course of intervention. This helped them to develop a better understanding of his fire setting behaviour, with the effect that they stopped blaming him for his actions. He incorporated the strategies learnt through therapy into his risk management plan and shared it with his parents so that they could look out for warning signs preceding fire setting. They had initially censured him for "letting them down", but became more supportive of him the more involved they were in his treatment. When tempted to set fires, Wally would invoke memories of the guilt he felt for letting his parents down.

DISCUSSION

Arson is legally defined as the intentional destruction of property via fire for unlawful purposes (Williams, 2005), whereas pyromania is a psychological condition involving fire setting behaviour. Hence, not all instances of arson are associated with pyromania. It has been clearly documented that illegal fire setting is problematic across many jurisdictions. In 2005, for example, 329,000 illegally set fires were recorded by US fire departments; this led to 490 deaths, 9,100 injuries, and property destruction amounting to more than one billion dollars (Hall, 2007). In Australia 40% to 50% of structural and vegetative fires are deliberately set (Bryant, 2008), some of which have devastating impact on the environment, human lives and property.

Unfortunately, we do not have data pertaining to the characteristics of the illegal fire setters within the Singaporean context. No epidemiological studies have examined the prevalence of illegal fire setting or pyromania in Singapore. At the moment, any intervention with illegal fire setters is largely dependent on research findings in western societies. There have been anecdotal, isolated incidents of fire setting in Singapore; these episodes are often similar in description to this case. Despite the seemingly low frequency of fire setting in Singapore, and, in the case of Wally, the absence of intent to cause interpersonal harm, it remains important to address illegal fire setting behaviour because of the potential devastation, injury or death it can engender.

Research in western societies has revealed that fire setters are more likely to be male than female (6:1 ratio; Bourget & Bradford, 1989; Stewart, 1993). Apropos of developmental features and associated traits, Wally did not have many of the reported associated features for pyromania, such as being subject to a neglectful parenting style (Showers & Pickrell, 1987), having suffered physical and sexual abuse (McCarty & McMahon, 2005; Moore, Thompson-Pope, & Whited, 1987), or having come from a financially impoverished family (Bradford, 1982; Heath, Hardesty, Goldfine, & Walker, 1983). However, he had exhibited symptoms of anxiety, low self-esteem,

Fact Box 10.3. Five Different Trajectories Have Been Hypothesised for Different Types of Fire Setters (Gannon et al., 2012).

1. Antisocial Cognition: Their critical risk factor is their antisocial cognitions, scripts, value. Such persons are typically involved in antisocial and criminal behaviour. They are unlikely to be fascinated by fire and engage in fire setting as a means to an end (e.g. for financial gain, to threaten rivals and to eliminate evidence for other crimes).

2. Grievance: Their most prominent risk factor relates to problems with self-regulation. These fire setters usually have trait aggression and are easily provoked by real and perceived slights. They are not interested in fires per se, but use fire to send an authoritative message, or to indirectly exact revenge against those who have wronged them.

3. Fire Interest: Their interest in fire is their main risk factor. For some of these persons, fire setting is intrinsically exhilarating and stimulating. For others, fire has arousal-reducing properties. Such individuals create fires when under high levels of stress as a coping mechanism.

4. Emotionally Expressive/Need for Recognition: Problems in communication are their primary risk factor. *Emotionally expressive* fire setters use fires to draw attention to their emotional needs when overwhelmed by stressful situations, or as a form of self-harm, or suicide. *Need for Recognition* fire setters use fires to gain social attention or status, but usually remain anonymous.

5. Multi-faceted: Their critical risk factors are fire interest and offense-supportive attitudes/antisocial cognitions. Early adverse experiences, such as abusive experiences and interactions with highly antisocial peers, coupled with a childhood curiosity towards fire results in fire setting being used later in life to send messages, to cope with stress and to achieve sensor and affective stimulation.

impulsivity, poor frustration tolerance, and poor communication skills (Canter & Fritzon, 1998; Grant & Kim, 2007; Jackson, Glass, & Hope, 1987a; Räsänen, Puumalainen, Janhonen, & Väisänen, 1996; Rice & Harris, 2008; Swaffer, Haggett, & Oxley, 2001).

That said, we have noted that much extant literature is focused on Caucasian samples from Western cultures. Therefore, it is important to consider how cross-cultural and cross-jurisdiction issues may affect the psychopathology of fire setters in Singapore. If, as we hypothesise, fire setters' experiences in early childhood and adolescence lead them to develop psychosocial deficits that prompt fire setting behaviour later in life, studying the differences in the contextual and societal factors of these early life experiences would help researchers and clinicians appreciate the differences in aetiology.

A number of theories seek to explain the development and perpetuation of fire setting behaviour. These include single factor theories (e.g., psychoanalytical, biological, and social learning), and multifactorial theories (e.g., Functional Analysis Theory (Jackson, Glass, & Hope, 1987b) and Dynamic-Behaviour Theory (Fineman, 1980)). In addition, what is also useful is the Multi-Trajectory Theory of Adult Fire setting (M-TTAF; Gannon, Ciardha, Doley, & Alleyne, 2012), which integrates current theory, typology, and research knowledge to arrive at a comprehensive aetiological theory of fire setting that attempts to explain its maintenance and desistance as well. Wally's presentation fits with the Fire Interest trajectory according to the M-TTAF classification, with inappropriate fire interest/scripts being his critical risk factor (*see* Fact Box 10.3). Understanding fire setting from a theoretical perspective forms an important part of the assessment process, and it also helps us to conceptualise and plan for the subsequent therapeutic intervention.

Lastly, interventions for adult fire setters are typically cognitive behavioural in nature, and conducted in psychiatric settings (Swaffer et al., 2001; Taylor et al., 2002; Taylor, Thorne, & Slavkin, 2004), but there have also been reports of behavioural aversion therapy (Royer, Flynn, & Osadca, 1971) and social skills treatment (Rice & Chaplin, 1979). Some of the common treatment goals include targeting coping skills, conflict resolution and problem solving, reflective insight, relapse prevention and education about fire danger. In addition, it has been suggested that repetitive fire setters may also benefit from behavioural interventions that focus on fire factors—early socialisation with fire, fire interest/reinforcement, fire as part of self-identity, attitudes supporting antisocial behaviour using fire, and fire education—as well as general treatment that relates to antisocial behaviour, such as violent or general offending (Gannon & Pina, 2010). Fire setters with high fire interest may also benefit from covert sensitisation (Clare, Murphy, Cox, & Chaplin, 1992), or physiological arousal conditioning. In Wally's treatment, a combination of the aforementioned methods was used to good effect.

In conclusion, Wally's regular attendance, cooperation with the requirements of therapy, and motivation to change were beneficial to therapeutic progress. His family's eventual involvement in his rehabilitation plans not only provided him with the support to overcome his pyromania, but also promoted their better understanding of his condition. Finally, through his therapist's encouragement to take ownership of his therapeutic goals, and her clear implementation of therapy, Wally's sense of self-efficacy was strengthened and he was able to make significant positive lifestyle changes. To date, he has managed to stay offence-free and his family has remained supportive of his rehabilitation efforts.

DISCUSSION QUESTIONS

1. Wally's psychologist used two psychological models—the Good Lives Model and the Risk-Need-Responsivity model—to guide the formulation and treatment of Wally's presenting issues. What might be the rationale for using each of these models for Wally?

2. The DSM-IV diagnostic criteria of pyromania include a fascination with fire and pleasure, gratification, or tension relief following the fire setting. If you were to assess someone who presented with fire setting behaviour, how would you elicit the relevant information to make a diagnosis? For example, what questions would you ask and what measures would you use?

3. When is treatment required for people who are fascinated with fire, *but* do not show any fire setting behaviour?

4. How would you reconcile the usage of Western measures of pyromania, such as those used with Wally, with the Singaporean context? What alternative measures could you recommend be used in the case in the Wally?

5. Fire setting has been found to be comorbid with alcohol use disorder, marijuana use disorder, obsessive-compulsive personality disorder, and various antisocial behaviour (Vaugh, et al., 2010). As a therapist, how would you determine the treatment priority and therapy goals?

6. Adolescent and adult fire setting may be expressive and/or instrumental in nature. What are some possible themes that might underlie an individual's fire setting behaviour?

CHAPTER 11.

SELF-HARM TO SELF-MASTERY

Borderline Personality Disorder

NG SUE YING ADALINE

INTRODUCTION

Sally was a 26-year-old Chinese inmate at the Changi Women's Prison (CWP) serving a three-year sentence for drug consumption and attempted suicide. She was referred for psychological intervention because she presented with a history of maladaptive behaviours such as self-harm and poor interpersonal skills. Her personal supervisor, the officer assigned to oversee her, reported that Sally frequently quarrelled with her cell mates. As a result of these conflicts, Sally would behave aggressively towards others or engage in self-harm, for example scratching or cutting herself. Sally complained that she was unable to control her emotions and "cannot stand stress". She was also prone to bad moods, acting out whenever she felt unable to manage her distress. This was especially so when she was housed alone as she found it difficult to be by herself. Not surprisingly, these difficulties adversely affected her time in prison and her relationships in general; she got into trouble often and had difficulty establishing friendships. She was receptive towards the treatment, and expressed eagerness to learn skills that could help her manage her emotions and behaviours.

BACKGROUND

Prior to incarceration, Sally lived at home with her parents and an older brother. Sally also had an 18-year-old sister who had stayed with her grandmother since young; hence they were not close. Sally shared a good relationship with her mother and brother. Her mother worked as a coffee shop assistant and "did everything for the family", taking care of all their needs. She was closest to her elder brother who was working as a beer distributor. She found that she could relate well to him because he had also been in prison. However, Sally reported a hostile relationship with her father. She explained that her father "drank and gambled a lot", "didn't care about the family", and would often quarrel with and hit her mother when he was drunk. She resented her father as he had reported her to the police for her drug use, resulting in her current incarceration. She did not understand why her father "would do such a cruel thing to his own daughter".

Sally had dropped out of school at Secondary Two despite her good grades because she had wanted to earn money and marry her then-boyfriend, Andy. She had "really loved" Andy, even though they had dated for less than a year. She described Andy, who was three years older, as "perfect" for her. To support both their lifestyles, Sally had worked mostly in karaoke bars and nightclubs—jobs that provided her with sufficient and "fast" money. Similar to her other intimate relationships, her relationship with Andy had been characterised by numerous verbal and physical altercations. However, she explained that these previous relationships had been brief and superficial because she had entered into them when she felt "bored" and "empty".

Sally's maladaptive behaviours of drug abuse, binge eating, and self-harm began in her adolescence, after she had dropped out of school. The nature of her work exposed her to substances such as inhalants, amphetamine-type stimulants (e.g., "Ice", "Ecstasy", and ketamine), buprenorphine ("Subutex"), and anti-depressants ("Upjohn", and "Erimin"). What began as experimentation led to the use of drugs to cope with her negative emotions, such as feelings of rejection. When under the influence of drugs, Sally would experience hallucinations and paranoid delusions about her relationships (e.g., Andy cheating on her).

Sally had been incarcerated twice before, at the age 19, and again at 20. At 19, she had been charged with "creating a nuisance in public", by "shouting at strangers and kicking the dustbins", while under the influence of substances. In addition, she had resisted arrest and assaulted a police officer. She received a three-month sentence for her disorderly and violent behaviours. For the second conviction, at the age of 20, she had tested positive for hallucinogens (ketamine) and was sentenced to one year imprisonment. At 21 years of age, and not wanting to be incarcerated again for drug consumption, she managed to stop her drug use. During this two-year period however, she began binge eating "from morning till night", in a bid to cope with her feelings of being "very inferior". Within four months, Sally had gained 20kg. Feeling distressed at how "fat" she was, and believing that drug abstinence was to blame for her weight gain, Sally slowly slipped back into her old lifestyle of drug abuse.

Sally had started engaging in self-harm at the age of 14. Her self-harming behaviours included cutting herself with a penknife and burning herself with lit cigarettes. The injuries she inflicted on herself were occasionally serious enough to warrant professional medical treatment. Sally's maladaptive behaviours were usually triggered by interpersonal difficulties, such as conflicts with Andy. She would also threaten to hurt herself when she felt rejected or was unable to resolve her interpersonal problems. She felt that by "scaring" others with the threats, they would understand "how bad" her distress was and "do whatever I wanted". She described having threatened to jump off a five-storey building during a heated argument with Andy. In her agitation, she had lost her footing on the parapet and fallen from the building, fracturing both legs. Fortunately, she managed to regain full mobility after recovery. On a separate occasion, she had threatened to jump from her apartment window to avoid arrest when police raided her house for drugs. It was this incident that led to her being charged with attempted suicide.

In contrast to her previous two incarcerations, her current sentence was "very difficult" for her. She found it extremely difficult to accept being in jail for three years, especially when it was her father who had reported her to the police. Sally also experienced numerous conflicts with her cellmates. For example, she often perceived their actions to be geared towards ostracising her. This led to misunderstandings with her cellmates, who labelled her "sensitive". This often left her feeling angry and sad, because she felt that such a label invalidated her experiences. Unable to suppress these distressing thoughts and emotions, she would turn to injuring herself and hurting others.

ASSESSMENT

An initial assessment of Sally's personal history, presenting problems, and treatment motivation was conducted over two sessions. The focus of the assessment was to obtain a personality profile of Sally and her sense of identity, perceptions of how relationships operate, aggressive tendencies, adaptive coping (especially when experiencing anxiety), and values. Given the interpersonal difficulties Sally experienced across contexts (e.g., family and romantic relationships) and time, it was hypothesized that certain personality traits of hers were responsible for maintaining her difficulties. As such, the self-report measure, Inventory of Altered Self-Capacities (IASC) (Briere, 2000) was used as part of the assessment. This is a 63-item self-report measure of an individual's psychological functioning in three areas: a) capacity to form and maintain meaningful relationships, b) capacity to maintain a stable sense of personal identity and self-awareness, and c) capacity to modulate and tolerate negative affect. This measure was chosen as the three assessed areas were similar to the difficulties that Sally presented with. Findings from this assessment highlighted problems in Sally's relationships with others, and a tendency to dramatically change her opinions about significant others. She rated highly on IASC items such as "becoming upset with a lover or a friend" and "looking up to people then becoming very disappointed by them". Her turbulent relationships with her past boyfriends lent evidence to this. Furthermore, she felt that she often misjudged others and noted that "angels can change to devils".

Sally was assessed to be sensitive to perceived or actual abandonment by significant others, often expecting the termination of important relationships. For instance, she had not only taken on two jobs to support Andy but had also paid off his car loan. She often made threats of self-harm to her boyfriends, viewing their reactions to her threats as assurance of their concern for her. Her negative expectations of abandonment were reflected in her strong endorsement of IASC items such as "doing just about anything to keep someone you care about from leaving you" and "feeling afraid that someone you cared about might leave you".

Sally had difficulty maintaining a coherent sense of identity and was highly susceptible to influence; she felt that she did not know "who [she] was" when left to herself and easily "lost [herself]" when in an intimate relationship. This was highly consistent with the IASC items she endorsed (i.e., "losing your identity when you are in a relationship" and "being easily influenced by others").

Sally's responses were also indicative of significant problems in emotion regulation and control. Sally reported that she had a "bad temper" and "got upset easily", especially if others were unable to meet her demands. When in distress, Sally would cope through self-harming, substance abuse, and/or binge eating. She would also "throw temper" at those around her.

Sally's risk of self-harm and violence towards others were assessed to be high. She had a history of aggressive behaviours towards herself and others that were easily triggered by interpersonal conflicts and negative emotions. Furthermore, the likelihood of her encountering these triggers was high. However, as she was in a secured environment, which greatly limited her access to objects that could cause fatal injuries, the severity of her aggressive behaviours was unlikely to be high. Also, she had no access to illicit substances while she was in prison.

DIAGNOSIS

Based on the DSM-5, Sally met diagnostic criteria for borderline personality disorder (BPD). One of the key symptoms that Sally presented with was that of chronic feelings of emptiness—she was fearful of being alone and would often resort to frantic efforts to avoid real or imagined abandonment. She also had a history of unstable interpersonal relationships in which her sense of self was easily influenced by her partner. She would also idealize her partner, only to be disappointed subsequently.

Fact Box 11.1. DBT Acronyms

Some of the Dialectical Behaviour Therapy (DBT) skills have easy-to-remember acronyms. For example, the various interpersonal skills can be recalled via the acronym DEAR MAN, GIVE FAST. Distress tolerance skills can also be remembered with acronyms IMPROVE and ACCEPTS. To find out more about DBT skills, go to www.dbtselfhelp.com. It is an extensive website written primarily by individuals who have been through DBT.

Another symptom she presented with was potentially self-damaging, impulsive behaviours, such as substance use and binge eating. She would also repeatedly hurt herself physically and make suicide threats when in distress. Her emotion regulation and affective stability were also poor, consistent with BPD.

Apart from BPD, Sally also presented with substance use disorder (American Psychiatric Association, 2013), evident from her persistent poly-substance use despite an awareness of their serious social and psychological consequences. While she had a reported history of binge eating, she currently did not present with any form of eating disorders. She also did not present with indications of affective disorders (e.g., depression).

INTEGRATIVE FORMULATION

A referral for intervention was made for her emotion regulation and interpersonal difficulties, and the following preliminary formulation was proposed for her presenting problems:

Predisposing Factors

Sally's experience of her father as undependable and abusive could have resulted in her belief that it was in others' nature to reject her and to be untrustworthy. Although she perceived her mother in a positive light, her lack of involvement in Sally's life, which "left [Sally] to face consequences alone", may have also contributed to her view that others were unreliable and that she was inherently bad and unlovable. The domestic violence that Sally witnessed—poor parental role-modeling of emotion regulation—possibly led to her own experience of relationship instability. These experiences shaped her beliefs about relationships and set the stage for her current difficulties.

Precipitating Factors

Sally's incarceration precipitated her presenting problems. Her experience of anger and sadness could be attributed to the unexpected police report made by her father and the duration of her sentence. Given that Sally was unable to cope through her usual method of drug abuse and binge eating inside prison, acting out became her way of coping with stress. This resulted in challenging altercations with her cellmates.

Perpetuating Factors

Sally's unresolved resentment towards her father and her current sentence length contributed to her tendency to experience negative moods. Coupled with her limited ability to tolerate distress, her bad moods increased her probability of getting into conflicts with others. Because she was highly sensitive to interactions with her cellmates, she would first ruminate over perceived problems and then react by behaving aggressively towards them or engaging in self-harm. Together, these factors resulted in a vicious cycle in which her intrapersonal experiences led to negative interpersonal experiences, further worsening her mood.

Protective Factors

Sally was highly motivated to seek treatment as she was keen to improve her relationship with her cellmates and "not get into trouble anymore". She was generally engaged during assessment and therapy sessions and was receptive towards feedback. She clarified her doubts when necessary and was open about her issues, which facilitated her progress in therapy. In addition, she was conscientious in completing her homework assignments, applying the skills and concepts learnt to the actual problems she faced.

PROGNOSIS

About 75% of individuals with BPD will be able to function at a close to normal level by the time they are about 35 to 40 years old, and about 90% of them by age 50 (Paris & Zweig-Frank, 2001). Research suggests that about 70% to 75% of them have a history of self-harm with varying lethality, and about 10% die from suicide attempts (Linehan, 1993a; Paris, 2005). Given Sally's age, it was likely that she would continue to experience BPD-related difficulties, including self-injurious behaviours. Other than the risk of a fatal suicide attempt, Sally was also at risk of returning to prison if she continued to use drugs to cope with her stressors after she was released.

Dialectical Behaviour Therapy (DBT), has been found to be a promising treatment for individuals with BPD both in the community (e.g., Linehan, Comtois, Murray, Brown, et al., 2006) and in prison (e.g., Nee & Farman, 2007), as well as for individuals with comorbid BPD and substance use disorders (Bornovalova & Daughters, 2007). DBT is a treatment approach that infuses behaviour therapy with mindfulness practices. Rather than emphasizing dichotomous thinking, it explores clients' contradictory patterns (e.g., wanting acceptance by others but behaving in ways that lead to rejection) and establishes a synthesized middle ground for these contradictions. The therapist also attempts to balance the acceptance of clients' experiences while encouraging change (Dimeff & Linehan, 2001). DBT was expected to help Sally improve her emotion regulation and interpersonal skills, which would lead to a reduction in her use of self-harm to cope.

TREATMENT

As the client's own safety and that of others are vital in any treatment, it was agreed with Sally that her treatment goals were to reduce her aggression towards herself and others. At the heart of her aggression were her emotional vulnerability and interpersonal problems. Hence, it was important to equip her with skills to better manage these issues.

Individual therapy sessions took place once a week. Sally was introduced to DBT skills related to core mindfulness, interpersonal effectiveness, emotion regulation, and distress tolerance (Linehan, 1993b). She agreed to refrain from self-harm and to instead utilize the skills taught and social support available to cope with her frequent personal crises. Her therapist and personal supervisor also engaged in weekly discussions of Sally's use of DBT skills. This helped her personal supervisor to provide Sally with the necessary support and to reinforce Sally's use of DBT skills between sessions.

Although Sally was receptive towards treatment, her tendency to ruminate over many issues was apparent from the start. She had problems focusing during her initial therapy sessions as she was often distracted by thoughts of her father's "betrayal" and the extended length of her sentence. She was also deeply unhappy about her housing arrangement—while she felt anxious about residing alone in a cell, she worried that being housed with other inmates would give rise to conflict. As a result, Sally was often observed to lose focus during sessions and to suddenly interrupt her therapist with a question on, for example, her housing arrangements.

Core mindfulness skills, the first set of skills Sally was taught in therapy, thus came in handy in helping her to focus her attention. Using this technique, Sally would imagine that her thoughts were clouds in the sky, which came and went as her own thoughts came and went. She would also imagine ocean waves, which would rise and fall in synchrony with her emotions. This means of monitoring her thoughts and emotions, not only increased her awareness of her cognitive and emotional patterns, but allowed her to experience them without reacting as strongly to them as before. Sally's practical application of core mindfulness skills during therapy helped to balance her acceptance of her experience, while encouraging new behavioural responses.

Once Sally had become more aware of her thoughts and emotions, she was taught how to improve her interpersonal skills. Increased mindfulness enabled Sally to identify obstacles that limited her interpersonal effectiveness (e.g., cognitions such as "It is devastating if I don't get what I want from others") and to encourage herself with new strategies (e.g., positive self-talk such as "I can stand it if others cannot give me what I want"). She learnt to pick up skills that calibrated her behaviour in social situations. For example, instead of demanding that others pay attention to her whenever she wanted them to, she would ask herself a series of questions (e.g., "Is the other party busy with something?", "How important is it that I get the person's attention now?") to determine the appropriate intensity of her behaviours.

Despite having been taught these alternative coping skills, Sally continued to be preoccupied with her housing arrangement, a topic that dominated therapy sessions. Instead of focusing on how her skills could be applied to difficult interpersonal situations, Sally often digressed and frequently requested that her therapist speak to her supervisor about changing her housing arrangement. This was at times frustrating for the therapist as treatment progress was hindered by the same issues from session to session. Nonetheless, it was important for the therapist to validate Sally's experiences while facilitating change. Thus, instead of skills application as the main focus of therapy, the therapist focused on her stressors, and introduced relevant skills and concepts when appropriate.

At weekly case discussions, Sally's personal supervisor expressed her difficulties in managing Sally and also appeared frustrated with her repeated questions about her future housing arrangements. Her personal supervisor was thus taught to validate Sally's concerns with statements such as, "You seem very worried about this", and to encourage the use of the skills taught by following up with questions such as "What skills do you think you can use now to make you less worried?"

Midway through treatment, Sally was housed with three other inmates. Consistent with research on BPD (Zeigler-Hill & Abraham, 2006; Russell, Moskowitz, Zuroff, Sookman, & Paris, 2007), she felt socially rejected by her cellmates. Sally's therapist thus introduced her to ways of regulating her emotions (building mastery, focusing on positive events). This reduced her vulnerability to negative emotions and, as she was observed to have "become more patient with others", conflicts with her new cellmates were also less frequent.

Near the end of treatment, Sally experienced a personal crisis. During one of her regular visits, Sally's mother mentioned Sally's father, causing Sally to immediately lash out at her verbally. Despite feeling extremely guilty about it afterwards, Sally was unable to make amends till her mother's next visit. Sally's therapist used this incident to teach her distress tolerance skills, one of which was to evaluate the pros and cons of controlling her reaction. Sally applied this to her situation and was able to cope adaptively with her guilt, by using the time between visits to properly plan her apology to her mother for the next visit, instead of hurting herself, or acting out. This further empowered her and increased her sense of self-mastery.

As Sally demonstrated improvement in her interpersonal skills, emotion regulation, and distress tolerance, a consensus to gradually terminate treatment was reached between her and her therapist. Given Sally's fear of abandonment, it was important that she had ample time to adapt to functioning without the support of therapy. When it was proposed that her remaining four sessions be held fortnightly instead of weekly, Sally appeared frantic and tried to negotiate for more therapy sessions on a weekly basis. Her concerns over the impending termination were discussed and her other sources of support (e.g., her supervisor) highlighted to reassure her of continued help.

Because the last few sessions were aimed at facilitating the termination of therapy, they focused on reinforcing Sally's progress and honing skills that would be useful in managing future crises. Although she encountered several challenges during this period (e.g., a misunderstanding with her cellmate), her reactions were less intense than before. Sally expressed happiness at being able to "get along better with others" and reported that she had "matured a lot" and did not act as impulsively as before.

Information from her supervisor also corroborated with Sally's account. She noted that Sally was better able to get along with her cellmates and could cope with negative experiences more effectively. Furthermore, Sally had not incurred any institutional charges for problem behaviours, such as self-harm, for the entire duration of the intervention. This was the longest period that she had maintained good institutional behaviour. Therapy was thus terminated.

DISCUSSION

About 80% of persons diagnosed with BPD are women (Skodal, et al., 2002). Within the prison system, there is an over-representation of female offenders with BPD—approximately 20% as compared to 2% in the general population (Singleton, Meitzer, Gatward, Coid, & Deasy, 1998; Swartz, Blazer, George, & Winfield, 1990). However, there are at present no studies on the prevalence of BPD in Singapore and Asia. While there are no specialist clinics for the treatment of BPD in Singapore, there is increasing recognition for professional development in this area. This is because individuals with BPD are often in treatment for their comorbidities, (e.g., eating disorders) and mental health professionals need to know how to treat their comorbid issues in the context of BPD.

Early studies on the effective treatment of BPD have focused predominantly

Fact Box 11.2. Therapy Components of DBT

The "standard" DBT is typically delivered in an outpatient setting, where there are four primary treatment modes, all provided concurrently. The four treatment modes are individual psychotherapy, group skills training, telephone consultation, and case consultation for therapists. Individual psychotherapy is usually conducted on a weekly basis, where factors that limit effective behaviours and reinforce maladaptive behaviours are the key focus. During these sessions, the individual learns to integrate new skills into his/her daily life. The skills training component is usually conducted in a psycho-educational, group format. The four main types of skills taught are Core Mindfulness, Interpersonal Effectiveness, Emotion Regulation, and Distress Tolerance. Telephone consultation provides an avenue for DBT clients to access support when they are in crisis between sessions. Finally, case consultations for therapists are necessary to minimize therapist burn out, as treating individuals with BPD is a stressful task (Linehan, 1993a).

on psychodynamic therapy, which has showed limited effectiveness. For example, Skodol, Buckley, and Charles (1983) found a treatment dropout rate of 67% for BPD individuals within three months of psychodynamic treatment. These traditional psychodynamic treatment approaches also appeared to be unsuccessful in reducing suicide risk of individuals with BPD (Paris, 1993; Adams, Bernat, & Luscher, 2001).

Recent research studies have supported the effectiveness of DBT in treating individuals with BPD. Randomized controlled trials have shown that compared to usual community treatment, DBT led to better treatment retention, fewer days of hospitalisation, and less para-suicidal tendencies. These treatment benefits were also sustained one year post-treatment (Linehan, Armstrong, Suarez, Allmon, & Heard, 1991; Linehan et al., 2006). The application of DBT on the offender population has had promising results as well. For example, Nee and Farman (2005) piloted DBT for female offenders with BPD in three British female prisons. They found that treatment completers showed improvements along measures of BPD symptoms, locus of control, emotion regulation, and impulsivity. Sally herself demonstrated improvements in similar areas, with no incidents of self-harm during the treatment period.

The application of DBT in the case of Sally was influenced by factors unique to the context of the prison setting as well as her ethnicity and religious beliefs. The DBT approach encourages the acceptance of emotions and situations rather than trying to change them, and this is rooted in Zen Buddhism (Linehan, 1993a). Sally's ethnicity and Buddhist beliefs likely minimized resistance towards specific concepts and skills of DBT, and facilitated her grasp of DBT skills and knowledge. For example, she was open to learning mindfulness skills and was not put off by the references to Eastern meditation practices, which might not be expected from an individual with different religious origins (Linehan, 1993b).

While it was expected that the security-oriented and spartan environment of a prison would limit the provision of treatment, surprisingly, it facilitated Sally's therapy. Within the constraints of a prison, certain skills could not be practised as intended. For example, Sally was taught an emotion regulation skill that required her to build on pleasant daily experiences based on a list of enjoyable activities. However, the prison context rendered more than half the list inappropriate (e.g., going to a movie in the middle of the week, going on vacation, going home from work) and limited the creation of more appropriate activities. Nonetheless, the prison context also contributed therapeutic benefits. The presence of supportive officers meant that Sally had a support system to fall back on in the event that her self-regulatory skills were ineffectual.

The prison context also meant that Sally could not avoid interpersonal situations that were challenging for her (i.e., being housed with individuals whom she was uncomfortable with). Coupled with the structure and routine of prison, which prevented her from engaging in maladaptive coping strategies (e.g., binge eating, substance use), these conditions provided her with ample opportunities to practise the skills she had learnt during therapy and possibly contributed to her motivation to use the skills.

Therapy with individuals with BPD also requires addressing transference/counter-transference issues. In the case of Sally, "the rescuer" and "the victim" roles were evoked during therapy, and Sally was often observed to adopt a helpless ("the victim") stance. The therapist had to be careful not to adopt a rescuer role as Sally could have become dependent on her (Chatziandreou, Tsani, Lamnidis, Synodinou, & Vaslamatzis, 2005). For example, when Sally was preoccupied with her housing arrangement at the early stages of therapy, she would often complain of her high levels of distress and request that her therapist speak to the prison officers on her behalf. It was important for the therapist to empathise with Sally, while encouraging her to take the initiative to independently discuss her concerns with her supervisor. This was to avoid infantilizing Sally, which could otherwise lead to her therapist taking an inappropriate amount of responsibility for Sally (Linehan,1993a), and ultimately reinforcing Sally's perception of helplessness.

Another challenge faced when working with individuals with BPD is that of therapist stress and burn-out (Perseius, Kaver, Ekdahl, Asberg, & Samuelsson, 2007). Individuals with BPD present with several challenges that may negatively impact therapists (e.g., invalidating their treatment, causing them to blame their clients and themselves). This is because this client population engages in the three most stressful client behaviours: suicide attempts, suicide threats, and hostility. They also reinforce ineffective therapeutic behaviours by their tendency to focus on their feelings rather than maladaptive behaviours (Linehan, 1993a). This was reflected in Sally's case: her focus on her distress, rather than the behaviours contributing to her distress, was salient throughout the course of the treatment. Her therapist's stress was further multiplied by the ever-present risk of her engaging in parasuicidal behaviours should she be unable to manage her crisis in between sessions. This was particularly so early on in treatment, before Sally had learnt to manage her distress. These challenges highlight the importance of therapist self-care and supervision in order to minimize the possibility of burn-out during the course of the intervention.

While Sally benefited from the intervention, there were other issues that might have required further work—Sally's relationship with her father and the application of DBT skills to help with her substance abuse problem. If the intervention duration had not been constrained by her imminent release from prison, further exploration on Sally's relationship with her father would have been carried out, if she was willing. Resolving Sally's anger with her father was a pertinent issue as Sally was easily affected by him and thus liable to impulsive behaviour. Although Sally demonstrated improved adaptive coping over the course of the intervention, it was uncertain if she was able to utilise the DBT skills to prevent a relapse into drugs. As Sally was not under jurisdiction to attend mandatory substance use treatment upon her release from prison, she was given a list of agencies that provide community counselling services and was encouraged to utilise these sources of support.

1. Although Sally made therapeutic improvements, do you think she would still require professional help for her Borderline Personality Disorder when she is released? If so, what are some areas that she would need help in?

2. The prison officer who was Sally's Personal Supervisor had some difficulties managing her. What might they have struggled with and what can be done to support prison officers managing inmates with Borderline Personality Disorder?

3. Linehan (1993a) found that 71% of BPD clients met diagnostic criteria for major affective disorder and 24% met criteria for dysthymia. Research by Swartz, Blazer, George, and Winfield (1990) indicated that 22% of individuals who met the diagnostic criteria for BPD presented with alcohol abuse and dependence, while 50% of them had a long history of drug use problems. As a therapist, how do you determine the focus of your treatment for a BPD client with comorbid disorders?

4. DBT is based on the principles of Eastern philosophy and Zen Buddhism. What are the potential difficulties in using DBT for clients with a different religious and cultural orientation?

5. Part of the interpersonal effectiveness skills of DBT requires the client to be assertive when making requests. To what extent will these skills be effective in the local context, especially being assertive towards individuals who are more senior than the client?

6. DBT has been found to be effective in reducing self-harm incidents. How does DBT inform the therapist to address such behaviours?

CHAPTER 12

DIFFERENT DAYS, DIFFERENT PLACES—A DIFFERENT ME

Autism Spectrum Disorder in Adulthood

ELAINE LI-YING SUM AND ILIANA MAGIATI

INTRODUCTION

Christine was a 31-year-old Singaporean Chinese woman, who referred herself to the psychology clinic because she was experiencing low mood "for no apparent reason" and high stress levels at work. She wanted to see a mental health professional as she noticed herself doing and feeling things she could not explain or understand. For example, she had recently felt an urge to dig her eyeballs out, but stopped immediately as soon as she felt some pain when her finger touched her eyeball. She said she often felt "confused" about what she did and why.

Christine talked about how she had been finding it difficult to sleep in the last four months and how stressed she had been feeling at work and at home. She felt pressured to support her parents financially and often argued with her mother. She had neither friends nor colleagues she could talk to, and did not go out or spend much time with other people. She shared that she had little interest in hobbies or activities outside of work. Her energy to be often fluctuating and she found it difficult to concentrate at work at times. She described having difficulties "getting in touch with" and understanding how she felt. This often made her feel confused about herself and her feelings, as if "my different selves did different things at different times".

Before coming to the clinic for the intake appointment, Christine had searched the internet for some explanation or description of her difficulties. She had read the diagnostic criteria for borderline personality disorder (BPD; American Psychiatric Association, 2013) and told the therapist that this disorder might describe her, given her recent impulsive urges and unstable, often tense relationship with her mother.

BACKGROUND

Christine had consulted a psychiatrist a few years prior to the present referral, as she had found herself engaging in checking rituals (i.e., repeatedly checking if the lights or household appliances had been switched off before leaving the house) and experiencing an inexplicable low mood. She was diagnosed with depression and obsessive-compulsive disorder and her symptoms were managed with medication. Christine noticed that her difficulties seemed to improve during her years of undergraduate and postgraduate studies. She had also received a diagnosis of mild dyslexia some time ago in adulthood, but she was not able to provide more detailed information about this.

Christine lived at home with her retired parents and her older brother, who had had a diagnosis of high-functioning autism since primary school and who was currently in full-time employment. She had always lived with her parents and had never moved out to live independently, except for one year when she studied abroad. When Christine was growing up, her mother had attended more to her brother largely due to his diagnosis of autism. Although she understood why her mother needed to be more attentive to her brother, she sometimes felt and continued to feel less attended to by her parents. Christine thought her mother had "long-term low mood", but as far as she knew had neither received a formal diagnosis of depression nor sought professional help. There was no other known psychiatric history in the family.

It was difficult to develop a good understanding of Christine's developmental history as a child and young person, because she was unable to recount many details. She also did not invite her parents to participate in these sessions, because she did not want them to know that she was consulting a psychologist. She said she did not want to be an added burden to her family, given her brother's diagnosis of ASD.

Within the first couple of sessions, it became apparent that Christine had experienced difficulties relating to other people since childhood. She had very few friends and did not maintain social relationships with others in school, work or other social settings. She would only meet up very occasionally with one tertiary school friend and with a small group of colleagues once a year. She had never been in a romantic relationship. Christine expressed a desire to be able to maintain friendships, however she said that she had no time or energy to text her friends or to keep in contact with them through Facebook. Christine appeared to have some insight into her difficulties in making and sustaining friendships; she confided that she felt she "damaged" potential friendships with her "high standards of morality", which she expected all her friends to adhere to. For instance, when a friend did not divide the food they had bought together equally between the two of them, she felt this to be "morally incorrect" and did not talk to that person again. She also acknowledged a number of difficulties in social skills, such as maintaining eye contact when interacting with people. She had tried to cope with this by reading widely about how to relate socially to others.

Christine had neither hobbies and interests nor participated in any leisure or social activities. She described her life as very "work-centered", working until 10 pm almost daily. Consequently, she did not have energy for leisure activities or to use the computer when she got home. She typically spent weekends on work for her company and household chores, which she always completed in a fixed order because "this was the most efficient way".

Despite her academic achievements—she held a master's degree in a science-related field and had been in full-time employment for two years after graduation—Christine reported experiencing considerable stress and difficulties at work. One such difficulty had to do with her fixed daily work routine. Every morning, after first checking her email, she would draw up a timetable and a to-do list, which comprised several goals for the day and various checkpoints at which she could stop to monitor her progress. As a result of trying to complete all her daily goals before going home, she frequently worked until very late at night.

Moreover, Christine set very high standards for herself and would spend hours redoing her work until she got it "right". Despite her heavy workload, she would be very reluctant to delegate any work to her colleagues and would leave detailed instructions for her colleagues before she went on leave. Upon her return however, she would redo her colleagues' work to ensure that it was done properly. Christine felt very strongly that her colleagues should also adhere closely to strict work protocols and rules. During lunch breaks, she preferred to have lunch alone and would often leave the food court to have her meal elsewhere if her colleagues were there. However, she often ruminated over what they might think of her, especially about her "not saying hi".

ASSESSMENT

At intake, Christine completed the self-report 21-item Depression Anxiety Stress Scales (DASS-21; Lovibond & Lovibond, 1995). The DASS-21 consists of three subscales that screen for negative emotional states of depression, anxiety and stress respectively. She obtained scores within the "normal" range for Depression, within the "mild" range for Stress and within the "extremely severe" range for Anxiety. However, when she completed the DASS-21 again at her third session, her depressive symptoms had increased to the "moderate" range; when asked, she attributed it to stress at work and not knowing her exact diagnosis.

The Structured Clinical Interview for Diagnostic and Statistical Manual of Mental Disorders-IV (DSM-IV) Axis II disorders (SCID-II; First, Gibbon, Spitzer, Williams, & Benjamin, 1997) was also used as part of the assessment process. The SCID-II consists of a 119-item self-report Personality Questionnaire and a clinical interview. The items Christine endorsed in the self-report Personality Questionnaire (which is designed as a screening tool to help clinicians identify specific difficulties and symptoms that are most relevant to the client to be explored in more depth in the SCID-II clinical interview) related largely to obsessive-compulsive personality disorder

(OCPD; American Psychiatric Association, 2013). Hence, the OCPD section of the SCID-II was subsequently used in the clinical interview. Christine appeared to meet criteria for a diagnosis of OCPD, as she scored in the clinically significant level for six out of eight criteria for OCPD, namely, preoccupation with details, rules, lists and schedules, perfectionism that interferes with task completion, excessive devotion to work, over-conscientious, scrupulosity and inflexibility about matters of morality, high reluctance to delegate work to others, and rigidity.

During the intake session and the four sessions that followed, the psychologist observed a pattern of rigidity in Christine's behaviour and difficulties in communicating and relating to her therapist. For example, Christine was often rather rigid in her attempts to follow and complete the agenda that was set at the beginning of each psychotherapy session. She was emphatic about sticking closely to the set agenda, even during a session that followed a distressing event in her life. She drew a detailed written timeline of her academic, occupational and psychiatric history, which she brought to the first session with the request that the intake interview be structured chronologically to ensure that no details were left out. It was very difficult for the psychologist to direct and structure the intake interview, as Christine was adamant on following her own timeline. She also corrected or interrupted the psychologist on a number of occasions. She was persistent in her request that the psychologist conduct therapy using a "transactional analysis" approach, which she had discovered on YouTube. Her psychologist found it difficult to communicate the importance and effectiveness of evidence-based intervention approaches to her.

Christine presented with a limited range of facial expressions and gestures during the sessions. Her intonation was also often flat and monotonous, and did not always accurately represent her mood since she used a similar tone when expressing different feelings such as sadness, stress or pleasure. She also seemed to be rather insistent on pinpointing her diagnosis.

Finally, she described having difficulties "getting in touch with" and understanding her emotions. She shared that she often only realised that she was feeling stressed when her body felt tense and started to ache— suggesting that she may have had to rely on her own physiological reactions to gauge what emotions she was experiencing. The psychologist's impression of Christine was a general bluntness in affect and difficulty in grasping what she was experiencing and feeling. Her expressed emotions and facial expressions would also tend to be incongruent with the magnitude of the distressing event she had experienced.

Because of her family history of ASD and the psychologist's observations of her rigid behaviour and poor communication and social skills, the psychologist considered the possibility that Christine's past and current presenting difficulties might be better explained by a diagnosis of autism spectrum disorder (ASD). ASD is a complex disorder characterized by impairments in communication and social interaction and by rigid, circumscribed behaviours and interests that can affect individuals of all ranges of intelligence (American Psychiatric Association, 2013). For this reason, Christine was instructed to complete the Autism-Spectrum Quotient (AQ; Baron-Cohen, Wheelwright, Skinner, Martin, & Clubley, 2001), a 50-item self-report checklist that provides information on behaviours, traits and symptoms associated with the autistic spectrum. The AQ can be completed by adults of normal intelligence and assesses five different areas: social skills, attention switching, attention to detail, communication and imagination (Baron-Cohen et al., 2001). Christine obtained an AQ score below 32 (scores higher than 32 are indicative of ASD). However, the results of screening tools do not constitute a diagnosis, and clinical decisions should not rest entirely on them. All screening measures are subject to measurement error and no screening tool has perfect accuracy. Furthermore, cut-offs for the AQ have not been determined for the local population. In Christine's case, there was strong and consistent historical and present information and observations to strongly suggest the possibility of ASD, despite an AQ score below the cut-off.

Christine denied any suicidal ideation or intent and any past or present self-harm. Although she reported acting on one of her impulses on one occasion (i.e., following her urge to dig out her eyeball), she denied any intention to hurt herself and had stopped herself upon feeling some pain. She did not have a history of drug or alcohol use. She was assessed to be at low risk of harming herself or others.

DIAGNOSIS

Based on Christine's family history, her recounted social history, and in-session observations, it was deemed highly probable that her presenting and historical difficulties could be explained by a diagnosis of ASD, with cognitive and verbal abilities in the non-intellectually disabled range.

Specifically, Christine appeared to meet the DSM-5 diagnostic criteria for ASD. She had persistent difficulties and impairments in social communication and social interaction across multiple contexts. In particular, she had trouble communicating with friends and colleagues and tended to avoid them during lunch. She also reported similar difficulties with peers in school and had no friends. She used very limited gestures and displayed a limited range of facial expressions and nonverbal communicative skills. She also struggled to develop and maintain relationships both at work and in social contexts. Christine often displayed inflexible adherence to routines (e.g., the fixed order in which she completed household chores, her fixed daily work routines, and her rigidity in performing work-related tasks). At the same time, Christine presented with anxiety and mood-related difficulties, which were considered secondary to her probable underlying social and communication difficulties. However, as Christine was reluctant to involve her parents in the diagnostic process, there was no information on the extent of these difficulties in her early developmental period.

As we were unable to conduct a full diagnostic assessment for ASD in our clinic, we were not able to completely rule out other diagnoses. For example, Christine appeared to meet six out of eight criteria for OCPD in the structured clinical interview that was administered. However, the presentation of preoccupation with routine, order and schedules, excessive devotion to work, inflexibility and rigidity seen in OCPD overlap to a great extent with symptoms of ASD. Moreover, a diagnosis of OCPD alone could not adequately describe or sufficiently explain Christine's persistent social communication and relationship difficulties. Therefore, a comprehensive assessment of ASD was recommended, as this would aid in understanding if Christine's behaviour and difficulties were better accounted for by ASD. Her presenting anxiety symptoms were likely co-occurring alongside her social and communication difficulties and related to increasingly more stress and social challenges at work. Anxiety disorders are very common in individuals with ASD (van de Steensel et al., 2011).

INTEGRATIVE FORMULATION

Predisposing Factors

As Christine has an older brother who has ASD, she may have been at higher risk for a diagnosis of ASD through genetic predisposition. Undiagnosed ASD could predispose her to the considerable anxiety and mood difficulties she had been experiencing throughout her life, and for which she had not found an explanation. In addition, Christine reported that her mother likely had depression, although not formally diagnosed. It was also possible that her mother's emotional difficulties had a negative impact on Christine through, firstly, a lack of modeling of adaptive coping strategies and emotional regulation in stressful situations; and secondly, by transmitting to Christine's unhelpful beliefs about herself (e.g., being unworthy of attention or care).

Precipitating Factors

Christine reported that long working hours, a stressful work environment and difficulties getting along with her colleagues precipitated her presenting concerns of low mood and anxiety. She had stopped talking to many of her colleagues and had reported a marked increase in conflicts with her mother, which added considerable stress. As her parents were retired, she had also begun to feel the added responsibility of having to support the family financially. The culmination of these stressors likely triggered Christine's presenting issues at that point in time.

Perpetuating Factors

Christine had very high standards and tended to be very particular and perfectionistic. These, together with her rigid routines, maintained and likely exacerbated the high amounts of stress she faced at work. In addition, as she appeared to have limited awareness of her own emotions and stress, she was less able to recognise and regulate her stress levels until cued by an intense physiological reaction. Her reluctance to delegate tasks also likely contributed to her stress at work. Lastly, Christine's social isolation may also have added to her worries about what her colleagues would think of her while concurrently depriving her of potentially positive social experiences with others.

Protective Factors

Christine was intelligent, committed and hardworking and managed to remain employed in the same company for two years, despite experiencing many challenges. She was focused and had good problem-focused coping skills—she believed that her good problem-solving skills were the main reason she was so persistent in pinpointing her diagnosis, as she felt capable of working to address these symptoms.

PROGNOSIS

ASD is a life-long, neurodevelopmental condition. As such, treatment is not focused on 'curing' individuals, but on strengthening skills, reducing problematic behaviours and helping them learn to better manage stress, anxiety and low mood. Christine's prognosis with regards to achieving her treatment goals was assessed to be good given her openness to seeking help, and her intelligence, willingness and motivation to understand and help herself. Specifically, targetting the long-standing nature of her difficulties in understanding and relating to other people would likely sustain improvements in her mood, stress levels and social/work life.

TREATMENT

Christine was keen to improve her social and communication skills, and in particular learn how to develop and maintain friendships. Her other treatment goal was to reduce her stress at work; she cited stress as the major reason she sought psychological help.

Christine attended a total of five sessions. While earlier sessions focused mainly on gathering information to make a possible diagnosis of ASD, the last two focused on beginning intervention for her anxiety and low mood symptoms. During these sessions, Christine identified her treatment goals and was provided with psycho-education on the rationale and main goals of cognitive behavioural therapy as modified for use with adults with Asperger's Syndrome (Gaus, 2007). She also started a mood/thought diary that would help her monitor her mood and identify stressful situations. When sufficient information had been gathered regarding Christine's social and communication difficulties and rigid patterns of behaviours, the possibility of Christine having undiagnosed ASD was discussed openly with her. When asked how she felt about this possibility, she said she was "okay" with this. She added that she really wanted to find out what was "wrong" with her, so that she could better understand her difficulties and receive appropriate intervention and support (Fact Box 12.1).

Although Christine appears to have met most of the diagnostic criteria for ASD, a more comprehensive specialist diagnostic assessment should be conducted for a formal diagnosis of ASD in adults. Unfortunately, the clinic where Christine was seen comprised of only psychologists. In addition, the staff were not trained to administer gold-standard diagnostic tools to assist in the diagnosis of ASD, such as the Autism Diagnostic Observation Schedule—2 (ADOS-2; Lord, Rutter, DiLavore, Risi, Gotham, & Bishop, 2012). For this reason, the provisional diagnosis of ASD without accompanying intellectual impairment was first discussed with Christine. With her consent, she was referred for a thorough multidisciplinary diagnostic assessment at a specialist adult neurodevelopmental service at a local psychiatric hospital. Christine decided to complete the ASD diagnostic assessment before continuing possible intervention at the psychology clinic; her explanation being that she wanted to find out the "true" cause of her difficulties first before delving into any intervention. At this point, therapy was thus terminated at the clinic.

For adults with ASD without an intellectual impairment, who have difficulties with social interaction, the UK National Institute of Clinical Excellence guidelines (NICE, 2012) recommends individual or group-based programs focused on improving social skills. NICE (2012) also recommends cognitive-behavioural therapy (CBT) adapted for individuals with ASD to help improve coexisting difficulties, such as anxiety or low mood. CBT for those with ASD should be more concrete and structured, focus more on changing behaviour than cognitions, with minimized use of metaphors,

---

Fact Box 12.1. Receiving a Diagnosis of ASD in Adulthood

Approximately 50% of adults referred for a possible diagnosis of ASD are self-referrals. Others are referred by a parent, other relative, a health care professional, partner, friend or teacher. Receiving a diagnosis of ASD in adulthood can be a complex experience, as many adults are often misdiagnosed with mental health problems, schizophrenia or personality disorders. Moreover, service provisions are often very limited past adolescence. Different people report a range of reactions following a diagnosis of ASD in adulthood: some report shock, confusion, sadness or anger at being misunderstood for so many years; many others report relief at finally understanding the "true" source of their long-lasting social difficulties as well as some of their strengths and finding a way to explain these to others. Ensuring non-judgmental understanding and appropriate post-diagnosis support is essential in improving their experience, reducing anxiety and depression and improving quality of life.

(Sources: Jones et al., 2014; National Autistic Society UK)

---

ambiguous and hypothetical scenarios and increased use of written and visual information or prompts (NICE, 2012; see also Gaus, 2007).

DISCUSSION

The assessment process presented several challenges for the psychologist. Christine was particularly anxious to know her diagnosis from the first session and repeatedly enquired about it, as she said she felt there was something "wrong" with her, but had been unable to pinpoint what exactly was "wrong". The therapist similarly found it difficult to ascertain Christine's main presenting issues, as she reported a wide range of symptoms, ranging from impulsivity to depression, anxiety, stress and social difficulties. Moreover, although Christine reported feelings of anxiety and stress, she did so in a rather "matter-of-fact" manner, and her facial expressions and flat affect were incongruent with the high amounts of stress and low mood she was experiencing. This made it harder for the psychologist to put her finger on what difficulties Christine was experiencing.

The male-to-female ratio for ASD diagnosis is approximately 4.3:1 (Fombonne, 2005). This gender imbalance has led to a disproportionate amount of research on males with ASD and to a male bias in terms of diagnostic criteria (Dworzynski,

Fact Box 12.2. What are some differences between males and females with ASD? Source: Kirkovski et al., 2013.

There is increasing evidence that the phenotypic profile of girls and women with ASD may be different to that of boys and men with ASD.

Females' greatest difficulty is often in developing and keeping peer relationships and friendships, particularly in adolescence and adulthood. At the same time, it has been reported by females affected by ASD themselves that they often observe and learn social behaviours from others. In other words, they "mimic" or "act out" socially appropriate interactions through observation and social learning rather than social intuition. This can often mask their true difficulties and thus escape being picked up by professionals.

Although findings from research studies are still somewhat inconsistent, females are generally reported to have fewer stereotyped behaviours and interests, although their routines can often be rather rigid and fixed. There are few differences in the rates or types of associated mental health problems experienced by both males and females with ASD.

Females with ASD may have higher rates of abnormal eating behaviours.

Ronald, Bolton & Happé, 2012). It is thus likely that females with high-functioning ASD remain underdiagnosed compared to males (Attwood, 2006; Fact Box 12.2 and 12.3). This may explain why Christine's brother was diagnosed with ASD, whereas her own symptoms were not recognised. Furthermore, Andersson and colleagues (2013) found that available screening instruments may be less reliable for identifying ASD in females, as these tools screen for impairments that are more prominent in males. This could account for Christine's score on the AQ, which was below cut-off.

Adult females with ASD typically present with fewer socio-communication difficulties as compared to males, as they are better able to compensate for their difficulties through observing others in social situations and adhering to social scripts (Lai et al., 2011; Willey, 1999). In other words, females may learn how to have reciprocal conversations and how to use facial expressions, gestures or eye contact for social communication. Christine, for example, was generally able to carry conversations and maintain reasonably good eye contact, but she shared that she had managed to do this by studying books and people in order to better understand what they meant and how to relate to them. Young girls with ASD appear on average to be better able to display complex emotions (Head, McGillivray & Stokes, 2012) and to produce more echolalic speech than boys, which can often lead to the misunderstanding

---

Fact Box 12.3. When should an assessment for ASD be considered in adulthood?

According to the most recent National Institute of Clinical Excellence guidelines for the recognition, assessment, diagnosis and management of ASD in adulthood (NICE, 2012), a differential assessment for possible ASD should be considered when an adult has one or more of the following:

- persistent difficulties in social interaction or communication;

- stereotypic, rigid and/ or repetitive behaviours, resistance to change or restricted interests;

AND one or more of the following:

- problems obtaining or sustaining employment or education;

- difficulties in sustaining social relationships;

- previous or current contact with mental health or learning disability services;

- a history of a neurodevelopmental disorder or mental health condition.

that girls have better language and communication skills (Knickmeyer, Wheelwright & Baron-Cohen, 2008). It could be that her "better" and "less obviously unusual" behaviours and skills masked Christine's more subtle, but still considerably impairing, difficulties when compared to her brother with ASD.

Females with ASD also have fewer inappropriate or eccentric special interests and activities (Attwood, 2007; Gould & Ashton-Smith, 2011) and display fewer aggressive and hyperactive behaviours compared to males with ASD (Gillberg & Coleman, 2000). Christine, for example, did not report any unusually intense or circumscribed interests or hobbies, although she did often behave in a rigid, fixed way in her work or home activities. Furthermore, girls with ASD who have social and communication difficulties and seem to be socially withdrawn may sometimes be mistaken as having a shy disposition (Wagner, 2006). Shyness can be associated with culturally valued characteristics such as "behaving modestly" or "not showing off" in the Chinese culture (Xu & Farver, 2008; Wu, 1996), which could further "mask" persistent social difficulties in individuals with undiagnosed ASD. This might have been the case with Christine—she may have been labelled a quiet, shy, slightly rigid young woman, rather than someone with undiagnosed ASD. The impact of culture on diagnosis has not been explored extensively, however, what is considered "typical" or "atypical" may differ depending on cultural norms and values. In fact, there has been some recent evidence of cultural differences in the expression and reporting of autistic traits in the general population (Freeth, Sheppart, Ramachandran, & Milne, 2013).

Many individuals with ASD, both men and women, also experience significantly higher levels of psychiatric difficulties, including anxiety and depression, than individuals without ASD (Rosenberg et al., 2011; White et al., 2011). Undiagnosed adults with probable ASD may often initially present to psychological services with such associated difficulties and, thus, careful attention should be paid to their history of social and communication development, as well as to the observation of their current behaviour and social interactions. Christine presented initially with stress, some anxiety and some symptoms of low mood, and appeared to meet some of the criteria for an OCPD diagnosis. Yet, a more in-depth assessment of her history and a careful observation of her current communication and interaction patterns with the therapist were strongly suggestive of possible ASD.

From our perspective, this case provides three important learning points. First, even though the client referred herself for therapy with a specific diagnostic "explanation" in mind (Borderline Personality Disorder), her initial presentation (anxiety and stress), her previous psychiatric diagnosis (OCPD) and her presentation during the sessions at the psychology clinic (which suggested ASD) were all different. This highlights the need for initial referral or triage information to be carefully investigated. However, the focus and direction of the initial assessment should continue to be comprehensive and broad in scope—rather than "narrowed down"—and should explore multiple areas of functioning and development. This case emphasises the importance of understanding each client's presenting difficulties in a wider context, by taking current and past issues into account and by considering neurodevelopmental and psychosocial "explanations". In Christine's case, for example, significant overlap exists between some symptoms of OCPD and those of ASD—clinicians should therefore be mindful that a client's fulfilment of a checklist's or screening tool's criterion symptoms does not equate to a clinical diagnosis.

Secondly, this case highlights the importance of making clinical decisions by integrating all information gathered together and using clinical judgment, and not just relying on screening measures. It is important to holistically integrate information from all sources, including direct observations of the client and relevant reported family and developmental history. Finally, it is important for clinicians to ensure that, despite their responsibilities and workload, they keep abreast of the latest research and empirical findings in their fields, as emerging developments—in this case, the diagnosis of ASD in adulthood and gender differences in the presentation of ASD—could change the way the client's presenting difficulties are understood and interpreted.

DISCUSSION QUESTIONS

1. What aspects of Christine's development in childhood and adolescence may point towards ASD being a more appropriate diagnosis for her compared to, for example, BPD or other diagnoses?

2. What do you think made it difficult for Christine to be appropriately identified with ASD at an earlier age? What "masked" her ASD-related difficulties?

3. In what ways do you think Christine's ASD symptoms (current and historical) may be contributing to her stress, low mood and anxiety?

4. Besides assessing for core symptoms of ASD, what should a comprehensive diagnostic assessment for ASD include?

5. Undiagnosed adults with ASD may initially present to mental health services with various mental health or psychiatric difficulties and may face considerable challenges in their adult lives. What could be some advantages and disadvantages of obtaining a diagnosis of ASD in adult life for these individuals, their families and their future? How can a diagnosis be raised and discussed with undiagnosed adults in a sensitive manner?

6. What cultural values or norms could possibly affect the expression or reporting of social and communication behaviours relating to autism (autistic traits) in the general population in different ethnic or cultural groups? Do you think these values and norms could affect the validity and reliability of autism diagnostic tools developed in the West when used with non-Western populations? How?

CHAPTER 13

THE THRILLS AND SPILLS OF PUBLIC MASTURBATION

Deviant Sexual Behaviour

GWEE KENJI

INTRODUCTION

Kenneth was a 21-year-old of mixed Asian ethnicity who was charged by the police for committing an "obscene act": he had exposed his penis and masturbated to a teenage female victim along a HDB corridor. After his arrest, Kenneth was sent for a psychiatric assessment to assist the courts in deciding on his conviction and sentence. He was diagnosed with a paraphilic disorder: an atypical sexual interest that causes dysfunction in life. Kenneth's sexual interest is considered unconventional to societal norms; dysfunction was evidenced from his criminal behaviour. The psychiatrist proceeded to refer Kenneth to a clinical psychologist, who could determine his suitability for psychological therapy, specifically for his behaviour of masturbating in public.

BACKGROUND

Kenneth was the average guy-next-door. Born through normal vaginal delivery and attaining normal developmental milestones, he grew up watching cartoons, playing with his younger brother, and trying his best at school. While he never shone academically, he completed his GCE 'O' Levels sufficiently well to qualify for further studies at a private institute. He did not mix with bad company, take drugs, drink alcohol, fight with others or play truant—his record was clean. In addition, he had no known serious medical conditions and was in fact quite healthy.

However, Kenneth had a dark secret. After stumbling upon his cousin's stash of porn during puberty, Kenneth began responding to his developing sexual needs in a dangerous way. At the age of 15, he started scouring his neighbourhood for female undergarments left on laundry poles to dry. At first, he would look at them. Before long, he began stealing them, holding onto them while masturbating at HDB staircases and corridors. He then "upped the thrill" by following young females around HDB estates before hiding in a corner and masturbating. He was only 16 years old.

One day, Kenneth was masturbating along a corridor in his neighbourhood again when his neighbour spotted him. After a complaint to his family, his parents sent Kenneth for a psychiatric assessment; he was diagnosed with fetishism, a disorder in which one experiences sexual arousal from objects. He was not treated with medication and his father, who appeared to have a dismissive attitude towards both Kenneth's behaviour and psychiatric input, did not see the need for therapy. While the diagnosis of fetishism was not appraised by Kenneth to affect him too much per se, he was happy to be let off with a warning, and was not charged in court for what he had done.

Unfortunately, for the next five years, Kenneth continued this habit, and kept it a secret from everyone. Whenever he felt bored at home, he would go on a "hunt" in his neighbourhood, following attractive and young females between the ages of 15 to 16, often ending his trips via sexual release by masturbating at HDB staircases and corridors. By then, he was already serving National Service.

While Kenneth had a rational understanding of the wrongfulness of his actions, he did not feel genuinely remorseful. He was "bored" and the excitement and sexual pleasure afforded by the habit overcame his moral inhibitions. It did not help that his father's talk to him had been brief and dismissive: "It's not right, so don't let me catch you doing that again!" Furthermore, his father's job required him to travel out of town frequently. The absence of an authority figure, the infrequency of enforced discipline, and Kenneth's mother's permissive parenting, gave Kenneth leeway to indulge in his misdemeanour. In fact, while his mother acknowledged that his behaviour was wrong, she felt that it was a "male issue" that should be sorted out between Kenneth and his father. Kenneth was not close to his younger brother, and they led largely independent lives, seldom engaged in shared activities and rarely communicated. There had been no history of psychiatric illness in the family.

In terms of his psychosexual development, Kenneth began puberty when he was 13 years old. He started using pornography when he was 15, egged on by his friends' constant discussion of it. He used the internet to access normal heterosexual pornography, and had not strayed into deviant types (e.g., bestiality, fetishistic or sadistic pornography). He would surf pornographic sites three times weekly, and masturbated to the same frequency. He had no girlfriend but had taken a fancy to females of his age when he was 14, and displayed interest in age-appropriate peers. He was clearly heterosexual in orientation.

When he turned 18, history repeated itself: he was spotted masturbating by a female occupant of one of the neighbouring apartment units. This time, the female victim made a police report. Although Kenneth managed to run away from the crime scene, the police tracked him down and came knocking on his door a couple of days later to formally press charges against him.

ASSESSMENT

Kenneth was first seen in a forensic ward after his arrest. He presented as a well-groomed young male of medium build. He was cooperative and forthcoming, providing details of his offence and past deviant behaviour. He was downcast and appeared resigned to his fate. When relating his offence, he was able to differentiate between cognition and emotion, which CBT practitioners typically deem a sign of suitability for CBT. For example, he confessed to feeling "great shame" that he had let his father down again. He was able to distinguish this feeling from the cognition that "This is the end of my life—my life goes down the drain here". He seemed accepting of his legal predicament and appeared to want to turn over a new leaf. Kenneth came across as less defensive and evasive as compared to other offenders whom the psychologist had seen, and seemed sincere in his willingness to change.

Significantly, Kenneth acknowledged that what he did was wrong. He attributed his actions to "thinking too much about sex", although these thoughts were short-lived, and he did not seem preoccupied with them. He perceived his behaviour as "not normal" and readily acknowledged its potential to jeopardise his future after NS, which involved pursuing a career in the food and beverage industry, which he already had some early investment in. Another impetus was his fear of letting his father down.

Mood or anxiety issues are complicating factors for therapy, and thus need to be assessed. For example, when depressed, a client might more readily seek deviant methods to alleviate depression than if he or she were not depressed.

Fact Box 13.1. In Vivo Exposure: Overcoming Arousal

In vivo exposure involves introducing the client to a real-life situation that evokes a sexual response from him. For Kenneth, being at HDB stairwells was one such situation, as his repeated acts of masturbation at these spots had conditioned him to be sexually aroused whenever he was there. The client begins by monitoring his degree of arousal when he approaches such real-life situations. The moment he feels aroused, he immediately engages in relaxation methods that have previously been taught and rehearsed during therapy sessions and practised at home. The principle underlying the use of relaxation methods is reciprocal inhibition—one cannot feel sexually aroused and relaxed at the same time. In other words, relaxation inhibits sexual arousal. After the client has consciously reduced his sexual arousal, he can leave the scene, and return later to repeat the exposure. The co-therapist's role is to serve as a safety net to prevent the client from acting on his impulses and reoffending should he fail to curb his arousal.

Anxiety symptoms may serve as a barrier to normal social interactions, which in turn can deprive one of meeting one's intimacy needs. Fortunately, Kenneth presented with no self-reported mood or anxiety symptoms, and there were no indications of any major mood problems in his past. Similarly, a client's level of intellectual functioning affects therapy as it determines the complexity and range of interventions appropriate for use, as well as the language used to explain them. For example, a therapist might employ more behavioural, rather than cognitive, interventions with clients of lower intelligence. In terms of intellectual functioning, Kenneth came across as being of average intelligence—no formal testing was carried out as it was not deemed critical given his otherwise normal presentation.

The severity of sexual deviance can also be indicated by an increase in the frequency of the use of pornography, an increase in the deviant nature of pornography material, and the presence of socially acceptable romantic and sexual relationships. Kenneth's use of internet pornography use had not altered in frequency or nature since he was 15. While he was not in any relationship, he was romantically interested in a female friend. He appeared defensive when talking about her, and it was difficult to ascertain his ability to socialise appropriately. However, no other sexually deviant behaviour was noted.

Kenneth's understanding of therapy was realistic and accurate—he thought that it would help him to have someone else to talk to in order to "find out how to control" his behaviour. In addition, he expressed a willingness to involve his father as a co-therapist should this be required (in Kenneth's case, a co-therapist can assist by being physically present while he performs in vivo exposure exercises (*see* Fact Box 13.1), which might involve controlling his urges in HDB corridors or corners that usually increase his sexual desires).

Lastly, but importantly, the risk that Kenneth posed to others in the community was manageable. Although he would follow women, he hid in a corner to masturbate rather than exposing or forcing himself on them. The non-contact nature of his offence, his fear of being seen when masturbating, as well as the salience of his recent arrest, suggest that he was not likely to escalate to pose greater harm.

Although not used with Kenneth, self-report questionnaires can provide valuable information for assessment of sexual offenders. For example, the Multiphasic Sex Inventory 2nd Edition (MSI-II; Nichols & Molinder, 2010) covers various aspects of sexual offending and can be used with sexual offenders, such as Kenneth. The MSI-II covers paraphilic preferences, psychosexual variables (e.g., aggression, treatment readiness and cognitive distortions), psychosexual history, and more variables of interest. Although relevant, the MSI-II was not administered as it required pay-per-use online submission to the test's publishers for interpretation, and such a practice was not established in the organisation of assessment. Instead, clinical interviews were used in lieu of structured assessment tools like the MSI-II.

DIAGNOSIS

Using the DSM-5, Kenneth was diagnosed by the psychiatrist to have paraphilic disorder, fetishistic disorder (302.81; *see* Fact Box 13.2). Specifically, his behaviour of following attractive females and masturbating while spying on them from stairwells was deemed atypical, against societal norms, and in opposition to the law. Additionally, he had expressed a preoccupation with female undergarments. While an interest in women in undergarments can be considered a typical male response, an exclusive fascination and sexual reaction towards female undergarments alone is considered fetishistic. He did not have any other affective conditions or comorbid diagnoses, and did not meet criteria for other paraphilias.

Kenneth's diagnosis of fetishistic disorder was more clearly related to his past preoccupation with female underwear than with his more recent acts of following girls and masturbating in public. However, treatment focused on the latter acts due to their immediacy and current relevance. While both behaviours were sexually driven, they are different in terms of abnormality and criminality. For example, one can argue that an interest in female undergarments may be an extension of a more normal

Fact Box 13.2. Criteria for Fetishistic Disorder

The criteria for Fetishistic Disorder in the DSM-5 remain largely unchanged from the DSM-IV-TR:

1. Over a period of at least 6 months, recurrent and intense sexual arousal from either the use of non-living objects or a highly specific focus on non-genital body part(s), as manifested by fantasies, urges, or behaviours.
2. The fantasies, sexual urges, or behaviours cause clinically significant distress or impairment in social, occupational, or other important areas of functioning.
3. The fetish objects are not limited to articles of clothing used in cross-dressing (as in transvestic disorder) or devices specifically designed for the purpose of tactile genital stimulation (e.g., vibrator).

A differential diagnosis of exhibitionism was considered. However, it was noted that Kenneth did not intend for himself to be seen. In fact, he avoided detection and panicked when spotted. Exhibitionism, on the other hand, involves intense sexual feelings brought on by exposing oneself. Additionally, as Kenneth had good school records and had not displayed other defiant or offensive behaviours, he did not qualify for a diagnosis of conduct disorder.

interest in women in underwear. Following girls and masturbating in public, while not having a formal diagnosis of its own, is deemed more unacceptable. As noted by Darcangelo (2007), the divide between unusual sexual preferences and psychiatric disorders remains ill-defined, and large variability exists in the continuum of sexual behaviour.

INTEGRATIVE FORMULATION

Kenneth's sexual experimentation of following girls and masturbating in public places went unpunished for five years and became a habit, which predisposed him to repeat such behaviours. A lack of close monitoring and the absence of a disciplinary figure in Kenneth's adolescence also served to tacitly reinforce his ability to get away with deviant behaviour. The first time he was reported to the police, he was given a warning instead of a heavier punishment. This diminished the consequences of his actions and may have further reinforced the notion that what he had done was not inherently bad. With repeated pornography use and the lack of more meaningful interpersonal relationships, meeting his sexual needs through the habitualised act of following girls became salient in Kenneth's life. His sensation-seeking personality, evidenced by his complaints of being "bored" and finding his actions thrilling, served as a further predisposing factor.

Kenneth's actions can be understood using an offence cycle, which depicts how factors trigger and maintain his behaviour:

FIGURE 13.1. KENNETH'S OFFENDING CYCLE

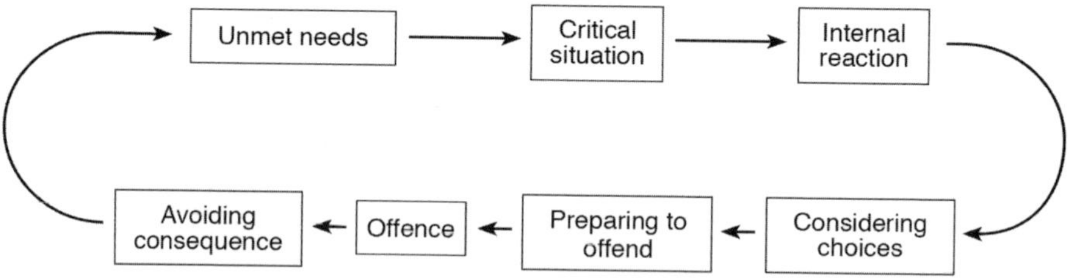

Kenneth's unmet needs, such as the lack of meaningful interpersonal relationships and limited daily excitement, made him more vulnerable to reoffending in certain situations. His primary trigger or 'critical situation' was seeing attractive females in HDB estates. He experienced an internal reaction, which included sexual excitement as well as the desire for intimacy. A decisional point would arise, and Kenneth could choose to pursue and tail his victim, or head home to meet his sexual needs on his own. When he opted for the former, he would get prepared to offend (e.g., he would look around to make sure that there were no witnesses or would follow the victim for a chance at physical proximity). He would then offend, usually by masturbating behind a wall while peeping at the victim. After the offence was committed, he would then avoid the consequences, by lying low to avoid being seen in the area. While this provided a temporary climax, his deeper need for intimacy remained unfulfilled, and the cycle would repeat.

Classical conditioning principles were also at play. By repeatedly pairing the highly pleasurable sensation of ejaculation with his behaviour of following girls and masturbating in HDB corridors and staircases, Kenneth created a conditioning that made tailing girls a pleasurable event. This undoubtedly perpetuated his behaviour. In addition, the danger associated with the possibility of being caught while doing these acts might have also heightened his arousal and accentuated the degree of pleasure he experienced.

PROGNOSIS

Kenneth possessed a few protective factors—good insight, motivation, impetus for change and the presence of supportive family and friends. As such, the prognosis for Kenneth was guardedly optimistic. Nevertheless, the lack of corroborative informants and the secrecy of his acts made it difficult to ascertain his degree of honesty. As such, motivating Kenneth became particularly important—it was germane to highlight to Kenneth how his actions threatened important things such as his future.

TREATMENT

Based on the formulation, Kenneth was deemed to be highly suitable for psychological therapy, which would be aimed at addressing his behaviour of following females, hiding in a corner and then masturbating in public. The recommendation to the Court was thus to have him receive psychiatric and psychological treatment. With the recent implementation of the Mandatory Treatment Order sentencing option, Kenneth was ordered by the Court to receive two years of compulsory psychiatric and psychological treatment as recommended by the psychiatrist. Thus began his journey of change.

At the beginning of treatment, the therapist provided Kenneth with psycho-education using the offence cycle and the Good Lives Model. The purpose of the offence cycle was to make Kenneth aware of his internal states that perpetuated offending, while the Good Lives Model highlighted the values and resources in his life that mattered more than his deviant behaviour, which would ideally motivate him to refrain from reoffending. Specific strategies like covert sensitisation would then be used to provide concrete behaviours at decisional points of offending. Once Kenneth had demonstrated a reasonable degree of gains from therapy, some element of relapse prevention would then be introduced to help maintain his gains.

Consistent with literature supporting the efficacy of combined pharmacological and psychological treatment for fetishism (Darcangelo, 2007), Kenneth received both psychiatric and psychological interventions. An anti-depressant was prescribed in low dosage by the psychiatrist to reduce Kenneth's sex drive, while psychological therapy focused on modifying his behaviour. Kenneth's two main goals of treatment were to control his sexual behaviour so as to avoid future run-ins with the law, and to engage in more meaningful activities such as work. As his deviant sexual behaviour was the focus of therapy, the approach adopted was primarily CBT for sexual deviance, informed largely by literature in the area of offending behaviour (e.g., Andrews & Bonta, 2010; Ward, Melzer, & Yates, 2007).

Early stages of therapy focused on helping Kenneth to develop a deeper understanding of his internal processes leading to offending, and building a conviction to change. The offence cycle (*see* Figure 13.1) was explained to him. Kenneth felt that he could relate to the cycle and that it made sense. For example, his *critical situation* was to be alone near HDB flats when transiting to and from home; when *considering choices*, he would usually consider going home to masturbate. Personalising the offence cycle helped Kenneth to realise that there were opportunities during his cycle to intervene. Prior to this exercise, he felt that he had run out of options to curb his deviant behaviour, but after the exercise "so many solutions were thrown up".

The Good Lives Model (Ward, Melzer, & Yates, 2007) was also used in the early stages of psycho-education to highlight the importance of other aspects of his life which he valued, and to identify his unfulfilled needs. This model proposes that if one can use healthy and adaptive ways to attain satisfaction in the following nine primary areas, then the need for antisocial outlets will diminish: 1) physical and sexual health, 2) knowledge, 3) mastery in work and play, 4) autonomy, 5) inner peace, 6) relatedness, 7) creativity, 8) spirituality, 9) happiness.

Kenneth's takeaway from this discussion was that he perceived himself to be "thrill seeking", which partially explained why he followed girls and masturbated in public. To fulfill this need for "thrills" in his life, he decided to invest his efforts in his F&B career, as this was something he was very enthusiastic about, and gave him a certain degree of excitement. While employment could not fully replace his need for his sexual thrills, it was the best Kenneth could come up with.

Covert sensitisation was then gradually introduced to Kenneth. The principle behind covert sensitisation is to increase the salience of negative consequences of deviant sexual behaviour. It is believed that, when the negative consequences of reoffending are prominent enough, individuals are less likely to commit such acts. To highlight these undesired consequences, individuals develop scripts of their typical modus operandi, which end in their arrest and amplifying the undesired outcome. A non-offending script is then developed to model a prosocial behaviour that leads to a non-criminal outcome (*see* Table 13.1).

<table>
<tr><td colspan="2">TABLE 13.1. KENNETH'S OFFENDING AND NON-OFFENDING SCRIPT</td></tr>
<tr><td>Kenneth's Offending Script</td><td>"When walking though the flats, I see an attractive girl. Just for fun, I follow her a while as she walks home. She looks sexy and I get more excited as I keep following her and watching her. When she reaches her floor, I wait at the stairwell and peep at her. There is no one around, so I start masturbating as I am very excited. After finishing, I head home, relieved. However, when there is a knock on my door a few hours later and my father opens the door to two policemen, I know that this is it. I feel scared and have disgraced my father. The sense of shame is overwhelming."</td></tr>
<tr><td>Kenneth's Non-offending Script</td><td>"When walking though the flats, I see an attractive girl. Just for fun, I want to follow her for a while as she walks home. I then remind myself of what happened the last time – my father's look, the strong sense of shame I felt, and the fear of my future being destroyed. I let her go without following her, but head home instead to masturbate. It's less fun, but I still feel good as I prevented a disaster."</td></tr>
</table>

Kenneth found these scripts useful as they evoked strong emotions—particularly shame—that served to deter him. However, Kenneth also wanted them to be physical reminders that could be accessed conveniently. With some improvisation and creativity, he designed a personalised wallpaper for his mobile phone that reminded him of his new girlfriend. Although they had only been together for a month and were not sexually active, she was privy to his offence and deviant sexual behaviour, and was accepting and supportive. As such, his phone wallpaper evoked strong reminders not to reoffend, and was effective in increasing his self-restraint.

While his father did not eventually participate as a co-therapist, he communicated more with Kenneth. In these father-son talks, his father acknowledged that sexual needs had to be met and did not totally dismiss Kenneth's actions. Instead, he highlighted the criminal implications, the impact on their family, and the repercussions on Kenneth's future. Notably, he spoke for the family and expressed support for Kenneth.

As Kenneth was motivated and engaged in therapy, he made early progress. He reported a drastic drop in his urges to reoffend, as well as his overall sex drive. He was taking his prescribed medication regularly and had not experienced any side effects. For six months there were no self-reported indications of deviant urges or behaviour. Specifically, he was asked at each therapy session if he had experienced urges to follow girls, and if he had acted on them. While it would have been easy for Kenneth to lie, the continuous emphasis of his life goals, his values, and what he stood to lose should he reoffend served as deterrents. Throughout the six months of therapy, motivational interviewing was used to spur Kenneth on to maintain his positive lifestyle changes.

By now, therapy had progressed to include relapse prevention and the concept of high-risk situations was discussed. As Kenneth was still serving NS, his time spent in camp prevented him from reoffending. Furthermore, his camp was quite inaccessible and lacked surrounding housing developments. However, Kenneth was able to identify moments just after sending or picking his girlfriend up from work and home as being of high risk. These moments placed him in close vicinity to HDB blocks, where his urges to reoffend were higher.

Throughout therapy, there was consistent monitoring of his sexual urges and intent (through his therapist and psychiatrist enquiring about them at each session). Although Kenneth constantly reported a very low or near absence of urges to reoffend, as well as a depressed sex drive, the tracking of changes to his libido was vital due to the nature of the disorder. All appeared to be going well and both his treating psychiatrist and psychologist were pleased by his progress. Then, six months from the commencement of therapy, Kenneth reoffended. He managed to zip his pants up before revealing himself, and although the police were involved, he was not charged. This event led to his increased motivation to change, as well as to his girlfriend's involvement in his journey of change.

As Kenneth completed NS and began his career, he continued therapy in the remaining months of his Mandatory Treatment Order (MTO) sentence. While the frequency and intensity of his sexual urges remained low, his high-risk situations changed somewhat as his exposure to HDB estates fluctuated as a function of where his work took him. He continued to be forthcoming about where he might "slip up". Over time, as he developed in maturity and motivation towards his career, his once deviant sexual behaviour became a struggle of the past.

Kenneth finally completed his two-year MTO sentence without further reoffence. Compared to a typical 16–20 sessions for such types of disorder in the context of MTO, Kenneth attended a total of 12 sessions. The shorter duration of therapy was due to his strong motivation and the support he received from his close friends and family, which, together, facilitated greater improvement. His career in the F&B industry was also in the works. In short, Kenneth had met his treatment goals. When asked what he found most useful from therapy, Kenneth identified the reminders of his decisional points and his high-risk situations. He also shared that "nowhere could [he] talk about such things" to the degree that he could during psychological therapy.

At the time of writing, Kenneth was scheduled to return for "booster sessions" twice a year. The goal of these sessions was to revise covert sensitisation by highlighting the consequences of deviant behaviour and emphasising decisional points in his offense cycle, and to monitor his urges, in light of the tapering off of medications that affected his libido.

DISCUSSION

Due to its secretive and shameful nature, rigorous epidemiological studies of fetishism have proved elusive. The best estimates of its prevalence range from 0.1–0.8% of adult psychiatric patients, and up to 3.4% of paraphilic sex offenders (Darcangelo, 2007). While these statistics indicate that fetishism may be very rare, the DSM-5 describes it as relatively common among paraphilic disorders. The strong sense of shame it entails is a barrier to seeking help, but can be used to motivate clients once therapy begins.

There have been no published studies on the prevalence of fetishism in Singapore. However, among those sentenced under the MTO, those with paraphilias (of which fetishism forms a part) make up only 15.3% of all MTO cases in 2011 (Koh et al., 2013). Unlike Kenneth, most of the offenders who received MTO sentences were diagnosed with psychotic illness (41.7%) or depression (31.9%).

In terms of accessing treatment, offenders who have been convicted and sentenced typically receive treatment from the Ministry of Social and Family Development (especially for those on probation), or the Institute of Mental Health (MTO program). Voluntary clients who readily seek treatment for fetishism in the absence of any forensic impetus are rare, perhaps attesting that the practice of fetishism can be a lifestyle choice not leading to any dysfunction under the right circumstances. When people do seek professional help, it is likely with private practitioners. The implication is that many persons who are assessed for MTO suitability may have been previously closet fetishists and may not have been particularly keen on therapy. The onus is thus on the psychologist to assess thoroughly their suitability for therapy. For the offender, it is a painful choice: to escape a jail term by entering the MTO program albeit having to admit to an embarrassing disorder, or to serve a sentence but to keep one's sexual deviance a secret.

Fact Box 13.3. The Continuum of Paraphilia

The DSM-5 distinguishes paraphilia from paraphilic disorder. Paraphilia refers to deviant sexual interests whereas a paraphilic disorder refers deviant sexual interests that cause personal or interpersonal dysfunction. As such, one can have the former and continue to lead functional lives, engaging in paraphilia as part of a sexual preference or lifestyle choice in a suitably contained fashion (e.g., having a consenting partner willing to share their interests), or not letting their sexual preferences affect their participation in other aspects of their lives. A paraphilic disorder, on the other hand, causes problems in the life of the individual, and as such, treatment is indicated.

Assessing the offender's suitability for therapy thus becomes an important and complex task. Psychologists can begin by adopting a simple framework of: (i) clinical factors (whether a treatment exists for the disorder), (ii) client factors (whether the client is keen and amenable to treatment), and (iii) supportive factors (whether there are resources in the offender's life that support the therapeutic alliance). Specific factors for consideration would typically include motivation to change, degree and chronicity of deviant sexual interests (How deviant and varied are his preferences? How long has he lived with them?), previous attempts to change (Has there been reasonable effort invested to change?), protective factors (Does he have a lot to lose due to his behaviour? Are there things more important than his deviance that can motivate him?), degree of support (Are his family members behind him?), and psychological mindedness (Is he aware of his internal processes? Will he be able to understand therapy?). Only when there are sufficient factors in favour should treatment begin.

The treatment strategies employed for Kenneth represent some of the typical approaches used for sex offenders: covert sensitisation, motivational interviewing, relapse prevention and the Good Lives Model. Despite appearing to engage well in therapy, Kenneth reoffended while undergoing treatment. Based on data from this therapist's workplace, approximately 10% of offenders who are undergoing treatment, such as Kenneth, are caught reoffending within two years of legal sanctions (Unpublished data, 2014). Of note is that his conviction to change appeared catalysed by his reoffence and a reinforcement of his fears of legal punishment. This may suggest that while the clinical strategies for working with behaviours related to sex offences may be important, legal factors such as the salience of prosecution or client factors may account for substantial change. Accordingly, a clinical psychologist working towards effecting change in others needs to ensure clinical strategies are appropriately and efficiently delivered, while also keeping tabs on the client's legal situation.

Should the therapist attempt strategies like covert sensitisation and in vivo exposure, a few notes about these approaches are in order. While in vivo exposure can have a large impact on the client given the reality of the situation, it is in practice more effortful to effect. Firstly, there is the issue of risk that must be addressed: what safety mechanisms are in place to prevent actual reoffending, since the client is being introduced to a high-risk situation? The availability and ability of a co-therapist varies between clients. Secondly, clients usually find the naturalistic setting challenging as other situation-specific factors (e.g., crowd volume, availability of preferred victim types, etc.) may be beyond their control. Lastly, the repeatability of such exposure sessions tends to be a challenge as the schedules of both client and co-therapist as well as the environmental variables have to be aligned. As such, covert sensitisation is preferred given its ease and privacy of use. However, keeping tabs on whether the client actually performs the mental processes for covert sensitisation is impossible.

As in fetishism, or other paraphilias that are often kept as a shameful secret, the honesty of the client is critical to recovery. Given the strong gains from lying—escape from the full force of the law—the therapist has to help the client to gain perspective of what he stands to lose if he does not address his maladaptive behaviour. For example, these behaviours stand in the way of the client achieving a meaningful life, being independent in a job, and having a normal romantic interest. As the therapist works together with his or her client towards achieving these normative goals, the rapport built between the therapist and client will encourage more honesty from the client.

In retrospect, Kenneth's success in therapy was likely due to the threat of punishment from reoffending, which he had previously assumed would be overlooked again. Being on the brink of completing his National Service and embarking on a career in F&B made Kenneth more cognizant of the salient consequences of a reoffence. The risk of being at the centre of a media storm due to the public nature of his future employment and the strong local stigma against sex offences acted as strong deterrents to his deviant behaviour. Furthermore, Kenneth had previously promised his father that he would not reoffend and "bring the family problems". His second reoffence probably drove the consequences of his actions home.

The use of anti-depressants for Kenneth can be interpreted as controversial. As some anti-depressants have the side effect of suppressing libido, certain studies have highlighted their efficacy in reducing the sex drives of sex offenders (Garcia, Delavenne, Assumpcao Ade & Thibaut, 2013), which, in effect, reduces recidivism. However, the efficacy of pharmacological treatment with sex offenders remains mixed, as other studies found limited utility of such treatment (Baratta, Javelot, Morali, Halleguen, & Weiner, 2012). Another issue of concern is the increased risk of suicide from anti-depressant use, which led the Food & Drug Administration (FDA, 2007) in the United States to issue warnings about the potential lethality of antidepressant medication, particularly in the 18–24 age band. Certainly, for someone like Kenneth who did not exhibit any mood or anxiety symptoms and presented with a low risk given the non-contact nature of his offences, the necessity of an antidepressant prescription was questionable, therefore gaining informed consent from Kenneth when prescribing psychotropics was particularly important.

Fortunately, the use of anti-depressants, together with psychological interventions, allowed for a satisfactory resolution to Kenneth's case. Although he had a shorter length of therapy and one incident of reoffending, he managed to effectively use the skills and methods he had learnt from therapy to reach his goal of not running afoul of the law again. Without the use of psychological treatment strategies, or the presence of a supportive therapist who allowed him to openly talk about his socially unacceptable sexual behaviour, Kenneth would most likely have reoffended earlier and more frequently. For the therapist, however, what stood out and made the difference was Kenneth's own conviction and eventual determination to change.

1. Identify the treatment strategies that were used with Kenneth. How did each strategy help him?

2. Identify some protective factors to include in Kenneth's integrative formulation. How exactly might each of these protective factors improve his prognosis? As a psychologist, how would you best use these protective factors in treatment?

3. Sexuality has a wide range of behaviours, and those considered normal or mainstream in one culture can be considered deviant in another. Take for example, homosexuality, which was once considered a psychiatric disorder. Are there any sexual disorders that are affected by the variability of culture and time?

4. Given that there is large variation in sexual behaviour, why do you think some behaviours (e.g., fetishism, paedophilia and exhibitionism) are considered mental disorders?

5. Some critics of the DSM have pointed out the circularity of definition where paraphilic disorders are concerned—the diagnoses for such disorders are based on the demonstration of the behaviour itself. In other words, as long as one performs those behaviours, one has the disorder. From a legal perspective, this is particularly troubling—do all such offenders then have disorders, given that they have demonstrated those behaviours? How can one distinguish a mentally disordered individual who offends because he has an affliction, from an offender who conveniently gets diagnosed with a disorder because he offended and hence exhibited those behaviours?

6. The literature supporting the efficacy of sex offender treatment to reduce re-offending is mixed at best. Given that there is no clear evidence that treatment for sex offending prevents future reoffending, should one still treat sex offenders, such as Kenneth? What would be an alternative?

CHAPTER 14.

YOU LEAD, I'LL FOLLOW. YOUR HANDS HOLD MY TOMORROW

Major Depression and Paranoid Personality Disorder

JASMIN KAUR

INTRODUCTION

Pete, a 34-year-old Chinese man sentenced to nine months of incarceration for motor vehicle theft, was referred for assessment and intervention by an intake counsellor at Singapore Prison Service after verbalising thoughts of suicide. Within the span of two months before imprisonment, he had made three attempts to end his life, and was currently planning to end his life after release from prison.

Pete had first tried to kill himself at the age of 33. He had swallowed 150 codeine tablets and washed them down with Chinese wine before phoning a friend, who had managed to admit him to a hospital in time for treatment. A few months later, he was arrested for his current offence, and diagnosed with major depressive disorder (MDD) at the Institute of Mental Health (IMH). Just after leaving IMH, Pete had tried to take his life again by ingesting more codeine tablets. However, he managed to regurgitate them through induced vomitting. His final suicide attempt took place just a few weeks prior to his prison sentence. He had lit a charcoal stove at night to suffocate himself in his sleep, but had woken up in the morning. Pete had wanted to end his life in a "peaceful manner", which was reflected in the methods he chose, aimed at achieving a "clean death rather than a violent one".

A year prior to his current imprisonment, Pete's godmother, Madam Lim, passed away from cancer. This was a difficult period for Pete. Although he had performed her funeral rituals and set up an altar for her in his home, the guilt he experienced for his earlier mistreatment of her and his regret for his inability to fulfil her last wish—to pass away in her own home—had haunted him since her death.

From the early age of seven months, Pete's parents had placed him under the care of Madam Lim. In the beginning, they had paid her for his upbringing. However, when payment ceased a few years later, Madam Lim continued looking after him for free, and she eventually adopted him legally. In addition to Pete, Madam Lim had also adopted an older boy named Henry.

Pete's mother had severed ties with him when he was young, causing him extreme emotional hurt. His father also visited him infrequently during Pete's childhood, which did not provide much consolation either. To Pete, his father's visits seemed to be driven more by the ulterior motive of borrowing money from his godmother than any real concern for his son. During one such visit, his father brought him to his brothel as part of an "outing". Pete's strong feelings of rejection due to his birth parents' lack of care were further compounded by his mother's remarriage and the marked difference in her care of his step-siblings. Pete expressed disappointment at his parents' inability to finance his expenses and he had felt like a burden to Madam Lim. Moreover, he did not believe that Madam Lim felt genuine concern for him as a person, and "had no choice" but to raise him once his own parents' financial provision ended.

Fact Box 14.1. Suicide in Singapore

While research on suicide in Singapore has been sparse, there are some findings that are of value in understanding the aetiology of suicide in Singapore. Based on the data available from the Samaritans of Singapore (SOS), the suicide rate for 2012 was 10.27 per 100,000 persons. Chia and Chia (2010, 2012) have identified certain factors that appear to result in higher rates of suicide.

Demographics (age/ethnicity/gender). Older Chinese males and younger Indian individuals were more likely to attempt suicide. The rate of suicidal behaviour for Malay individuals is relatively low, comprising only 4% of those who committed suicide in 2012 (SOS, 2012).

Socioeconomic Status. The loss of a marital partner appears to be a key stressor that can lead to individuals attempting suicide. Unemployment was also clearly found to be related to suicidal behaviour.

Psychiatric History. Schizophrenia and depression have been found to be more prevalent in individuals who commit suicide as compared to a matched comparison group (Thong, Su, Chan & Chia, 2008).

Wanting to support himself independently, Pete had left school after his GCE 'O' levels, completed National Service, and joined the Singapore Armed Forces for approximately four years. He was subsequently employed in various contract delivery positions. Despite being gainfully employed throughout his life, he did not gain much satisfaction from work. He attributed this to his limited interest for his work and his unwillingness to form strong relationships with others.

Pete had stayed with Madam Lim throughout his growing years and into his adulthood. After her diagnosis with cancer, Pete had expressed resentment and anger over his need to care for her. He had even lost control of his emotions on one occasion and physically abused her, shoving her till she fell down. He had felt extremely guilty after this and had subsequently engaged a domestic helper to help look after her. Pete's resentment over Madam Lim's helplessness did not subside and he eventually sent her to stay with his adopted brother, Henry. This, he said, was to prevent possible future abuse towards her. Madam Lim passed away in the hospital after her illness took a turn for the worse.

Pete's psychosocial functioning had deteriorated after Madam Lim's death. Minimal contact with his adopted brother coupled with shallow relationships with colleagues and friends had increased his social isolation. While earlier thoughts about suicide had been fleeting, he started to contemplate suicide in earnest, and made three attempts to take his own life. Because he felt responsible for his godmother's death, ending his own life seemed to be the only fitting form of self-punishment. In fact, contemplating or attempting suicide gave him a "sense of relief", as he felt that it could make up for his loss of self-identity and unfulfilling relationships. He was a staunch Buddhist and his belief in reincarnation meant that after death, he could "recreate [himself] as someone else".

Without social support, Pete coped by retreating into a fantasy world in which he belonged to a closely knit family that cared for him. He shared that his coping strategy had proved to be useful in dealing with challenging life events. For example, when faced with difficulties, he sometimes imagined dying and being reincarnated as a wealthy individual with a loving family. In reality, Pete described his relationships with others as "superficial and manipulative". He would only keep in contact with others when he needed something from them, and made no attempts to maintain a relationship with them otherwise. He was uncomfortable interacting with others in a group and would quickly lose interest in friends with different interests. Furthermore, he rationalised that keeping a distance from people would "protect" him from future hurt and abandonment. Consequently, he had ended previous intimate relationships when he felt unable to cope with higher levels of commitment.

Prior to his incarceration for stealing a motor vehicle, he had been convicted twice for the same offence. These had resulted in jail sentences of less than a month on both occasions. He felt unable to hold back: "it was so thrilling to ride different bikes despite having my own bike. Nothing else gives me so much pleasure".

Pete was assessed through clinical interviews which were partially structured on two assessment tools, the Suicide Risk Assessment Questionnaire (SRAQ; Singapore Prison Service, 2004) and the Adult Attachment Interview (AAI; Main & Goldwyn, 1998). In addition, Pete completed the Personality Assessment Inventory (PAI; Morey, 1991) to gain a better understanding of his personality structure in order to determine the treatment approach.

The SRAQ is commonly used as a guide in assessing suicide risk factors and augments the information gleaned from a structured interview to provide an estimated rating of an individual's risk of suicide. This instrument was developed within the Singapore Prison Service. It takes into account factors such as the presence and frequency of symptoms, past suicide attempts, current suicide plans, and resources or support available to the individual.

Assessment using the SRAQ concluded that Pete was at high risk of suicide—his most recent suicide attempt had been within the last two months, and he had specific plans to end his life within two weeks of his release from prison. He also had the means

---

Fact Box 14.2. Suicidal Behaviour Disorder

There is currently insufficient evidence for suicidal behaviour disorder to be recognized as a disorder in DSM-5. The following represents a proposed set of criteria which requires further research:

- Within the last 24 months, the individual has made a suicide attempt

- The act does not meet criteria for non-suicidal self-injury—that is, it does not involve self-injury directed to the surface of the body undertaken to induce relief from a negative/cognitive state or to achieve a positive mood state

- The diagnosis is not applied to suicidal ideation or to preparatory acts

- The act was not initiated during a state of delirium or confusion

- The act was not undertaken solely for a political or religious objective

- Specify if:

    1. Current: Not more than 12 months since the last attempt

    2. In early remission: 12–24 months since the last attempt

to carry out his suicide act—access to codeine tablets. Although overdosing on codeine was not specifically lethal, it had the potential to cause death.

AAI is an interview protocol that provides a current assessment of a client's childhood experiences with caregivers (Hesse, 1999). It was used to gain insight into Pete's current view of his attachment to his birth parents and godmother. Relationships were always significantly challenging for Pete in his growing years. It was hypothesised that this was due to a lack of secure caregivers, coupled with rejection by his birth parents. The results confirmed the presence of resentment and poor relationships with his natural parents who barely maintained contact with him. His childhood experience of abandonment by his parents and his dependency on his godmother were likely causes for Pete's fear of relationships and being close to others.

The PAI is a self-report assessment that allows for an in-depth understanding of an individual's personality features and current stressors. It has been found to be useful in deciphering challenging clinical presentations that are prevalent in the criminal justice system (Ruiz & Ochshorn, 2010). The results of the PAI were consistent with a depressive profile with evident suicide ideation. In addition, they indicated the possible presence of a paranoid personality disorder. Individuals with paranoid personality disorder are characterised as being mistrustful, hostile and abrasive in their interactions with others. Additionally, they are likely to hold rigid views that can instigate arguments with others (Strack, 1999). These characteristics were highlighted in Pete's strong endorsement of items such as "I have to be alert to the possibility that people will be unfaithful", "People have to earn my trust", and "People around me are (not) faithful to me".

DIAGNOSIS

Using the DSM-5, Pete met diagnostic criteria for major depressive disorder (MDD, moderate severity) and paranoid personality disorder. It was important to differentiate Pete's diagnosis of MDD from a normal grief response towards his godmother's death. This is especially since bereavement as an exclusion criterion for depression has been removed from the DSM-5. The key features of grief include feelings of emptiness and loss while a major depressive episode is characterised by persistent low mood and the inability to anticipate pleasure. Another key distinction is that grief is usually associated with a preoccupation with thoughts and memories of the deceased, whereas MDD is usually associated with self-criticism and negative rumination, which was more consistent with Pete's presentation.

INTEGRATIVE FORMULATION

Predisposing Factors

Pete's early experiences were a key predisposing factor of his current difficulties. His relationship with his birth parents had been highly unstable while his attachment to

Madam Lim had been ambivalent. A lack of important relationships in early childhood can cause stunted development in terms of emotional closeness to others in adulthood (Scroufe et al.,1999), and the rejection from his birth parents consequently hampered his ability to form secure relationships.

Individuals with secure attachments seek emotional support from persons close to them during a distressing event. In contrast, those with an avoidant attachment style often had childhood experiences that intensified their social isolation, which causes them to experience a decrease in self-worth whenever they require assistance from others, and when they feel restricted in their ability for emotional closeness (Scroufe et al., 1999). Pete, for example, was unwilling to seek social support as it would demonstrate a "lack of control over my life". His mistrustful personality further increased his aversion towards relationships and interpersonal conflict. He was unable to maintain close relationships with others as he oscillated between suspiciousness of the motives of those around him and the desire to be close to others.

Precipitating Factors

Pete's suicidal behaviour was precipitated by his unresolved grief after the death of Madam Lim. According to Worden (2001), abnormal grief reactions usually arise from a survivor's dependency on the deceased. While Pete claimed not to be close to his godmother, he revealed that they were dependent on each other. His abnormal grief reactions may have been further complicated by inadequate early attachment engendered by parental rejection. Such an attachment can increase the likelihood an individual will experience depression when important relationships are lost later in life (Scroufe et al., 1999). In this instance, Pete's depression was directly related to his extreme guilt for abusing his godmother and for not fulfilling her last wishes. This, coupled with a lack of social support, further compromised his self-worth and worsened his depressive thoughts, and led him to consider ending his life.

The factor which most immediately precipitated his attempt to kill himself was his arrest for motor vehicle theft. His encounter with law enforcement reinforced his increased sense of hopelessness and futility to live. To Pete, it was a confirmation that he "did not deserve to live". Death was a "better option" than a guilt-stricken life.

Perpetuating Factors

Individuals with paranoid personality disorder often do not form close relationships with others. Another key characteristic of such individuals is an unwillingness to check the validity of their thoughts and impressions. They often hold strong convictions that their beliefs are universal truths without engaging in reality testing (Millon, 1999). This was congruent with Pete, who was unshakable in his erroneous belief that suicide was the only way to improve his "karma". Because he found it extremely difficult to accept alternative explanations or viewpoints, he would constantly argue with the prison's Buddhist monks and counsellors to justify his beliefs. Pete also held very rigid perspectives. He viewed any form of dependence on other person as a sign of weakness. When it was pointed out that the idea of over-dependence rather than dependence was problematic, he shared that he had never seen the difference previously.

Two other prominent features of Pete's difficulties in forming relationships were his tendency to be abrasive and argumentative in his interactions, and his warped perspective of relationships. His past relationships had always been tenuous and were simply a means to an end. Thus Pete would not hesitate to take advantage of persons close to him to further his personal gains (Millon, 1999). Despite this, Pete yearned for supportive relationships and often fantasised about being a successful individual with a loving family in a bid to experience some semblance of a positive connection with other human beings, which persons with paranoid personality disorder do crave (Millon, 1999).

Pete's poor self-image and fluctuating self-perception also maintained his suicide ideation. His perception of himself varied from one of self-recrimination and harsh self-criticism to one of an inflated sense of self-confidence (Millon, 1999). At one moment, he would feel like a "nobody" and express resignation at having to "get through the day without anyone talking to me". The next moment, he would claim to have chosen to limit his levels of social interaction with others because they "were not good conversation partners" and were not "stimulating" enough for him. One moment, he was a lone motorbike rider, whom no one deigned to notice, and his work was menial and inconsequential. The next moment, he was a thrill-seeker who lived life on the edge, and who did not associate with people who were "inferior" to him at work. It was this former image which supported his depressive thoughts and encouraged his suicidality.

Protective Factors

While it was not mandatory for him to attend counselling in prison, his high risk of suicide and his suicidal ideation necessitated the need for engagement in therapy and duty of care. Although Pete had expressed doubt and cynicism towards the benefits of treatment, he was willing to give it a try. His openness toward therapy was essential for progress during treatment; his strong faith in Buddhism was also deemed to be an area of strength for him.

PROGNOSIS

Pete's reduction in suicide ideation and depressive symptoms was only expected if he engaged in treatment. It was anticipated that progress would be slow and difficult, and that gains made in therapy could easily be undone because of Pete's rigidity of thought and suspicious personality features. Helping individuals with challenging personality features involves raising their awareness of the maladaptive aspects of their personality disorder and teaching them to manage it in order to live a more fulfilling life. This generally requires long-term psychotherapy between a motivated client and a skilled therapist. A good prognosis for Pete was thus limited by his ambivalent motivation and the short duration available for therapy.

TREATMENT

For suicide treatment to be successful, Berman (2006) emphasised reducing the acute risk for suicide and any underlying suicidal thinking. Therefore, Pete's therapist's first act was to ascertain whether crisis intervention was required. That Pete did not verbalise any immediate plans to commit suicide and was under heightened monitoring within the prison system mitigated his immediate physical safety.

Given the complexity of suicidal behaviour and the varied reasons for an individual's suicidal ideation, many clinicians adopt a mix-and-match approach towards treatment. However, this can result in increased confusion for the client (Rudd, 2000). It is thus important to have a clear treatment approach grounded in theory and research. While current literature on therapy targetting suicidal behaviour is sparse, Comtois and Linehan (2006) have advocated the use of cognitive behavioural therapy

Fact Box 14.3. Attachment Styles

In a simple study, Hazan and Shaver (1987) provided participants with three descriptions of attachment styles (see below) and asked them to rate which was characteristic of the way they behaved in intimate relationships. The majority of participants rated themselves as secure (60%), while the rest rated themselves as avoidant (20%) and anxious (20%) respectively.

Secure Attachment Style. I find it relatively easy to get close to others and am comfortable depending on them and having them depend on me. I don't worry about being abandoned or about someone getting too close to me.

Avoidant Attachment Style. I am somewhat uncomfortable being close to others; I find it difficult to trust them completely, difficult to allow myself to depend on them. I am nervous when anyone gets too close, and often, others want me to be more intimate than I feel comfortable being.

Anxious Attachment Style. I find that others are reluctant to get as close as I would like. I often worry that my partner doesn't really love me or won't want to stay with me. I want to get very close to my partner, and this sometimes scares people away.

(CBT) as an effective treatment. Pete's therapist chose CBT treatment because it would allow Pete to challenge his maladaptive and depressive thoughts.

Because of his mistrustful and paranoid nature, rushing the initial phase of establishing a therapeutic alliance would have caused Pete to quickly disengage from treatment. His therapist thus spent their first four sessions on rapport building and assessment. Rather than challenging his suicidal tendencies from the outset, she reframed thoughts about ending his life as a coping mechanism in the presence of unbearable pain (Jobes, 2000). Validating his views and beliefs about suicide prevented him from feeling as though she was attempting to assert control over him. Futhermore, discussing suicide as an unhelpful coping strategy gave him the opportunity to consider alternative, helpful coping methods (Jobes, 2000). To ensure his immediate safety, she made a no-suicide contract with him, in which he agreed to inform her or his prison officer of any drastic increase in suicide ideation. Pete also agreed not to harm himself throughout his prison stay. These initial steps were vital in keeping him engaged in later sessions.

FIGURE 14.1. ADAPTED FROM THE CBT MODEL OF SUICIDE BY MATTHEWS, 2012

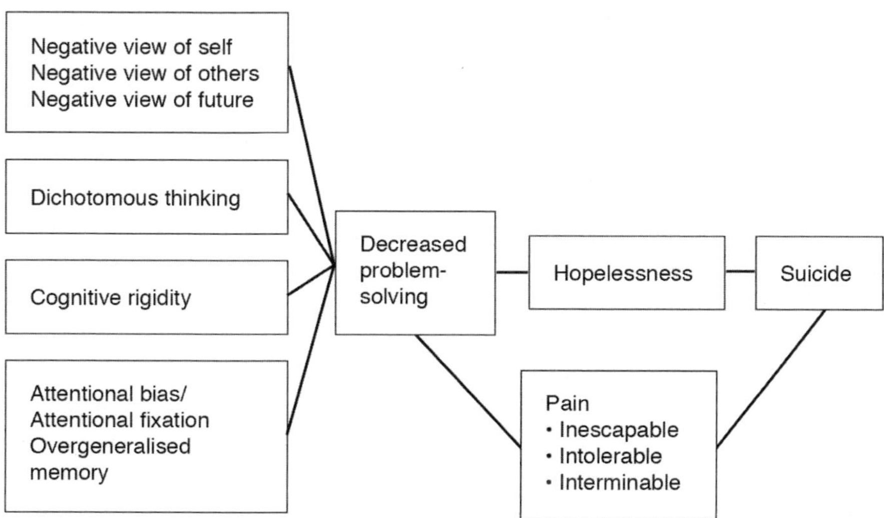

In order for CBT to be most effective, an intensively collaborative approach was adopted. Pete thus worked with his therapist to come up with treatment goals: to reduce his suicidal intent and increase his will to live. He was sceptical about attaining these goals however. He also agreed to work on maladaptive thoughts related to his godmother's passing. Pete's treatment plan was designed according to the principles of CBT for suicidality. The suicidal belief system is characterised by hopelessness and supported by three core beliefs, namely, unlovability ("I don't deserve to live"), helplessness ("I can't solve this") and poor distress tolerance ("I can't stand the pain anymore") (Rudd, 2000). The specific areas addressed in Pete's treatment plan were adapted from the CBT model of suicide (*see* Figure 14.1).

Pete's prison sentence was relatively short. Thus psychological treatment was brief and focused on the alteration of suicidal intent. As individuals with paranoid personality disorder require time to feel safe within a therapeutic space in which they can process issues discussed with greater openness (Millon, 1999), ten bi-monthly sessions were planned for Pete's therapy. Having a fortnight between sessions also allowed him sufficient time to absorb the material taught and to apply the techniques learnt outside of therapy. These CBT sessions included the following treatment components—psycho-education, cognitive restructuring, behavioural experiments and affective awareness. After each component was broadly introduced, Pete was given homework that aimed at reinforcing alternative, adaptive thinking and reducing suicidal intent. Throughout therapy, care was taken not to dismiss or prejudge Pete's views.

A major feature of CBT treatment was tackling Pete's thoughts about living and dying. While earlier sessions simply explored Pete's suicidal motivations, later sessions were aimed at increasing his ambivalence towards suicide through explorations of the costs and benefits of living and dying. Together with his therapist, he learnt to identify his reasons for living and to challenge his maladaptive thoughts about death. Helping him to understand his relationships with others was another important focus of treatment as Pete's primary difficulties arose from a lack of secure relationships. Pete was encouraged to examine his thoughts and beliefs regarding his relationships with his godmother, his birth parents and others. This allowed him to resolve some of the loss he experienced following his godmother's death. Finally, behavioural training involved improving Pete's ability to engage his fellow inmates positively. Pete's therapist guided his evaluation of these interactions and worked with him to devise solutions to address the challenges he faced in relating to people. It was necessary to focus on relationships in suicide intervention to encourage alternatives to suicide, which can be considered the ultimate rejection of all relationships (Jobes, 2000).

Various challenges arose during treatment. Firstly, because of Pete's abrasive and argumentative nature, there were times when he would disagree vehemently with his therapist, even when he did not have any strong basis for his arguments. So, when a day came during which that he doggedly persisted in his claim that he made decisions through "careful consideration" and the "weighing of the pros and cons", his therapist set him homework—to revisit how he made decisions. Pete returned to the following session, acknowledging that he did, in fact, make decisions impulsively. Secondly, Pete tended to focus primarily on his guilt and negative affect and failed to see positive nature of events such as rekindling his relationship with his brother. Despite her awareness of his personality features and depression, his constant cynicism and negativity could be draining to his therapist.

By the end of treatment, Pete's suicide risk, as measured by the SRAQ, had been reduced from High to Moderate. Pete shared that his suicide ideation had decreased and that he was hopeful of making positive changes to his life. While his fantasies still involved creating a warm and loving family, he envisioned them happening in this life, upon his release from prison, rather than in his "next life after reincarnation". His relationship with his adopted brother, Henry, had also improved. Despite overcoming his conviction that Henry's visits were a form of obligation, he continued to assume that other people's positive acts stemmed from ulterior motives. However, he was no longer as adamant that suicide was the only "way out". As he became less rigid in his thought, he also became more willing to consider living as an option. This upward trend was predicted to continue as long as Pete reached out and engaged in forming relationships with others despite the possibility of being hurt.

Pete was encouraged to voluntarily seek treatment at a Family Service Centre near his home after his release from prison, in the hope it would strengthen his will to live and bolster his ability to deal with his past difficulties. His adopted brother was also informed about Pete's suicide ideation and they were both provided a list of available mental health and support resources and contact information.

DISCUSSION

Suicide is a challenging issue for clinicians as it involves potential death. Collaborative effort between a therapist and client is important as the client has to learn to take responsibility for his life from the beginning to facilitate treatment efficacy (Meichenbaum, 2005). For the therapist, training in assessing and managing suicide risk is vital as this is a common challenge in clinical settings. Although intervention with individuals whose suicide risk is extremely high and uncontrolled can be managed through enforcing restraints and involuntary admission, this does not encourage the formation of positive relationships—especially between family members and their clients—due to the restriction of visits and contact. Especially challenging for clients in the prison system is the building up of social support options while they are incarcerated. Besides family members, clinicians need to form a good working relationship with suicidal clients, as positive relationships are a primary protective factor for people who are suicidal (Jobes, 2000). In Pete's case, a good therapist-client relationship was essential as he did not have other significant relationships at that point of time.

Pete's strong belief in Buddhism was initially thought to be a strong protective factor and was thus targeted to provide support towards living. However, he was convinced that his suicidal intent was in line with his faith and was willing to argue with his religious counsellors over it. While his therapist understood that his personality features and rigid cognitions contributed to his beliefs, her lack of familiarity with Buddhist faith and practices made it difficult for her to address his maladaptive thoughts as they related to his religion. Given Singapore's multicultural and multireligious society, the use of culture and faith as reasons for maladaptive behaviour has to be manoeuvred with caution during psychotherapy. It may be necessary to work together with religious or spiritual leaders in formulating a treatment plan for individuals who view religion as important in order to provide the most useful intervention to the client.

Although the intended focus of treatment was to increase Pete's options for living, it was inevitable that the issues underlying his personality structure came to the fore. For example, the use of CBT techniques to increase alternatives to suicide and to boost his reasons for living also helped create doubt in Pete's mind with regard to the validity of his paranoid or maladaptive beliefs. This highlights the dynamic nature of therapeutic interventions as it is impossible to target one specific problem, such as suicide ideation, without uncovering other problem that seemed equally important to address. A therapist thus has to remember to keep track of the treatment goals at all times so as to keep from taking on more than what was initially agreed upon with his or her client.

One key learning point for the therapist handling this case was the need to control some of her natural reactions at various points during the sessions. Overreaction or the desire to abandon the client has been reported when dealing with a difficult-to-treat client with suicide ideation (Berman, 2006). An understanding of Pete's interpersonal conduct allowed the therapist to manage her emotions in situations where his interactions would have normally incurred anger and exasperation (Millon, 1999). Any adverse reaction would have further cemented Pete's thinking about the futility of making connections with others. A therapist's loss of hope for a client who is resistant or demonstrating any improvement can negatively impact the therapeutic alliance and indirectly fortify the client's decision to end his life (Berman, 2006). While Pete's therapist did experience hopelessness at times in light of his impending release date, therapy supervision was instrumental in ensuring that she remained objective. This allowed the therapist to target her interventions in a more precise manner.

This case emphasises that an important feature of intervention with suicidal clients is helping them to develop a sense of responsibility for their decisions. The therapist's role is to facilitate their client's development of the ability to think, reflect and feel that their life is important and worth saving—though the final decision remains the client's (Gormley, 2004). As in Pete's case, the presentation of a personality disorder in a client contemplating suicide adds to the complexity of treatment and challenges the treatment process. However, regular and careful reflection under the continued support of her supervisor allowed his therapist to make progress in terms of increasing Pete's ambivalence towards suicide.

Two years after the end of intervention, Pete made contact with his therapist to share that he still looked forward to life. Although he continued to face challenges with law enforcement, he was no longer suffering from depression or suicidal ideation.

1. Considering Pete's background and personality, how could the assessment of his condition be improved? Clearly state your rationale and limitations for your chosen assessment methods.
2. What are your own beliefs of suicide and how would this affect your conduct of an assessment/therapy with a client, such as Pete, presenting with suicide ideation?
3. Is there research evidence that points to suicidal behaviour as a disorder? How do you think it should be classified?
4. What are some of the key features of this therapist's treatment of Pete that allowed a positive outcome? What more could have been done?
5. What are some cultural or social features of suicide intervention that need to be considered in a Singaporean context? How would you reconcile suicide as a criminal offence when intervening with individuals who display strong suicide ideation?

CHAPTER 15.

THE GAME IS OVER. SO AM I.

Gambling Disorder

JULIA CY LAM AND MUNIDASA WINSLOW

INTRODUCTION

Evelyn was a 44-year-old, married, Chinese insurance agent with a gambling habit. A year ago she had allegedly committed an offence that had led to her recent charge of "assisting in the contravention of unlicensed moneylending activities". While on bail, she was referred by her lawyer to a private psychiatric clinic, to assess if she had any psychological conditions that might have compromised her judgement in the lead up to her offence, to evaluate if her reported symptoms of depression and insomnia were associated with any psychological condition, and to determine which factors could facilitate her treatment and rehabilitation if this was later deemed necessary.

BACKGROUND

Evelyn had a tough and lonely upbringing. She was the eldest of a family of six children, all of whom lived in a small, rented room and shared cooking and bathroom facilities with the flat's other tenants. She spent most of her time taking care of her younger siblings as her mother needed to work. Her father was an alcoholic as well as a problem gambler, and there were frequent bouts of domestic violence towards the children. He left the family for another woman when Evelyn was 13 years old. This threw her mother into depression and she resorted to drinking, which further alienated her from her children.

Evelyn never felt loved by her parents, and received little attention from them. She felt obliged to take care of her younger siblings, and was resentful that she could not enjoy her childhood and do things other girls her age could do. She was close to and confided in her second sister. However, her sister committed suicide after a failed romantic relationship when Evelyn was 20.

After completing her GCE 'O' levels, Evelyn worked in the service industry, at first as a sales assistant and later as a waitress. She met her Korean husband, Hae Yong, at a friend's gathering when she was 20 and they married the same year, shortly after her sister's passing. She was "in a hurry" to marry because she could not wait to leave her overcrowded family home to start a new life. Immediately after their marriage, the couple moved to Korea for six years before returning to Singapore because of Hae Yong's work. They had two children, each with very different needs. Jonathan—18 years old—was gifted and currently serving his National Service. Crystal—8 years old—was the child of an unplanned pregnancy and had Down Syndrome. She was attending a special needs school for children with intellectual disability. Caring for Crystal gave Evelyn a lot of "stress and sadness", especially since Evelyn felt that she was the only person who understood Crystal. The differences between the two children led to great disharmony within the family.

Evelyn had begun hearing voices and "seeing things" in her teens. Her auditory hallucinations had become more frequent in the past two years, and Jonathan and her colleagues had occasionally observed her talking to herself. During her intake assessment, she disclosed that she had previously been bullied and touched inappropriately by persons living in her neighbourhood. However, she had never told anyone about these experiences. To deal with the chronic low mood, insomnia and migraines she had experienced since her teens, Evelyn had sought treatment from a psychiatrist when she was in her early 20s. She was prescribed anti-depressants and Valium (a benzodiazepine / hypnotic) to manage her mood and sleep. However, these medications had "slowed her down", so she had stopped taking them. She regularly self-medicated when she had migraines, but when these became unbearable, she would take an excessive dose of painkillers and sleeping pills to help her fall asleep and to "numb herself". At times she would drink a whole bottle of wine to calm her nerves, to sleep and to feel happier.

Over the past ten years, Evelyn had visited multiple GPs for prescriptions of sleeping pills. The main consequence of her chronic use of these pills was an increased tolerance, which further disrupted her sleep. Even if she had been able to fall asleep the night before, she always felt terrible the next morning—lonely and depressed. She had been hospitalized four times in the last five years for overdosing on sleeping pills. Nobody had visited her each time.

Evelyn had become a full-time, licensed insurance agent in 2005. She loved and excelled in her work, which was the "only source of hope and satisfaction" in her life. Her work was more productive when her mood and sleep were better, as was her ability to take care of her children. As for her husband, his job required him to be stationed in Korea and he only returned home once every three months. When he was back in Singapore, Hae Yong would occupy himself by watching TV and did not appear to show any concern for her or for their children. Most of the time, Evelyn described her marriage as "plain water and cordial". However, when she tried to talk with Hae Yong they usually wound up quarrelling. The couple's sex life had ceased after Crystal's birth eight years ago. Four years later, Evelyn found out her husband had been having an affair overseas. She had subsequently overdosed on sleeping pills and was hospitalized.

Evelyn described herself as stubborn, impulsive and straightforward. She had trained herself to be strong and autonomous as there was "nobody I can count on in life". Apart from giving her mother a monthly allowance, she had no other contact with her family of origin. Although she put on a lively and outgoing front, she confessed that she was lonely and depressed. She tended to keep things to herself and could not recall when she had last felt happy. She considered her three cats her only "friends" who would keep her company. Evelyn had no hobbies until the opening of the Resorts World Sentosa (RWS) casino in 2010, which introduced her to the world of gambling. She began frequenting the casino most evenings and soon became a regular customer. Despite her aversion to crowded places, she found refuge in the casino, where she could "be herself" without anyone caring about what she did. She could sit alone, smoke and drink freely. In fact, she only ever smoked and drank in the casino. Apart from work, playing baccarat became her only interest in life. She also spent a lot of time on jackpot machines, mesmerized by their sounds and images. Preoccupied with her games, she did not have time to think about her problems.

However, gambling had its pitfalls. As Evelyn's gambling bets increased, she became more preoccupied, frequented the casino at irregular hours after putting Crystal to bed with the domestic helper, and usually stayed at the casino for at least six hours each time. She lost more often than she won. Although she had begun by gambling alone, she soon met some new gambling friends. They offered her companionship, and seemed to share a common interest—to conquer the games at the casino tables and to have a good time. Egged on by her "friends", Evelyn started chasing her gambling losses. She eventually lost all her income and savings, had to sell the family house after a year of gambling, and had to move her family into a rented HDB flat. Her husband was alarmed, but did nothing about the move. Her losses were significant, totalling about $300,000. She went on to pawn most of her jewellery, including her wedding ring and a Titus watch her husband had given her. She approached her relatives and colleagues for loans, until she ran out of goodwill.

As her gambling escalated, Evelyn became suicidal after big losses and had overdosed on 30 sleeping pills each time. Out of guilt and desperation, she had applied for Voluntary Self-Exclusion with the National Council on Problem Gambling (NCPG) to ban herself from entering casinos after her discharge from the hospital. Without gambling, however, she began to rely more on alcohol and sleeping pills to cope with the stressors in her life. Occasionally, when her resolve weakened, she would go on cruise ships to gamble. After the expiration of her one-year Exclusion Order, she glued herself to casino tables and jackpot machines once again. Her gambling problem worsened and she began to chalk up higher debts.

Two years into heavy gambling, Evelyn's gambling debts hit new highs and she began to borrow money from five to six unlicensed, illegal moneylenders (also known as "loansharks" locally). Initially, she was able to make payments to them as she was still earning an income as an insurance agent. However, her gambling soon went out of control. She became "another person" when she gambled—someone who had no fear about losing. Gambling put her in a "numb and hypnotic-like" state. She did not feel any pain in parting with her money. Winning was the means of prolonging her game, whereas losing her hard-earned money was justifiable punishment of herself and her family for their lack of attention towards her.

Evelyn eventually fell into the trap of one of the loansharks who kept depositing money into her bank account without her permission and charging her interest. He then pressured her into opening a new bank account, and into giving him her ATM card and Personal Identification Number (PIN). Two months later, she was approached by police officers, asking her to assist in their investigations. She was subsequently charged with "assisting unlicensed moneylenders' activities".

ASSESSMENT

A thorough clinical interview was conducted across two days, for a total of four hours. A talkative Chinese lady who appeared guarded and defensive, Evelyn was a woman of average weight and height, who looked much younger than her actual age, was well-dressed and appropriately groomed. Her eyes were swollen from crying and a lack of sleep. She was forthcoming about events that led to her arrest, and understood the rationale for a psychological assessment. However, she could not understand how her emotions had affected her gambling behaviour to result in her current plight.

Her assessment provided an opportunity to a) gain information about Evelyn's current presenting problems and background; b) assess her strengths, weaknesses, and support systems; and c) identify triggers to her gambling and enrol her in a gambling counselling program. Techniques of Motivational Interviewing and the Stage of Change Model (Prochaska and DiClemente, 1982) were adopted to assess Evelyn's readiness to change her gambling behaviour. Motivational Interviewing focused on how important it was for Evelyn to change her gambling behaviour, as well as how confident she felt about doing it. The Stage of Change Model was used to identify which stage (i.e., Pre-contemplation, Contemplation, Preparation, Action, Maintenance or Termination/Relapse) she was at in order to match treatment strategies. She was assessed to be at the Stage of Contemplation.

Involvement of family members in therapy facilitates the process of a client's behavioural change. Despite Hae Yong knowing about Evelyn's legal issue, however, he refused to get involved in her therapy. Evelyn did not tell her children about her offence and charges. She was also evasive when asked if her siblings or colleagues could be interviewed.

The Diagnostic Interview on Pathological Gambling (DIPG) was used to collect information about Evelyn's gambling problem (Table 15.1) and to determine if she met diagnostic criteria for a Gambling Disorder (Table 15.2). Her frequency and quantity of alcohol and sleeping pill use were also assessed. She was also administered the Beck Depression Inventory (BDI-II) and Beck Anxiety Inventory (BAI) to gauge both the baseline level and the severity of depression and anxiety symptoms. Findings from the assessment indicated that she suffered from a Gambling Disorder, and that she used alcohol and sleeping pills to medicate her low mood. Her scores on both BDI-II and BAI were in the severe range, which were consistent with her clinical presentation.

DIAGNOSIS

Evelyn's presentation was consistent with DSM-5 criteria for Gambling Disorder (formerly known as "Pathological Gambling" in DSM-IV) at the time when she committed the offence, meeting all the diagnostic criteria (Table 15.2). The Diagnostic Interview On Pathological Gambling (DIPG) was developed as a structured assessment of different aspects related to the history and evolution of a person's gambling problem). She met criteria for the category of an "Escape Gambler", who gambles to escape/avoid facing life problems (Lesieur & Blume, 1991).

Section	
1	Motives for consultation
2	Games that lead to a partial or complete loss of control
3	Information on the development of gambling habits
4	Information on current gambling problem
5	DSM-IV Diagnostic Criteria
6	Consequences of the gambling problem
7	Suicidal ideation
8	Current living conditions
9	Other dependencies (present or past)
10	Mental health—prior experiences
11	Strengths and available resources
12	Comments

TABLE 15.1. DIAGNOSTIC INTERVIEW ON PATHOLOGICAL GAMBLING (DIPG)

Evelyn had a history of clinical depression, suicidal attempts and insomnia, and these difficulties had been exacerbated by her severe financial problems following her gambling problems. She was diagnosed with Major Depressive Disorder of moderate severity. Considering her vague suicidal thoughts, sense of hopelessness and ongoing prescription of sleeping pills, she was assessed with a moderate risk of self-harm. Although she frequently used sleeping pills (benzodiazepines) and had also overdosed on sleeping pills in her past suicidal attempts, she did not meet the criteria for Hypnotic Use Disorder.

<table>
<tr><td>

TABLE 15.2. DSM-5 DIAGNOSTIC CRITERIA FOR GAMBLING DISORDER (312.31; APA 2013)

</td></tr>
<tr><td>

A. Persistent and recurrent problematic gambling behaviour leading to clinically significant impairment or distress, as indicated by the individual exhibiting four (or more of the following in a 12-month period:

1. Needs to gamble with increasing amounts of money in order to achieve the desired excitement.
2. Is restless or irritable when attempting to cut down or stop gambling.
3. Has made repeated unsuccessful efforts to control, cut back, or stop gambling.
4. Is often preoccupied with gambling (e.g., having persistent thoughts of reliving past gambling experiences, handicapping or planning the next venture, thinking of ways to get money with which to gamble.
5. Often gambles when feeling depressed (e.g., helpless, guilty, anxious, depressed).
6. After losing money gambling, often returns another day to get even ("chasing" one's losses).
7. Lies to conceal the extent of involvement with gambling.
8. Has jeopardized or lost a significant relationship, jobs, or educational or career opportunity because of gambling.
9. Relies on others to provide money to relieve desperate financial situations caused by gambling.

B. The gambling behaviour is not better explained by a manic episode.

</td></tr>
</table>

INTEGRATIVE FORMULATION

Predisposing Factors

Evelyn grew up in an environment where gambling and drinking were part of her parents' lives. Her father was an alcoholic and problem gambler. Her mother had a history of clinical depression and used alcohol to cope with life's adversities. Her second sister had committed suicide after a relationship breakup. It is possible she adopted the same behavioural patterns to cope with life stressors.

Evelyn's propensity to take care of others (her siblings when she was younger, and later, her daughter) and having to put others' needs and interests first led to a denial of her own needs and interests. Her chronic marital difficulties and a non-supportive husband led to ongoing feelings of unhappiness, emptiness and loneliness. Some of her core beliefs which contributed to these negative states were: "I am all on my own", "Nobody will be there for me" and, "I do not deserve love and attention". Coupled with her impulsive personality, when faced with overwhelming life stressors, she quickly found refuge in the casino. She discovered gambling to be a way to escape from her problems, and to free herself from the pain of these problems.

Precipitating Factors

The opening of the casino, the excitement of gambling and the opportunity of meeting new friends, all made gambling an attraction to end Evelyn's monotonous yet stressful life. However, snowballing gambling debts, having to sell the family house, and drying up financial resources from her family, relatives and colleagues, caused a recurrence in her depression and suicidal attempts, and an increased use of sleeping pills and alcohol to self-medicate her low mood.

Perpetuating Factors

Living with the chronic stressors of her daughter's Down Syndrome, overwhelming gambling debts, and boredom with little or no family support, Evelyn became more preoccupied with gambling, which allowed her to escape, albeit temporarily, her family and marital issues. She had limited coping skills when faced with stress, apart from self-medicating with alcohol, sleeping pills and gambling. She had little social support and no constructive hobbies to pass her time.

Similar to many gamblers, Evelyn harboured some cognitive distortions relating to her gambling. For example, she believed that if she continued gambling, she would be able to win back what she lost. She also had illusions of control and believed that she could control the jackpot machines she was using. Her daily visits to the casino, finding friendship and companionship at the casino, and the feeling that she was not alone but was surrounded by others of similar interest, reinforced her gambling habit.

Protective Factors

Evelyn had a limited number of protective factors. She had a resilient personality, having gone through a tough childhood where she had to both fend for herself and take care of others. Although she felt "very alone" as Crystal's sole caregiver, Evelyn felt that her daughter gave her a reason to continue living, and was her motivation to return to a non-gambling life.

Despite her difficulties, Evelyn had managed to maintain her job and had a good work record as an insurance agent. She took pride in her work and derived much satisfaction from her job. Her commitment to excel in her work motivated her to get well and to abstain from gambling as her insurance agent's licence would be revoked by the Monetary Authority of Singapore should she be convicted and have a criminal record. She saw her work as a source of hope and something that provided satisfaction in life. Her work was also the only means by which she could support her children financially, rebuild her family and reclaim her life.

Evelyn also demonstrated some insight into her gambling problem as she had previously taken the initiative to obtain a self-exclusion order from the casino. Her current Voluntary Self-Exclusion Order would hopefully fortify her determination to abstain from gambling.

PROGNOSIS

The prognosis of gambling disorder without treatment can be bleak and result in debilitating financial predicaments, interpersonal, occupational, emotional and behavioural problems. Many pathological gamblers end up engaging in illegal acts to finance their gambling behaviour or to repay gambling debts. Untreated gambling disorder is likely to jeopardize occupational functioning, particularly for someone like Evelyn who, other than possessing an insurance agent's licence, had limited work skills. A prison sentence would have a serious impact on the functioning of her daughter and family. Evelyn was motivated to abstain from gambling and had applied for a Voluntary Self-Exclusion Order.

Similar to an alcohol or substance addiction—which share features of tolerance and withdrawal but without obvious physical signs—pathological gambling is one of the most difficult behavioural addictions to treat. By the time a person is aware of the dangers of gambling, they would usually have already experienced severe financial repercussions, and impairments to their interpersonal relationships, work and leisure activities. Comorbidities like substance use, insomnia and depression are common (George & Murali, 2005). For Evelyn, continued gambling could result in another attempted suicide through an overdose of sleeping pills, gambling-related crimes like forgery, embezzlement and fraud, or working for loansharks to clear her gambling debts.

Factors that could improve her prognosis included regular attendance and compliance with therapy, a closer relationship with her family members, stable work, meeting new friends, developing new hobbies to fill her time and learning appropriate coping skills. It was also important to treat her comorbidities. Evelyn had a chronic history of undertreated depression. Depression without treatment can be lethal, as persons with this condition could resort to suicide to end their suffering. Evelyn's psychologist believed that she would benefit from medication to alleviate her mood. For her insomnia, learning proper sleep hygiene and engaging in regular physical exercise were introduced to replace her habit of relying on sleeping pills.

TREATMENT

Despite presenting as an Escape Gambler, who used gambling to self-medicate, Evelyn's gambling problems were secondary to her depression and relational issues. Her goals for therapy thus included abstaining from gambling, developing new coping skills, and maintaining a work-life balance with new hobbies. Three main areas were identified for targeted treatment: Evelyn's gambling disorder, major depressive disorder and insomnia/sleeping pill dependence.

While Evelyn readily accepted treatment for her depression by taking anti-depressants, she was reluctant to commence treatment for her gambling disorder. She reasoned that she had no more money left to gamble with and was thus not at risk of further gambling. However, when her psychologist pointed out that prior to her arrest, she had borrowed money from relatives and colleagues, as well as unlicensed moneylenders, Evelyn realised that if left untreated, she was likely to commit further illegal activities in order to finance her gambling. She stopped denying treatment for her gambling disorder.

Based on Evelyn's assessment and formulation, her psychologist proposed 10–12 weekly Cognitive Behavioural Therapy (CBT) sessions, in conjunction with brief family therapy and medical consultation. Her treatment goal was abstinence from gambling. CBT has been found to be an effective approach in treating female gamblers (Dowling et al., 2006). While gambling treatment was not mandatory, Evelyn was aware of the association between her gambling and unintended offending. She was motivated to stay away from further gambling, and was ready to examine some of the core issues and beliefs which led to her compulsive gambling behaviour.

At the time of writing, Evelyn had attended ten therapy sessions over a period of three months. She turned up for nearly all her sessions. Two sessions were cancelled due to clashes with Crystal's medical appointments. Evelyn was diligent in completing her homework, and filled out a Daily Self-Monitoring Diary to chart her urge to gamble, her perceived control and any actual gambling behaviour, including the time and money she spent on it.

Adopting a multidisciplinary approach, Evelyn was reviewed by a psychiatrist fortnightly to monitor her mood and sleep. Selective Serotonin Reuptake Inhibitors (SSRIs) were prescribed to help reduce impulsive and compulsive behaviour (i.e., her urge to gamble), as well as to regulate her mood. Her sleeping pill use was also slowly tapered off with better sleep hygiene and a weekly physical exercise regime. She responded well to the treatment and her new lifestyle without gambling.

Evelyn also attended Gamblers Anonymous (GA) meetings twice a week in a community setting. GA is a self-help group modelled on Alcoholic Anonymous. It

Fact Box 15.1. Acupuncture for Gambling Addictions?

There is currently no evidence for acupuncture treatment specifically for gambling addiction. However, because addiction shares some similarities to substance abuse in clinical feature and neuropathology, some propose that acupuncture may show similar effects for gambling. The most recent review by the World Health Organisation (WHO, 2002) of the effectiveness of acupuncture rated the evidence base for alcohol, opiate and tobacco dependences as 'Category 2': therapeutic effect has been shown but further proof is needed. Reviews conclude that while not free from serious adverse events which are rare, acupuncture is relatively safe (Birch et al, 2004).

Acupuncture is one of the key components of Traditional Chinese Medicine (TCM) and has been practised for thousands of years. Traditionally used to address a wide array of ailments, it works by stimulating specific points on the body using a variety of techniques, including insertion of thin metal needles through the skin to remove blockages in the flow of *qi* and to restore health. In recent years, it has been developed internationally as part of an integrated treatment program to curb addictive disorders.

Acupuncture treatment for addictive disorders, including pathological gambling, is now available in Singapore at the National Addictions Management Service (NAMS), Institute of Mental Health (IMH). NAMS promotes acupuncture as a method for aiding addiction recovery by reducing the severity of withdrawal symptoms, pain and cravings, as well as the symptoms of some comorbid disorders such as mood disorder and anxiety. It is not intended as a substitute for primary treatment programs which are the mainstay of treatment for patients with addictive disorders (e.g., pathological gambling, internet addiction and substance dependence), but is used to complement and enhance these existing psychiatric and psychological treatment programs.

For more about treatments in Singapore, *see*: http://www.nams.sg/resources/Documents/Services. For psychological treatments and their effectiveness among *Asian* problem gamblers, *see* Raylu, N., Loom J., and Oei, T. (2013). "Treatment of gambling problems in Asia: Comprehensive review and implications for Asian problem gamblers". *Journal of Cognitive Psychotherapy*, *27*(3): 297–322.

utilizes the 12-step recovery program and is adapted for people with a gambling problem. GA filled her need for social support, and taught her that she was not alone in her fight to stop gambling. She was further referred to Credit Counselling Singapore (CCS) for help in sorting out her finances and in setting up a debt management program. She attended her appointment with CSS and for the first time in many years felt in control of her life.

Although family therapy was built-in as part of Evelyn's treatment, Hae Yong declined to be involved. Evelyn came to acknowledge the futility of saving her marriage and initiated a divorce. As her husband was not contesting the divorce, she planned to have full custody of her daughter.

In her earlier sessions, Evelyn experienced a lot of inner struggle arising from her deep sense of shame and guilt. She found it difficult to forgive herself easily. She encountered the usual life stressors faced by most recovering gamblers. For instance, she worried that her licence to practise as an insurance agent would be revoked because of her court case, and how this would increase the burden on her and limit her resources to care for her daughter with special needs. Not surprisingly, she experienced mood swings despite being put on medication.

Evelyn's therapy comprised behavioural and cognitive interventions. Her earlier sessions were focused on "Discovery". Evelyn discovered a lot about her unresolved issues, her triggers to gambling, her sense of helplessness and powerlessness. She eventually understood how her low mood and sleep difficulties had exacerbated her gambling behaviour and vice versa. She was taught to acknowledge her inner strengths, such as her resilient personality, her passion and commitment to work. She learnt the steps of effective problem-solving, and had a better understanding of her cognitive distortions (e.g., her illusions of control about jackpot machines). She was asked to consider alternative responses in situations where she would be prone to gamble.

Her later sessions were focused on "Recovery". She learnt about gambling relapse warning signs and relapse prevention skills. She also learnt about using more appropriate coping skills such as goal setting, time management, reframing, assertiveness, and self-care, and was made to challenge her own avoidant coping style. Instead of avoiding her problems, she tried to identify them and either work on a solution or accept her inability to change the situation. She was given homework in the form of a diary to fill out and document her thoughts and feelings after each session. This was used for discussion and as a means of monitoring her treatment progress during treatment sessions. She also obtained support from fellow problem gamblers whom she met at her GA meetings.

Evelyn's mood and sleep slowly improved and stabilized. Once in a while, she experienced strong urges to gamble, but was able to distract herself with other activities. She strolled with Crystal in the neighbourhood park in the evening, picked up needlework as her new hobby, and focused on her insurance sales. For her court case, a forensic psychological report was prepared highlighting her mental state as well as the circumstances she was in around the time when she committed the offence, together with her amenability to change, risk of future re-offending and treatment and rehabilitation progress. Evelyn was given a "Discharge not amounting to an acquittal" (DNAQ) for 12 months. This meant she had to keep away from any illegal activities for a period of 12 months, or the charge would be restored. Evelyn was very relieved and grateful for the outcome as she could keep her insurance agent's licence.

DISCUSSION

Gambling in Singapore is generally illegal apart from a few authorized activities managed by Singapore Turf Club and Singapore Pools (Lim, 2009). It is an exceptionally popular pastime among the Chinese population (Loo et al., 2008; Wong & Tse, 2003). When Singapore's two casinos first opened in 2010, a daily average of 20,000 visits by Singapore citizens and permanent residents was recorded. Three years later, the figures dropped to 17,000 visits daily. The Singaporean government, through the Casino Control Act, has put in place a number of social safeguards: a S$100 levy of entry fees for every 24 hours and a S$2,000 annual membership on Singapore citizens and permanent residents and, casino exclusion orders (voluntary self-exclusion, family exclusion and third-party exclusion) issued by the National Council on Problem Gambling (NCPG).

Fact Box 15.2. Gambling in Australia.

In Australia, the prevalence of problem gambling in the psychiatric population was more than four times that of the general community; and depression and substance abuse were commonly occurring problems among people with gambling problems.

In light of these findings, the following recommendations were made by Victorian Responsible Gambling Foundation:

- Education about the need for screening clients of mental health services for gambling problems is warranted

- The referral of people with mental health and gambling problems to specialist problem gambling services is indicated to improve access to care and to reduce the time it takes for this access to occur

Source: http://www.responsiblegambling.vic.gov.au

The annual report 2012–13 of the Casino Regulatory Authority of Singapore (CRAS) noted that 7.7% of the local adult population had made more than one visit to the casinos in the past three years. A Gambling Prevalence Survey of NCPG in 2011 reported rates of 1.4% and 1.2% as "probable pathological gamblers" and "probable problem gamblers" respectively among Singapore residents.

One would normally think an adult male who bets on soccer matches and participates in online gambling as a typical picture of a "pathological gambler". From our clinical practice, we have noted two main groups of problem gamblers: Action Gamblers and Escape Gamblers (Blaszczynski, 2000; Blaszczynski & Nower, 2002). Action Gamblers are mostly men, who are interested in "games of skill" like cards, sports betting, horse-racing and stock. They usually have an early onset (e.g., teens) of gambling. They falsely believe that there are systems, formula and statistics which they can work out in order to beat the odds.

Escape Gamblers, on the other hand, are usually women who gamble to escape problems, negative emotions and relationship issues. They are interested in "games of luck" like electronic gaming machines (or jackpot machines), 4D, TOTO and bingo, and gamble to numb their feelings. Female gamblers usually have a shorter gambling history and accumulate gambling debts very rapidly (Tang et al., 2007). Winning is viewed as a means to be able to gamble longer. Those who seek treatment usually present with a variety of complex problems and needs (Holdsworth et al., 2013). The onset of the disorder is usually in their 30s or 40s, and they reach the addictive stage of gambling three times faster (i.e., within a shorter period of time) than male gamblers. About a third to half of all gamblers are women. The majority of them (89–95%) are "Escape Gamblers" who prefer electronic gaming machines. About half of this group grew up with a parent or parents who had gambling and/or alcohol problems, and have themselves been dependent on something (e.g., sleeping pills, alcohol) other than gambling at some time in their life.

Female gamblers, in general, are often perceived more negatively compared to their male counterparts as they contradict the idea of the traditional role of the submissive housewife, which may render them less likely to come forward to seek treatment because of the stigma associated with therapy. Accessibility of legalized gambling (e.g., opening of casinos) is an important factor that fosters and accelerates the process of a female gambler developing a gambling disorder. Gambling provides a number of incentives to a gambler: escape from problems, relief from negative moods, empowerment to boost low self-esteem, a sense of freedom, the promise of the fulfillment of dreams and release of endorphins. Once inside a casino, demands or expectations from others fade away, replaced by a sense of empowerment and regained control not experienced in the female traditional role, and a sense of accomplishment in successfully attaining emotional numbness and oblivion.

Evelyn always tried her best to fit what she perceived to be her traditional role—a filial daughter, subservient wife, and responsible mother. Through the years, she had bottled up lots of negative emotions, emptiness, loneliness, helplessness and powerlessness. Her introduction to the casino had initially "set her free emotionally"; within years, she had an enormous price to pay: unsurmountable gambling debts, involvement with loansharks, and ultimately, her unwitting participation in criminal activities. Without intervention, this would be the typical progression of a person with gambling disorder in Singapore.

The very fact that female gamblers do not fit the picture of a typical gambler presents barriers to treatment. For example, there is more perceived shame and guilt, a greater fear of being judged, and the need to keep gambling and its associated problems a secret from spouses and children. The majority of problem gamblers, regardless of gender, are usually in denial. It is not uncommon for their contact point with gambling treatment to be the criminal justice system, be it a forensic assessment with regard to sentencing, or a mandatory treatment order granted by the court.

It is doubtful if Evelyn would have presented herself voluntarily for an assessment of her gambling problem and commenced treatment, if she had not encountered the criminal justice system. The majority of pathological gamblers commit offences late after the onset of the disorder and these offences are typically gambling-related (Rosenthal & Lorenz, 1992). About 70% of female gamblers have been found to have used illegal means (e.g., forgery, fraud, theft, or embezzlement) to finance their gambling habit. In a prison setting, about 30% of women inmates have gambling or gambling-related problems (Abbott & McKenna, 2005).

Treatment for Escape Gamblers utilizes a variety of modalities, including individual/group, family, medication, psychoeducation, vocational and counselling (legal, financial and recreational). The core treatment modality of problem gambling is CBT. Dowling et al. (2009) found that self-selected goals of treatment, be it "abstinence" or "controlled gambling", worked equally well in CBT. Self-help groups like Gamblers Anonymous, were found to be helpful, as was the development of social and coping skills.

Psychiatric comorbidities are common in problem gamblers (Teo et al., 2007), in whom lower subjective well-being has also been reported. In Evelyn's case, in addition to having gambling disorder, she also suffered from depression, insomnia, occasional misuse of sleeping pills and alcohol, and had attempted suicide several times. While treating these comorbidities is important, other crises or pressing issues like legal and financial predicaments should not be overlooked. Evelyn's treatment for clinical issues, for example, took place alongside her legal and financial concerns. As she was receiving treatment from a multidisciplinary team, psychiatric consultation was integrated to help stabilize and maintain her mental wellness.

The findings of the 2011 National Council on Problem Gambling (NCPG) survey highlighted some emerging concerns about a small group of low-income and frequent gamblers, who have poorer self-control and were into heavier gambling. There has also been an increase in the number of Casino Exclusion Orders made with the NCPG, whether voluntarily, by family members or by third-parties. As of October 2013, there were about 12,000 individuals under a Self-Exclusion Order, and another 1,600 persons under Family Exclusion Orders. Realizing the financial and emotional harm she was doing to herself and her family, Evelyn had applied for a self-exclusion order on three separate occasions. While an Exclusion Order can bar a gambler from entering the casinos, it does not stop them from gambling via other means like visiting overseas casinos, gambling on cruise ships, betting on 4D, TOTO and online gambling.

With the advance of technology, there are increasingly diverse ways one can gamble in the virtual world. Maintaining behavioural change in this arena is thus a constant challenge; slips, lapses and relapses are common in addiction recovery. The process of overcoming a gambling disorder is a long one, and individuals usually will have to persevere through the Stage of Change Model a few times. Public education about effects of excessive gambling and the availability of assessment and treatment services is thus essential in stopping gambling from becoming a major public health issue in Singapore.

DISCUSSION QUESTIONS

1. Female gamblers are often considered a "forgotten group". What are the similarities and differences between male and female gamblers? How would these inform treatment and prevention?

2. There are two main treatment approaches in problem gambling—abstinence versus controlled gambling. How realistic is it for patients to opt for "controlled gambling" as a treatment goal?

3. Is Gambling Problem more an Impulse Control Disorder or an Addictive Disorder? Why was the criterion "has committed illegal acts such as forgery, fraud, theft, or embezzlement to finance gambling" taken out of the DSM-5?

4. Casino Exclusion prohibits an individual from entering casinos in Singapore. There are three main types of Casino Exclusion—Self-Exclusion, Family Exclusion and Automatic Exclusion by Law. How effective is Self-Exclusion? What does it take to self-exclude oneself?

5. Would we still have the same gambling problems if there were no casinos in Singapore?

CHAPTER 16

KEEP CALM, IT'S NOT A HEART ATTACK

Panic Disorder

NISHTA GEETHA THEVARAJA AND GWEE KENJI

INTRODUCTION

Linda, a 36-year-old Chinese woman, sought treatment at a hospital for panic attacks after being troubled by them for a year. Upon consulting her psychiatrist, she was prescribed anti-anxiety medication. Because she was hoping for more ways to deal with her panic symptoms, Linda was subsequently referred to outpatient psychotherapy services for cognitive behaviour therapy (CBT).

At her first session, a visibly distraught Linda reported experiencing sudden panic attacks without any obvious trigger. She described being suddenly assailed by palpitations, cold and numb hands and feet, tingling feelings on her back, hyperventilation, choking feelings, feeling faint at times and an overwhelming dread that something bad was going to happen to her (e.g., a heart attack). She had panic attacks about twice a month, each lasting for about 30 minutes to an hour. At other times, she had experienced some panic symptoms, which did not develop into a full-blown episode.

Linda's first panic attack took place at home, late at night when everyone was asleep. She was suddenly beset by heart palpitations, cold sweat, numbness in her limbs and a feeling of choking. The thought arose that no one would be able to help her before she lost consciousness. She was in a state of shock and did not know how to deal with her unprecedented and overwhelming bodily sensations. Terrified, she woke her mother up in the midst of her panic attack, which only abated after an hour. Following this alarming experience, Linda grew very concerned about her health, especially her heart condition. As her father had experienced heart complications, she immediately assumed that her panic symptoms were indications of a potentially critical heart condition. Faced with Linda's distress and health-related complaints, family members often had to reassure her, reminding her to "relax", "take it easy" and not to "worry herself sick".

In therapy, a tearful Linda admitted that her health worries resulted in her constantly checking on her bodily symptoms, as she felt that these could alert her to a potential heart malfunction. For instance, she would check that her heart rate was even and without palpitations. She would also monitor the colour of her palms, soles, lips and fingernails, to ensure that they were not pale. When doing housework, she noticed that she would sometimes pant excessively. This caused her to feel exhausted and exacerbated concerns for her health. Shortly after her first panic attack, Linda went for a host of cardiology assessments and medical checks to evaluate her heart condition and numbness in her legs. No abnormalities were detected and she was given a clean bill of health. Her therapist ruled out other comorbid mental health conditions.

Because of her panic symptoms and her reading of religious scriptures with death-related content, Linda feared sleeping alone in her bedroom. As a result, she started to sleep on the couch in the hall. When asked if her condition was affecting her social life, she said that she had been dating someone exclusively for a few months, but had not "tortured" him with details of her health concerns for fear of putting him off. Linda enjoyed social interaction and talking to others. Interestingly, she was able to pinpoint with certainty that her panic attacks or symptoms never occurred when she was in conversation with others or giving talks at work, and only occurred when she was alone.

BACKGROUND

Linda described herself as an anxious individual, comparing herself to her family members. She had always feared death. For example, she recalled entering a room with a low ceiling and immediately feeling "like I was in a coffin". She experienced shortness of breath and felt like she was suffocating. She also had an "overly active imagination", and was capable of mentally recreating scenes and situations based on what she read in books and newspaper articles. Her family members would often tease her for being "dramatic", because she would fuss over and exaggerate details of her daily experiences. In therapy, Linda accepted that her imagination played a key role in "exaggerating" her panic symptoms to the extent that she genuinely believed that she was suffering from a heart condition.

Linda's father was her pillar of strength and role model. However, he was diagnosed with a chronic heart condition when she was in her late teens, and he passed away when she was 21 years old. As the eldest sibling of three younger brothers, Linda had to take on more responsibilities and provide for the family. Linda had been very close to her father. She would forlornly talk about how he had always wanted her to be independent. Linda looked up to her father as a "confidante" and "guide" and was often "impressed by his wisdom". She felt "safe and protected" when he was around because he often reassured her when she felt insecure or unsure about decisions she had to make. Although she had sought reassurance from other family members during and after her panic attacks over the past year, she felt that other family members would not be able to take the place of her father, as they were not as "credible". Months before his passing, Linda had constantly checked if her father's blood circulation was normal. She checked his palms, the soles of his feet and his fingernails to ensure that they were not pale. Perhaps due to how much he meant to her, her preoccupation with his bodily functions and vigilance about his health generalized into an acute awareness of her own bodily functions, which contributed directly to her panic attacks.

Linda was still confused as to how such frightening "heart attack–like" symptoms could not be indicative of an underlying heart-related condition. With much apprehension she heeded the advice of an Accident and Emergency consultant to seek psychiatric help because he had suspected that her symptoms and multiple hospital visits were the result of panic attacks.

Linda joined government services after graduation. Although she was thoroughly passionate about her work, she had resigned three years prior to psychological consultation. This decision was motivated by stress at work and her desire to explore other employment opportunities. Soon after, Linda set up her own private company, which afforded her flexible working hours. Following her panic attack however, she reduced her working hours to only 5–10 hours a week. Her earnings were variable and, despite the simple life she led, barely sufficient for her needs and expenditure. During therapy, Linda shared that she hoped to find full-time work that was more fulfilling, which would assure her of constant income and incentives. However, she felt that her anxiety problem and her potential health condition were holding her back.

ASSESSMENT

At her first intake session, Linda appeared to be friendly, eloquent and forthcoming. She was cheerful, chatty and very expressive as she related her experiences of panic attacks. Whilst she expressed anxiety over these attacks, it was very apparent that they

Fact Box 16.1. DSM-5 Changes to Diagnosing Panic Attacks

In the DSM-IV-TR (2000) there were 3 types of panic attacks: situationally bound/cued, situationally predisposed, and unexpected/uncued. In the new DSM-5 panic attacks are categorised into 2 types: expected (due to specific fears) and unexpected (out-of-the-blue, sudden, no external cue). There are no changes to the criteria; panic attacks largely remain unchanged from the DSM-IV-TR to DSM-5.

did not lower her mood for extended periods. Her response to them did not suggest any psychotic features either.

Based on her presenting concerns, the following self-rated measures were administered to Linda at the beginning (*see* Table 16.1) and end of therapy. The results of these were shared with her to create a sense of self-awareness for her presenting concerns and to help her better understand her physiological, cognitive and emotional states in relation to what was considered normative. Additionally, they provided objective evidence on her overall progress, instilled hope in recovery, and encouraged her continued practise of the skills and strategies learnt upon termination of therapy.

Throughout the course of therapy, Linda was assessed to be at minimal risk of self-harm and harm to others. She did not report any suicidal or homicidal thoughts or intent. She also denied having resorted to drinking alcohol or using drugs to cope with her panic attacks. Despite her anxiety, she generally appeared euthymic and cheerful during sessions. She was motivated and hopeful that therapy would help her manage her panic attacks more effectively.

DIAGNOSIS

Based on her history of presenting concerns of unexpected panic attacks (Table 16.2) and limited symptom attacks over a course of a year, Linda exhibited the defining features of a panic attack and met the DSM-5 Criteria for panic disorder (Table 16.3). Panic disorder is characterized by recurrent and unexpected panic attacks (American Psychiatric Association, 2013). For Linda, her panic attacks seemed to "come out of the blue", which was congruent with literature on the experience of unexpected episodes. She experienced both full-blown attacks (four or more symptoms) and limited symptom attacks (three or fewer symptoms; American Psychiatric Association, 2013), without the presence of agoraphobia (anxiety related to feeling uncomfortable in certain environmental situations, such as crowded places or open spaces) (*see* Fact Box 16.1 for information on the types of panic attacks*)*.

Although it was likely that Linda had unresolved grief-related issues that were related to her panic attack symptoms, neither comprehensive assessment nor therapy was carried out with respect to grief. She did not meet criteria for post-traumatic stress disorder (PTSD), which can also cause similar symptoms of panic. Therapy remained focused on providing Linda with short-term therapy for her panic attacks, in line with her own goals of therapy.

TABLE 16.1. LINDA'S MEASURES AT THE BEGINNING OF THERAPY

Monitoring panic attacks (frequency/ duration)

Typically, Linda experienced full-blown panic attacks twice each month and intermittent panic symptoms. In fact, she had one panic attack on the morning of her first intake session. This lasted for five minutes.

Monitoring general anxiety levels

The Depression, Anxiety and Stress Scale (DASS; Lovibond and Lovibond, 1995), a 42-item self-report questionnaire designed to measure three negative emotional states, was used to capture Linda's general anxiety levels. Linda's self-reported emotional states at intake using the DASS indicated that her depression and stress levels were within "normal" ranges and that her anxiety was within the "moderate" range.

Believability in thought statements related to panic attacks

When innocuous bodily symptoms are interpreted catastrophically, they can induce a panic attack. For example, when Linda experienced somatic symptoms, she immediately thought that she was going to have a heart attack. This inevitably increased her panic symptoms. Therefore, Linda's thought processes/beliefs associated with panic symptoms were monitored with the Agoraphobic Cognitions Questionnaire (ACQ; Chambless, Caputo, Bright and Gallagher, 1984). The ACQ comprises of a list of statements individuals under a panic attack might endorse. Respondents are required to rate their degree of believability in each statement from 0% ("I do not believe in this") to 100% ("I am completely convinced this is true"). Linda's highest rating of 90% was for the statement, "In a panic attack, I will suffer serious physical or mental harm". She further elaborated that she felt that she might die when experiencing her panic attack because she perceived it as a heart attack.

Fear ratings of panic-related bodily sensations

Linda also completed the Body Sensations Questionnaire (Chambless et al., 1984), in which she rated sensations she found particularly disturbing on a scale of 1 ("Not frightened by this sensation") to 5 ("Extremely frightened by this sensation"). The three bodily sensations Linda found most distressing were Heart palpitations (4), Numbness in legs/ arms (4) and Feelings of shortness of breath (2).

<table>
<tr><td colspan="2">TABLE 16.2. DSM-5 CRITERIA FOR PANIC ATTACK (AMERICAN PSYCHIATRIC ASSOCIATION, 2013)</td></tr>
<tr><td colspan="2">An abrupt surge of intense fear or intense discomfort that reaches a peak within minutes, and during which time four or more of the following symptoms occur. The abrupt surge can occur from a calm state or an anxious state:</td></tr>
<tr><td>1</td><td>Palpitations, pounding heart, or accelerated heart rate</td></tr>
<tr><td>2</td><td>Sweating</td></tr>
<tr><td>3</td><td>Trembling or shaking</td></tr>
<tr><td>4</td><td>Sensations of shortness of breath or smothering</td></tr>
<tr><td>5</td><td>Feeling of choking</td></tr>
<tr><td>6</td><td>Chest pain or discomfort</td></tr>
<tr><td>7</td><td>Nausea or abdominal distress</td></tr>
<tr><td>8</td><td>Feeling dizzy, unsteady, lightheaded, or faint</td></tr>
<tr><td>9</td><td>Chills or heat sensations</td></tr>
<tr><td>10</td><td>Paresthesias (numbness or tingling sensations)</td></tr>
<tr><td>11</td><td>Derealization (feelings of unreality) or depersonalization (being detached from oneself)</td></tr>
<tr><td>12</td><td>Fear of losing control or going crazy</td></tr>
<tr><td>13</td><td>Fear of dying</td></tr>
</table>

<table>
<tr><td colspan="2">TABLE 16.3. DSM-5 CRITERIA FOR PANIC DISORDER (AMERICAN PSYCHIATRIC ASSOCIATION, 2013)</td></tr>
<tr><td>A</td><td>Recurrent unexpected panic attacks</td></tr>
<tr><td>B</td><td>At least one of the attacks has been followed by one month (or more) of one or both of the following:</td></tr>
<tr><td></td><td>1. Persistent concern or worry about additional panic attacks or their consequences (e.g., losing control, having a heart attack, going crazy).</td></tr>
<tr><td></td><td>2. Significant maladaptive change in behavior related to the attacks (e.g., behaviors designed to avoid having panic attacks, such as avoidance of exercise or unfamiliar situations).</td></tr>
<tr><td>C</td><td>The Panic Attacks are not restricted to the direct physiological effects of a substance (e.g., a drug of abuse, a medication) or a general medical condition (e.g., hyperthyroidism, cardiopulmonary disorders).</td></tr>
<tr><td>D</td><td>The Panic Attacks are not restricted to the symptoms of another mental disorder, such as Social Phobia (e.g., in response to feared social situations), Specific Phobia (e.g., in response to a circumscribed phobic object or situation), Obsessive-Compulsive Disorder (e.g., in response to dirt in someone with an obsession about contamination), Posttraumatic Stress Disorder (e.g., in response to stimuli associated with a traumatic event), or Separation Anxiety Disorder (e.g., in response to being away from home or close relatives).</td></tr>
</table>

INTEGRATIVE FORMULATION

Predisposing Factors

Linda's father's death 15 years ago due to a heart condition had a significant impact on Linda, as she feared having an underlying, undetected heart condition herself, which could account for her heart palpitations, shortness of breath, tingling feeling down her back and the numbness in her hands and feet. Linda's anxious predisposition likely exacerbated her fears of having such a heart condition.

Precipitating Factors

Linda did not report any obvious life event-related or specific triggers to her condition. Her panic attacks were sudden and unexpected. Although she had been suffering from panic attacks for a year, she only sought psychiatric help after undergoing a host of medical assessments to rule out medical causes for her panic symptoms.

Perpetuating Factors

The factors that perpetuated Linda's problems could be explained by the CBT model of panic (Figure 16.1). For instance, when faced with sudden heart palpitations, numbness in legs and arms and shortness of breath, Linda perceived these bodily sensations as being life-threatening (panic symptoms), spiralling her into full-blown panic attacks. Linda's worry that her somatic symptoms were similar to heart attack symptoms and her belief that this indicated a heart condition similar to her father's (*see* Fact Box 16.2) increased catastrophic thinking and worsened her panic during an attack. Her vivid imagination perpetuated these symptoms as she was able to visualise the worst happening (e.g., having a heart attack). In frantic attempts to cope, Linda tended to take short and fast breaths in and out through her mouth, which made her pant. The auditory input of panting, together with the reduced volume of oxygen being inhaled, functioned to exacerbate her bodily sensations.

Linda's constant body monitoring of her physiological state (body scanning) increased the likelihood of her panicking. Because her tracking of her physical symptoms was carried out so automatically and unconsciously, the occurrence of her panic attacks always seemed unexpected. After her first panic attack, her anticipation of the next attack resulted in a heightened sense of anxiety, paving the way for more panic attacks. Seeking reassurance from family members by constantly asking them about her symptomatology and talking about death only induced more fear and uncertainty about life. This increased her chances of misinterpreting bodily symptoms as threatening and reinforced her erroneous beliefs that she was going to die from them.

Protective factors

Linda had good insight into her panic symptoms and demonstrated good motivation to seek help for them. She also was receptive to the suggestions of professionals working with her.

PROGNOSIS

Linda's acceptance of her condition as panic disorder, as opposed to a more detrimental health condition, also meant that the prognosis for therapy was hopeful. She was also compliant with instructions from the psychiatrist, taking her medications as prescribed. She was prescribed an anti-anxiety medication, which could be taken amidst a panic episode. She called it her "miracle pill". While she had yet to use it, she admitted that just having it made her feel safe.

Additionally, Linda did not have agoraphobia or other comorbid mental or physical health conditions that would be a barrier to treatment prognosis. For example, a person with moderate levels of depression experiencing panic symptoms may have been less energized to participate in therapy. In the absence of such complicating comorbidities, which would require attention, Linda's therapy was brief and specifically focused on alleviating her panic symptoms. CBT targeted for panic disorder, which has been shown to be effective (Taylor, 2000; Craske & Barlow, 2000), was used in her therapy. On the whole, the prognosis for Linda's treatment was positive.

TREATMENT

Brief CBT was offered, with six sessions arranged weekly or bi-weekly depending on her schedule. Therapy included psycho-education and relaxation exercises, as well as challenging dysfunctional beliefs (cognitive restructuring) and reassurance-seeking behaviours and contemplating the possible effect of delayed grief in maintaining her panic attacks. Through therapy, Linda hoped to better manage her panic attacks and find quicker relief from panic.

One of the main aspects of Linda's therapy was psycho-education. Linda was taught about her panic attacks and the panic cycle using Clark's (1986) model (*see* Figure 16.1). Together with her psychologist, a model was built using details of Linda's most recent episode. As homework, Linda was required to independently create her own panic model based on most of her panic attack episodes. Psycho-education helped Linda better understand the nature of her condition and how her problem was maintained. Awareness of her panic cycle led to an increased acceptance that her panic attacks were due to an anxiety problem and not to a life-threatening medical condition.

Fact Box 16.2. The Comorbidity of Anxiety and Heart Conditions

Symptoms of panic attacks have been found to mimic a cardiovascular disease, acute coronary syndrome (ACS). In fact, when panic attacks were first described during the American Civil War, they were given names such as "functional cardiovascular disease" and "cardiac neurosis". However, having a panic attack is not mutually exclusive from having coronary heart disease (CHD). Anxiety disorders have recently been found to have a moderate to strong association with coronary heart diseases, with rates of comorbidity ranging from 11 to 27%. Panic disorder has also been implicated (in separate studies) in sudden death in men, and in CHD in women with no history of cardiovascular disease.

For more information on the studies mentioned above, *see* Soh & Lee (2010).

Being able to distinguish the severity of her attacks (full-blown versus limited symptom attacks) meant that she could adjust her expectations as to how successful her attempts to overcome her panic during those attacks should be.

Linda was curious to understand why her panic attacks were sudden, with no obvious triggers. It was explained that for most individuals with panic attacks, it was normal for their first attack to be sudden and unexpected. Additionally it was explained that Linda's hypervigilance to her bodily symptoms and the monitoring of her regular bodily functions (body scanning) were so automatic that it was likely that her body was preconditioned to unconsciously pick up the physiological symptoms of panic.

FIGURE 16.1. TRIGGER STIMULUS (INTERNAL OR EXTERNAL)

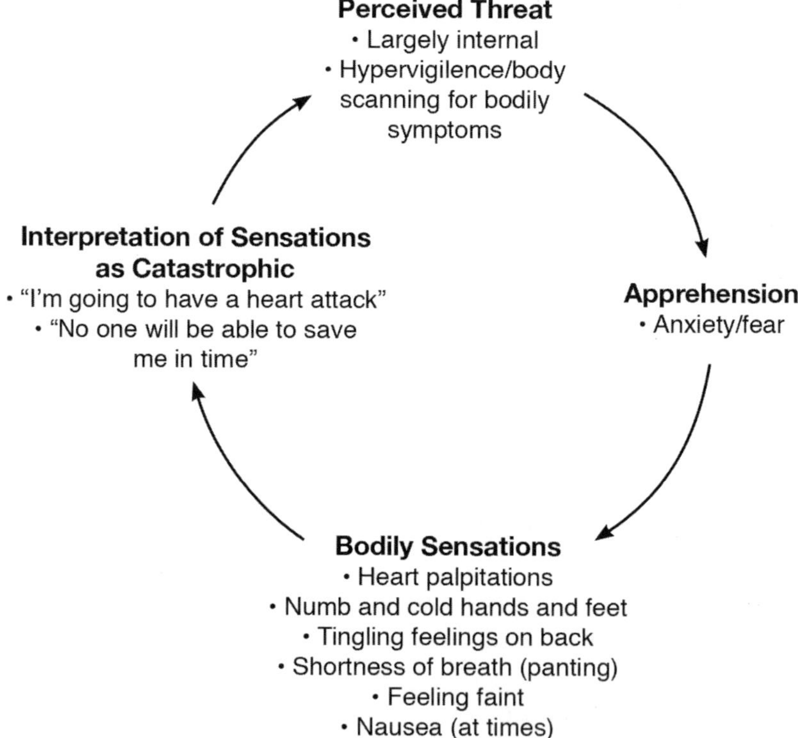

Linda realised that she never experienced panic attacks when she was busy at work or at family gatherings. She shared that at such times her focus was on other people and conversations (external) rather than checking on her bodily symptoms (internal). It was then highlighted that a medical condition could occur at all times, whereas her symptoms fluctuated with her levels of preoccupation and activity. Subsequently, Linda was encouraged to increase her focus on the external environment/

conditions (e.g., conversations with others, details of external objects) rather than on internal conditions (e.g., changes within bodily symptoms). For example, she was asked to summarise conversations with the therapist whilst in session, and to describe the sights and sounds of the therapy room. Through such practice, she was later able to focus more successfully on the external environment in her daily life, outside of therapy sessions.

Psycho-education also addressed Linda's anxious predisposition, raising her awareness that she had a tendency to judge neutral situations as potentially threatening. Linda agreed that this was typical of her personality as her family members had noticed this about her and that she was often in need of reassurance. Discussing her anxiety helped Linda understand that while it was a natural reaction to danger and threats, when it became overwhelming, it could affect daily experiences.

Another significant aspect of therapy was relaxation exercises. Specifically, Linda was taught the practice of deep breathing. She quickly learnt that taking slow, deep breaths rather than fast, short breaths helped her feel more relaxed and calm. She quickly adopted this technique on a daily basis at home. Linda's panting and how it was contributing to her panic cycle was discussed. She understood that not only did panting limit oxygen intake to her brain and make her feel faint, its accompanying "panicky" sound also exacerbated her panic symptoms. The psychologist likened Linda's experience to watching a horror movie with the background music switched on at maximum volume: it was the background music that usually augmented the scariness of a movie. Linda found that she could relate to this analogy. Recalling this analogy helped her make a conscious effort to exercise deep breathing. Panting versus deep breathing was practiced during therapy session, to reinforce healthier breathing techniques. Linda also sought her family members' opinions on which breathing techniques they found more calming, by asking them to attempt both hyperventilation and deep breathing. She developed a practice of deep breathing exercises in the morning with her mother, who also found the exercises relaxing.

As is common in those with anxiety/panic, Linda openly shared that she could not master deep breathing because she was too focused on breathing in the correct manner, resulting in her often feeling dizzy while trying to achieve this. Linda was thus asked to try to breathe the same way she did when she jogged—in through her nose and out through her mouth. She soon found a rhythm to her breathing, which enabled her to feel more relaxed. Linda also raised concerns that she had sometimes stopped jogging if she anticipated a panic attack. Therefore, if she suddenly started to have catastrophic thoughts while jogging ("I am going to die", "No one will save me"), she made a conscious efforts to focus on her external environment (surroundings and people) instead of her internal bodily symptoms, reducing her tendency to body scan.

Progressive Muscle Relaxation (PMR) is a technique that involves tensing and relaxing various muscle groups to raise awareness on how to reduce whole body tension (Bourne, 2000). Linda was taught PMR techniques to address the numbness and tingling feelings she experienced down her back, shoulders, hands, back, thighs and feet. Linda often felt numbness in her thighs and feet when seated on the couch after watching television for more than an hour. It was explained that that this was normal, and that most people would get "pins and needles" if they did not stretch intermittently. To verify her psychologist's claim, she asked several family members and friends, most of whom had similar experiences from having sat for hours in the same position to watch a movie at home, at the cinema or on long-distance flights. As therapy progressed, Linda began to take mini-breaks to move her legs while watching television at home, as she realised that they reduced numbness. Linda also shared that over time, she was more convinced that her prolonged seating position was likely the cause of numbness in her limbs.

Challenging Linda's dysfunctional cognitions was another important facet of therapy. Throughout therapy, Linda's catastrophic misinterpretations of her bodily experiences and symptoms were challenged. Questions were asked to facilitate Linda's consideration of the practicality and feasibility of her fears materializing (e.g., "How have you managed to survive these attacks so far?", "Why have the cardio-tests not revealed any problems?", "Why are your heart palpitations reduced when you talk to someone, especially if it *is* a heart attack?"). Linda was taught to use self-talk to independently challenge her cognitive misinterpretations. For example, she would say to herself, "This is not a heart attack. If it is, why does it become better when I am distracted?" She was encouraged to question the credibility and practicality of experiencing a heart attack, especially since the series of cardio-assessments and medical check-ups she had undergone had not revealed any cause for concern.

Finally, therapy aimed to address Linda's reassurance-seeking behaviour and delayed grief response. At a later session, her psychologist facilitated the exploration of her the relationship with her late father. Fearing that she would die from heart-related complications, Linda often sought assurance from her family members that her bodily symptoms were not precursors of a heart attack and that she would not pass away in a manner similar to her father. However, she was unable to find comfort in their words.

Linda felt that no one could replace her father. Her psychologist thus encouraged her to reflect on her experiences with her father and to put into practice the lessons she learnt from him and the words of wisdom he had imparted. She was also prompted to incorporate his words (e.g., "Believe in yourself", "Even if I am not always by your side, I am always there with you in spirit", "Try and if you fail, failure only makes you stronger") and his vision of who she could be (independent, confident, and emotionally strong and resilient) into her self-talk statements. Linda was moved to tears, but felt that this discussion gave her new-found strength to overcome her panic attacks.

Finally, Linda understood that talking to her family members about health problems and death was counter-productive to overcoming her condition, as it fed into her panic cycle and made her symptoms worsen. She thus made a conscious effort to talk about neutral or light-hearted topics with others.

After learning to better manage her panic symptoms, Linda was agreeable for discharge. She appraised her condition as being attributed to a combination of factors such as life circumstances (her father's death) and personal attributes (anxious personality traits). Through therapy, she came to understand how she tended to misinterpret neutral cues as threatening or catastrophic and cited learning to challenge these unhelpful perceptions as crucial to her progress.

Recommendations were made for Linda to continue practicing the techniques she had learnt. Linda was motivated to do so as she intended to stop taking medication for her condition in the long-run. At discharge, some possible future stressors (such as marriage and pregnancy), which could result in a re-emergence of her panic attacks, were discussed. Linda also recognised that these were situations in which she would be more attuned to her bodily condition as she would be less preoccupied with work and have more free time. However, she was hopeful of "mastering" techniques taught to her to better prepare for potential life stressors.

Towards the end of therapy, Linda was confident enough to move back to her bedroom at night. A better understanding of her bodily symptoms helped her to have the courage to sleep alone. At discharge, Linda reiterated having initially held off full-time work as she wanted to identify the root cause of her somatic symptoms. However, she had since realised that she had a reduced tendency to experience somatic symptoms when she was occupied at work and distracted. She was thus convinced that her panic symptoms were unlikely to impede her work. However, she was still hesitant about taking on a full-time job.

At discharge, Linda had not experienced any full-blown panic attacks for 1.5 months. She still experienced some panic symptoms such as palpitations, feeling like she was choking, breathlessness and nausea, which were considered to be milder, limited symptom attacks. The DASS was re-administered to capture Linda's general anxiety levels at discharge. Her general anxiety level at intake was within the moderate range and this had returned to the normal range at discharge.

Her degree of belief rating for the statement "In a panic attack, I will suffer serious physical or mental harm" was 10% at discharge, a remarkable drop from her 90% rating for the same statement at intake. Linda also shared that she was less disturbed by sudden heart palpitations and numbness in her legs and arms. Her subjective ratings of these were consistent with her verbal account. Her fear ratings for heart palpitations and numbness in legs/arms had dropped to from 4 to 2 at discharge, while her fear rating for shortness of breath remained at a low of 2/10.

DISCUSSION

To date, no epidemiological studies have explored the prevalence of panic disorder in Singapore. The most recent study by Chong and colleagues (2012), only explored the prevalence rates in Singapore for two anxiety disorders, obsessive-compulsive disorder and generalized anxiety disorder. The lifetime prevalence rates for unexpected panic attacks range from approximately 1% to 4% (American Psychiatric Association, 2000; Wittchen et al., 1998). Lifetime prevalence rates have been demonstrated to be consistent around the world (Weissman, et al., 1997; Ayuso-Mateos, 2012). Based on overseas estimations, the typical age of onset for panic disorder is between 15 and 19 years or between 25 and 30 years (American Psychiatric Association, 2000; Ballenger & Fryer, 1996). It also has been noted that women are diagnosed with panic disorder twice as often as men (Weissman et al., 1997; Ayuso-Mateos, 2012).

As evident in Linda's therapy, psycho-education can be considered a form of patient empowering training (Wood, Brendtro, Fecser & Nichols, 1999). This is a very powerful therapeutic tool, which empowers clients to work towards strategies to overcoming their conditions. Awareness of the causes and effects of their problem often leads to improved self-efficacy, which enhances self-control (Wood et al., 1999). Therefore, helping clients understand their experience of panic and portraying an accurate, yet detailed depiction of their panic cycle is a critical step in CBT for panic disorder. This is especially so if clients are as motivated as Linda. Although there are similarities in how panic attacks are experienced for most clients, understanding each individual's unique experience with panic attacks is important for therapy to be meaningful for them. For Linda, the sudden and unpredictable nature of her panic attacks made her distressing experience all the more bewildering. Therefore, she found much relief in understanding how her anxious predisposition, personal experiences (father's death due to a heart condition), physical symptoms of panic and maladaptive thought processes ("I am going to have a heart attack") combined to produce a profoundly disturbing experience.

Psycho-education could also take place at various junctures within therapy, to clarify doubts and to enable the client to personalise the CBT model for panic disorder, using their own unique experiences and set of symptoms. For Linda, and many others with panic disorder, to convince them that panic symptoms are indicative of an anxiety problem as opposed to a health problem is essential for therapy to progress. For example, Linda noted that her panic symptoms were often not experienced when she was engaged in conversation or at work, which largely supported the fact that her panic symptoms were unlikely to be linked to a medical condition.

Acceptance of a diagnosis of panic disorder is another important factor for therapeutic prognosis. Often, individuals suffering from a panic attack would believe that they are experiencing a life-threatening illness and would thus first seek services to rule out medical conditions. Linda was no exception, having been through several medical examinations before turning to psychiatric help as a last resort. Therefore, she was less resistant towards accepting she had an anxiety problem, which helped her to take a more proactive stance throughout therapy.

The tendency for clients to disclose more information over the course of therapy due to increasing trust in their therapeutic relationship sometimes brings about new challenges. For instance, Linda only opened up about her reassurance-seeking behaviours, her grief related to her father's death, and fear of dying at later sessions. As disclosure only took place at later sessions, her psychologist had to make clinical decisions as to whether and to what extent these matters should be addressed by revisiting Linda's initial referral question. As such, reassurance-seeking behaviours and grief-related issues were only very briefly touched on by the psychologist, and only when they were related to Linda's panic attacks. The focus of therapy therefore, was primarily on her panic symptoms.

At later sessions, Linda was advised to explore grief work (psychological or religious/spiritual) if she felt the need to seek closure on the loss of her father. However, her psychologist's willingness to listen to her thoughts about her father's death and its implications on her own health concerns facilitated a more personalised approach for therapy. For example, through understanding that Linda found her late father's words of wisdom reassuring, her psychologist encouraged Linda to create self-talk statements using his words, from which she could draw strength to overcome her panic.

Often, sharing good rapport with clients can put them at ease. When Linda said that breathing techniques did not suit her, her psychologist was willing to explore other means of modifying her breathing habits (e.g. attempting to reduce the sound from panting which would exacerbate panic). Modifying recommended strategies or providing alternative strategies based on client feedback kept Linda hopeful not only for the outcome of therapy, but for long-term progress as well.

Culture can also play a role in the manifestation of a panic attack. Lewis-Fernandez, et al. (2011) suggested that certain panic attack symptoms may be more prevalent or commonly reported in certain cultures, due to their beliefs about how the body works. For example, Cambodian beliefs about a wind-like substance in the body that is associated with neck soreness and tinnitus may predispose Cambodians to emphasize such symptoms when reporting panic attacks. While there is no observation in Singapore about how local culture leads to certain symptoms receiving more emphasis than others, Linda's case highlights the familial context associated with the development of her symptoms. It remains possible that culture affects the etiology or representation of panic attacks, and consequently should be considered in psychological formulation and treatment.

DISCUSSION QUESTIONS

1. Explaining the panic cycle to Linda helped her understand that she had an "anxiety condition" and not a "medical condition". For Linda, how would you deliver psycho-education about her panic cycle? Take into consideration how you would appropriately explain psychological jargon.
2. Other than CBT, what other therapeutic approaches and/or interventions could have been considered for Linda's case?
3. Linda often reminisced better times with her father and often compared her panic experience to her father's medical condition. Would it have been useful for the

psychologist to address grief-related issues in an in-depth manner during therapy meant for Linda's panic attacks?

4. Mental health conditions can significantly impact upon overall functioning (academic, social and occupational). Linda initially wanted to put off her job hunt, until she had received help for her panic symptoms. Why do you think Linda showed reluctance to engage in full-time work?

5. It is common for people suffering from panic attacks to seek assurance from family members. How would this seeking of assurance from others manifest itself in an Asian society, where levels of collectivism are relatively higher than that of Western cultures? Would there be more assurance seeking, or would family opinions be deemed more authoritative?

6. Using what you know about Singapore's culture and various ethnic beliefs, postulate ways that culture might have an effect on how panic attacks may manifest differently from patients in the local population.

CHAPTER 17.

WASH IT ALL AWAY

Obsessive-Compulsive Disorder

TAY SZE YAN AND GWEE KENJI

INTRODUCTION

Patricia was a 32-year-old Chinese woman who had previously undergone medical and psychological treatment for obsessive-compulsive disorder (OCD) and post-partum depression. More recently, she approached the psychiatric services at a tertiary hospital for her uncontrollable need to wash her hands and toilet taps, which interfered with her ability to complete her daily tasks and caused her considerable distress and frustration. She was referred to psychological services by her psychiatrist for treatment.

Patricia had ongoing OCD symptoms since the age of 22, and reported that she started to develop an extreme fear of germs and dirt a year ago. Her presenting complaint was her inability to share her kitchen sink with her flat-mates. She was concerned with her flat-mates' level of hygiene and had to constantly clean her kitchen tap in a particular manner whenever she felt that it was dirty. This usually occurred after her flat mates used the sink, and whenever others in the house used the sink after using the toilet. Her ritual involved cleaning the tap from three angles using a sponge and rinsing her hands up to eight times in a row. Patricia was also fearful of using the public wash areas, and tried to overcome her fear by not using the palms of her hands to press the taps. She described being worried about germs due to the number of potential illnesses in the world today. These worries and compulsions frustrated her and made her feel incompetent and "different". She was particularly distressed over her tap-washing behaviour as her tap needed to be replaced recently due to excessive washing and she was reprimanded by her husband for that.

The onset of Patricia's OCD symptoms followed the birth of her child when she was 22 years old. She remembered feeling extremely stressed and powerless at that time because her husband had "made me have the child". She vaguely recalled having an extremely low mood, during which her clearest memories were those of frequently washing milk bottles, taking long showers and feeling extremely frustrated by her family members' constant reprimands. Her symptoms waxed and waned from then on, and she reported many a time where she had difficulties leaving the house.

BACKGROUND

Patricia was born and raised on a small island in China. She completed only lower primary education, read and wrote only minimal Mandarin, and spoke in simple Mandarin. Her father left her family when she was very young, and her mother later left for Beijing to work. She had lived with her godmother (whom she felt disliked her) since the age of 10. She underwent "matchmaking" by her godmother and left for Singapore to get married in her early 20s. She had minimal contact with her own family members after that and was currently in conflict with her mother-in-law and sister-in-law. She recalled a history of psychiatric illnesses within her biological family but was unable to provide any details.

Patricia suffered from asthma and was frequently ill as a child. Due to the poor medical facilities in her hometown, she often had to suffer the course of her illness without proper medical treatment. She attributed her frequent illnesses to her hometown, which she described as "dirty and dusty". As a result of that, she became particularly and overly attentive to cleanliness in her own house, in a bid to prevent her and her children's current health from being affected in a similar fashion.

After dating him for two years, Patricia married her husband, when she was 20 years of age. He was a few years her senior and had a strong traditional mindset, believing that her role in the family was a subservient housewife. This resulted in marital conflict following the conception of her first child, who was delivered two years after their marriage. According to Patricia, she was not keen on having the child but relented after her husband threatened divorce should she abort the pregnancy. Patricia's OCD symptoms emerged amidst conflicts with her mother-in-law, and a lack of support from her husband, who became increasingly distant. He argued with Patricia over her performance in household chores, and sided with his mother and sister. After the birth of her second child two years later, her mood and OCD symptoms worsened again, and she finally sought treatment.

Patricia suffered from post-partum depression following childbirth and underwent psychiatric and psychological treatment. She received anti-depressants and anxiolytics (anti-anxiety medication), which were prescribed in increasingly higher dosages over the course of her 15-month-long treatment. While psychological therapy involving supportive counselling and behaviour therapy was offered, Patricia did not fully engage. In fact, she was admitted to the hospital partway through her period of therapy for a suicide attempt (drug overdose) as she was stressed out over her child.

At the time of current treatment, almost a decade after her last treatment, Patricia and her husband were sharing a rented flat with another family. She was distressed about her living arrangements as she disapproved of the other family's low standards of hygiene, and observed that their daughter was frequently ill.

Patricia had previously been employed in a number of jobs within both the food and sales industries. However, when she presented for treatment, she was unemployed and had left her previous jobs mostly as a result of stress or her OCD symptoms. Patricia and her husband had always barely made ends meet; he was employed in the industrial sector, and they had to rely on social assistance.

ASSESSMENT

A range of standardized self-report measures are commonly used in the assessment of OCD symptoms, including the Obsessive-Compulsive Inventory (Foa, Kozak, Salkovskis, Coles, & Amir, 1998), the Yale Brown Compulsive Checklist (Goodman, Price, Rasmussen, Mazure, Fleischmann, Hill, Heninger & Charney, 1989) and the Responsibility Attitude Scale (Salkovskis, Wroe, Morrison, Richards, Reynolds, & Thorpe, 2000). However, with the unavailability of Mandarin versions and the low literacy levels of some local patient populations, it can be difficult to administer these scales. Low literacy levels not only make it difficult for patients to read and fill out these print materials, but can also affect their ability to understand and make sense of all the information provided. During such situations, clinical interviews are often done

---

Fact Box 17.1. Different Types of Compulsive Behaviours

"Compulsions" are repeated behaviours that people feel they have to perform to reduce emotional distress or to prevent undesirable consequences. While people with OCD can engage in unique forms of compulsions, common types of compulsive behaviours are as follows: *Excessive washing or cleaning*—Persons are often afraid of contamination, and clean or wash themselves or their surroundings many times a day. *Checking*—Persons repeatedly check things (making sure that the oven is turned off, the door is locked, etc.) that they associate with harm or danger. *Hoarding or saving things*—Persons fear that something bad will happen if they throw anything away, so they compulsively keep or hoard things (such as old newspapers or scarps of papers) that they do not need or use. *Repeating actions*—Persons repetitively engage in the same action many times, such as turning on and off a light switch 20 times, or shaking their head 13 times. *Counting and arranging*—Persons are often obsessed with order and symmetry. They may have superstitions about certain numbers, colours, or arrangements, and seek to put things in a particular pattern, such as ensuring everything is symmetrical.

in lieu to gather details about the patient's symptoms, background and medical history, as well as the frequency and impact of OCD behaviours on their daily activities. This was the case for Patricia.

Patricia attended all the sessions alone. She was cautious in the initial sessions, but gradually revealed more information about herself as therapy progressed. While the clinical interview was done in a casual and conversational way in order to increase rapport, detailed aspects of her problem were focused on to make up for the lack of use of a structured assessment tool. Specifically, Patricia was asked about the nature of her OCD behaviours (hand washing, tap washing), the frequency of OCD behaviours, her appraisal of these behaviours (were they illogical, tiresome acts that she would rather not have, or welcome by her?), her confidence in controlling these behaviours, what typically happened after these OCD behaviours (sense of relief, feeling "right"), as well as her family and living situation. These aspects were explored both in the current as well as historical context, and information gained was used in the formulation and diagnosis of Patricia's case.

DIAGNOSIS

Patricia fulfilled the full DSM-5 criteria (American Psychiatric Association, 2013) for obsessive-compulsive disorder. She held recurrent and persistent thoughts of dirt, which she attempted to neutralize by repetitive washing and checking behaviours. These symptoms were causing her distress and were significantly affecting her functioning. While Patricia had a history of depression, she reported her mood as stable and denied experiencing any depressive symptoms. She did not meet DSM-5 criteria for depressive disorders. She indicated no suicidal, homicidal or self-harming ideations and was clinically assessed to be at low risk for self-harm.

INTEGRATIVE FORMULATION

Predisposing Factors

Patricia's case was conceptualized using Salkovskis's cognitive model of OCD (Salkovskis, 2007). This model postulates that obsessions happen when we perceive aspects of our normal thoughts as threatening to ourselves or to others, and we feel responsible to prevent this threat from happening. These misperceptions often develop as a result of our early childhood experiences. In Patricia's case, her childhood experience of living in a "dirty and dusty" area and her frequent and untreated asthmatic attacks probably led her to associate a lack of hygiene with suffering. While this association was probably rational in the context of her childhood environment, it can be argued to be unnecessary in a clean environment such as that in Singapore and is evidently maladaptive when taken to extremes. As a result of this association, she started to feel threatened when she saw the unhygienic behaviours of her flat-mates. Given her poor attachment to her godmother who raised her, and the absence of parents' supervision, she would have concluded, from a young age, that she was responsible for her own well-being. This likely led to the development of her belief that she was responsible for preventing her own suffering.

Precipitating Factors

Whilst the above factors made Patricia more vulnerable to developing OCD, it generally takes a critical incident to trigger an OCD episode or disorder. From Patricia's psychiatric history, the precipitating events of her OCD symptoms were situations in which she experienced a loss of control over her circumstances. Her initial OCD symptoms had manifested after she was pressured to go through with a pregnancy she felt unready for, while her most recent symptoms had surfaced when she had to share a rented place. Her OCD symptoms could have been triggered by her belief that she was responsible for the prevention of further suffering. They could also have been symbolic of her attempts to gain a sense of control over her difficult situations. Adding to her sense of helplessness were her high expectations for cleanliness. In both incidents, it is possible that she was concerned that her baby's or family's health would be compromised by her "unhygienic" environment, triggering her symptoms. In normal circumstances, caring for a newborn and having to share a house with strangers are situations that would trigger health concerns. As a result of feeling responsible for potential negative outcomes despite not having control over them, clients with OCD tend to develop a range of rituals in an attempt to neutralize their thoughts to prevent their perceived harm. This preoccupation often makes them extremely aware of stimuli of concern (e.g., focusing on the tap after flat mates have used it), which increases the occurrence of intrusive thoughts and heightens their level of discomfort, leading to an increase in neutralizing behaviours, thereby initiating a cycle.

Perpetuating Factors

Clients with OCD also often use their mood as an indicator to gauge when they should stop performing their rituals or compulsions (mood-as-input mechanism; Davey, Field & Startup, 2003). This usually perpetuates their OCD behaviour as they are often under high levels of distress. In Patricia's case, she was plagued by intrusive thoughts that her flat-mates were dirty and were contaminating the kitchen. As germs and dirt were threatening to her and were associated with suffering, she was extremely upset by these thoughts and images. She thus engaged in several neutralizing behaviours (e.g., cleaning the tap and washing her hands whenever she felt that they were dirty) to counter these threats and would continue performing these acts till she felt satisfied. Each time she engaged in her rituals, her distress would actually increase. This likely contributed to an elevated sense of anxiety and to the threat of further intrusions, perpetuating her obsessive-compulsive process.

Because Patricia likely paid close attention to environmental stimuli (for example, observing the behaviours of others in the house and keeping track of when others used the toilet), the chance of noticing situations that would trigger her intrusions and ritualistic behaviour were heightened, perpetuating her OCD process. While preoccupied with distressing emotions, Patricia was rendered even more susceptible to intrusions, which initiated and perpetuated the OCD process.

On top of neutralizing behaviours, she engaged in counterproductive strategies such as avoiding using the kitchen sink and cleaning the taps excessively. Together, they perpetuated her belief that these actions prevented harm, which provided her with a sense of control. They also kept her from the realization that even if she refrained from her rituals during these stressful circumstances, the outcomes might be no different from if she had performed her rituals.

Protective Factors

Patricia was a motivated individual who referred herself to psychiatric services for treatment of her OCD symptoms. Although these symptoms were persistent, previous psychological treatment had helped her.

PROGNOSIS

Despite her long-lasting waxing and waning symptoms, she had been able to hold down several jobs and to manage her household responsibilities, demonstrating her strength in coping with her symptoms and her potential for sufficient recovery. Based on the above formulation, the psychologist could thus extrapolate her pattern of behaviour and expect a good prognosis for functional improvement. Her low levels of literacy and education would, however, be a challenge, particularly for cognitive elements of the treatment. Adaptation of her treatment strategies would thus be required.

TREATMENT

As recommended by Salkovskis's (2007) treatment protocol for OCD, Patricia's treatment plan involved cognitive strategies of examining and restructuring the thoughts and interpretations maintaining her OCD symptoms in the initial stages of therapy, followed by Exposure Response Prevention (ERP) methods once she was able to understand and utilize these cognitive strategies. However, taking into consideration Patricia's low level of literacy and cultural background, ensuring flexibility in our approach and making necessary adaptations along the treatment process were required. In terms of the goals of therapy, Patricia hoped to be able to share the kitchen sink with her flat-mates without engaging in tap-washing behaviour. She also did not want her hand washing to interfere with her completion of household chores.

Patricia attended 17 sessions over a period of 11 months, each lasting between 60 to 90 minutes. Initial sessions focused on assessment and education. During these sessions, Patricia's case formulation was shared with her and the goals for treatment were discussed. Using terms she could understand, her psychologist highlighted certain pointers that appeared most prominent in her case. It was explained to Patricia that her OCD symptoms had psychological explanations ("problem with thinking and deciding"). Her actions were described as a response to her fear of contamination and to the importance she placed on cleanliness. She was told that intrusive thoughts were actually common and normal experiences but that unlike her, others would not act on them if they were deemed to be of low importance. Together with her psychologist, Patricia explored how she could either be less bothered by her intrusive thoughts or engage in something she enjoyed doing during these instances.

While cognitive factors likely contributed to her symptoms, it was difficult for Patricia to identify the dysfunctional thoughts and beliefs that perpetuated them. Several attempts were made to elicit these underlying beliefs through interviewing and Socratic questioning. However, Patricia's awareness of what motivated her behaviour was superficial (e.g., she related that she engaged in cleaning behaviour because of the fear of germs and dirt).

The first step of ERP—simply monitoring the frequency and pattern of her washing behaviours—was surprisingly effective. When she returned the following week, Patricia was delighted to share that she had been able to refrain from washing

Fact Box 17.2. What is ERP?

OCD was initially thought to be resistant to treatment until studies showed that a procedure known as "Exposure and Response Prevention" (ERP), based on behavioural theory, helped clients with their symptoms. The process of ERP requires the client to first create a hierarchy of their obsessive thoughts, identify the triggers that bring on their obsessions and compulsions, and rate their distress levels on each of these. A situation that causes mild or moderate distress is then chosen, and the client is then repeatedly exposed to their obsessive thoughts (exposure) while at the same time trying to resist engaging in any identified behaviours/rituals that they have been using to neutralise these thoughts (response prevention). Their anxiety level is tracked as they engage in the exposure exercise, and typically, anxiety levels subside over time and even without them needing them to act out their compulsions. The exposure will be repeated until the item on the hierarchy is no longer causing significant distress to the client, upon which the next higher distress-inducing situation is tackled in a similar fashion. An expected outcome of ERP is that clients realise that they can tolerate their obsessive thoughts without rituals, hence reducing the associated emotional distress as well as repetitive behaviours that characterise OCD.

her hands until after she had completed her household chores. She had been able to ignore her intrusive thoughts and rehearse what she had learnt from previous sessions: "no matter how many times you wash, still dirty". She was delighted with her progress as she could complete her chores more quickly. She noted smoother hands and more time to complete other chores.

A hierarchy of exposure was subsequently constructed and initiated. This is a list of anxiety-provoking items that incur increasing level of distress in a client. During ERP, a client is exposed to increasingly anxiety-provoking items on their list once they have overcome their distress for 'easier' items, till they eventually reach their goal (*see* Table 17.1). Patricia was thus gradually exposed to the items on her exposure hierarchy. As she habituated to increasingly distressing stimuli, she began moving up the hierarchy. She was eventually able to maintain her behaviour of sharing the kitchen sink with her flat mates and washing the tap only once a day. This gave her a boost in confidence; she felt she could cope independently with her symptoms and soon requested termination of therapy.

When her therapist explained to her that she was still experiencing OCD symptoms and advised against termination of therapy, Patricia acknowledged that she had not sufficiently recovered from OCD and decided to continue with therapy. Patricia and her therapist thus revisited the techniques successful in reducing her symptoms previously, such as externalizing her thoughts and using relaxation strategies.

It was at this point, however, that new OCD symptoms had arose. On further investigation, it was clear that in the process of conquering some of her OCD symptoms, others had emerged. This process is commonly experienced in therapy for OCD, in which client's anxiety can be simply transferred to alternative compulsions or safety behaviours. Patricia now shared she was checking her pillows compulsively every night to ensure that there were no insects on them, waking early to wash her bathroom pipe and sink, and rubbing her tap. She reflected that these compulsions increased whenever she was stressed and feeling helpless and low in confidence.

After ten sessions of therapy, Patricia's therapist left the service and her therapy was assigned to another psychologist. As such, Patricia took the initiative to summarize her progress in therapy. She recognised that she had benefited from ERP, but also observed that stress from the conflictual relationships with her in-laws affected her mood and moderated the success of ERP. Patricia's new therapist took over the work by revising ERP principles with her using simple Mandarin terms. They focused on two techniques: using simple, concrete behaviours to counter her OCD (e.g., aim to 'wash your hands only three times') and further building her confidence. The latter was achieved by normalising the effect of stress on OCD symptoms, and encouraging her to practice ERP on days when she was feeling more confident, and not feeling guilty for having difficulty on more stressful days.

Patricia's confidence grew. She appreciated the opportunity to share her perspectives, receive validation from her therapist amidst her challenges, and feel a sense of relief in sharing her 'load'. Instead of the anxious, subservient persona she previously had, Patricia reported confidence in change, her symptoms reduced, and she even became more assertive with her husband.

Besides increased motivation, Patricia displayed a greater sense of ownership of her problems by taking the initiative to modify the way certain exposures were done. She challenged herself to increase her exposure to more distressing situations without prompting. After her therapeutic gains plateaued around her 15th session, Patricia initiated termination of therapy. She was happy with her gains, was convinced that ERP worked, and appeared mindful about returning when needed. As she appeared more confident, and displayed relative stability of her symptoms without the emergence of new OCD behaviours, her decision to terminate therapy was supported by her therapist.

Three months later, Patricia's feedback to her therapist indicated that she had sufficient mastery over her OCD symptoms. Even though they were still present, they were at a significantly lower intensity; she was now able to function better as a homemaker and to interact with her family members more effectively. Typical of other patients with OCD, elimination of all symptoms was not a realistic outcome for Patricia. Instead, a good enough recovery is defined by the resolution of some symptoms to increase functioning in daily life. As such, Patricia was deemed to have been sufficiently "recovered".

TABLE 17.1. EXPOSURE HIERARCHY FOR PATRICIA'S TAP-WASHING BEHAVIOUR; GOALS SET FOR EACH SESSION	
Session 3	Maintain frequency of tap-washing (two times) without rituals
Session 4	Achieve lower frequency of tap-washing (once) without rituals
Session 5	Maintain frequency of tap-washing (once) without rituals and using tap together with tenant
Session 6	Maintain behaviours achieved from Session 5

DISCUSSION

Patricia's challenges with Obsessive-Compulsive Disorder (OCD) are typical of patients with this disorder, not just in Singapore, but also worldwide. Firstly, rates of OCD in Singapore are comparable with international rates. The latest lifetime prevalence rate of OCD in Singapore is 3.0% and the 1-year prevalence rate was 1.1% (Chong, Abdin, Vaingankar, Heng, Sherbourne, Yap et. al., 2012). These figures are comparable to international lifetime prevalence rates of OCD that fall between 1%–3%

and 1-year prevalence rates of 0.5%–2.1% in adults (American Psychiatric Association, 2000; Clark & Beck, 2010; Karno, Golding, Sorenson, & Burnam, 1988).

Patricia's treatment was based on evidence-based approaches for OCD. The development of effective treatment for OCD began in the last three decades (Riccardi, Timpano & Schmidt, 2010). Treatment guidelines for OCD have recommended the use of CBT with an ERP component; either alone or in combination with selective serotonin reuptake inhibitors, depending on the severity of the symptoms (National Institute for Health and Clinical Excellence, 2005). However, a majority of those afflicted either do not to seek treatment or delay their treatment; this could be related to motivational issues and poor readiness to accept these recommended treatments (Clark & Beck, 2010). Some of those in treatment have also been found to demonstrate poor response due to low compliance, and poor insight into their obsessions and OCD subtype (Clark & Beck, 2010).

Within the local context, while it is important to adhere to evidence-based treatment, consideration of cultural and ethnic factors is equally important for application of treatment in the most effective way. An American study of OCD in New York has suggested that black clients (including those of Carribean descent) with OCD are particularly secretive as compared to ethnically white clients, are often vague about their symptoms, fear the stigma associated with their behaviours and have limited information with regards to these compulsions (Hatch & Friedman, 1996). Working therapeutically with Chinese clients is similarly challenging because of their often lower levels of verbal expressiveness and discomfort in openly discussing and confronting their problems in the presence of others (Foo, Merrick & Kazantzis, 2006).

Low literacy levels can pose another challenge. This is not only because of difficulties clients face in reading educational handouts and filling out print materials used in therapy but also possibly because of their lower cognitive capacity to absorb all the information provided, which creates a need to adapt treatment methods in a way appropriate to their ability (Kuhajda, Thorn, Gaskins, Day & Cabbil, 2011).

In Patricia's case, her cultural background as well as low literacy hindered the application of CBT. Her therapists found it challenging to explain the cognitive aspects of her OCD symptoms to her. Several factors may have contributed to this. Firstly, Patricia had experienced OCD symptoms for many years thus it was possible that she was so accustomed to engaging in OCD behaviours when faced with triggers that she had forgotten the underlying function of her behaviours. Secondly, as she was from a culturally conservative background, it might have been difficult for her to express her personal thoughts and beliefs early in the therapy process. Furthermore, given her low education, she might not have been able to grasp the association of her cognitions and behaviours. Perhaps, if attempts made to elicit her cognitions had taken place later in the therapeutic process, a strong alliance with her therapist would have been established and she may have been more forthcoming and open to being taught to understand her cognitions better.

OCD has been described as a condition of chronic and unremitting nature, with symptoms disappearing and recurring over a lifetime in response to changing life stressors, making it an anxiety disorder with one of the lowest remission rates (Clark & Beck, 2010). Patricia's case clearly demonstrated this phenomenon, and was evidenced by a relapse of symptoms during moments of prominent stressors in her life. The multiple OCD behaviours that waxed and waned rapidly over the course of therapy posed a challenge to ERP techniques. Successful therapy for OCD requires close monitoring of symptoms, attending to emerging symptoms during the course of therapy, and ensuring that goals can be consistently achieved before the termination of treatment. In Patricia's case, the therapist emphasised and revisited successful strategies that helped her reach her goals to help her manage her new behaviours.

Close monitoring of clients' abilities to maintain their progress and tracking the emergence of other symptoms during treatment is pertinent. Also of importance to charting a client's progress is the acquisition of comprehensive and detailed information on his or her OCD symptoms, types of obsessive thoughts, compulsions, safety behaviours and related functional impact. While this is commonly achieved through the administration of self-report forms, it was not possible with Patricia due to her low levels of literacy and competency in English. Alternatively, therapists can employ the help of family members to give an objective view on a client's condition. Unfortunately, in Patricia's case, her family members did not participate in treatment.

While customising evidence-based techniques like ERP and helping Patricia increase her self-confidence were critical for improvement, the therapist's support and validation played an important role. It was possible that, with an unsupportive husband and chastising in-laws, Patricia's sole source of support was her therapist. As clients with mental illnesses rely tremendously on familial support (Jones, 2002), Patricia's therapists could thus have been filling this role in her life. In Patricia's collectivistic culture, in which the impact of familial support was even more important than in individualistic cultures (Teo, Graham, Yeoh, Levy, 2003), her therapists' support was probably paramount to her successful practice of ERP strategies. Without this moderating factor, therapy would probably have been less effective.

DISCUSSION QUESTIONS

1. Patricia's therapist had to explain psychological terms associated with her treatment. How would you explain terms such as cognitive distortions, graded hierarchy and hypervigilance, in layman's terms?
2. Consider the predisposing, precipitating, perpetuating and protective factors for Patricia's formulation. Which would you target for intervention and why?
3. How are OCD behaviours different, if at all, in other Asian cultures? Are there culture-specific approaches to dealing with this disorder?
4. How would Patricia's condition have been appraised differently, if at all, if she went back to her homeland?

PART 3.

OLDER ADULTS

CHAPTER 18

MORE MONEY THAN SENSE

Neuropsychological Assessment of Financial Decision Making

SIMON LOWES COLLINSON

INTRODUCTION

Mr Woo was an 88-year-old Singaporean man of mixed Chinese-Malay parentage who was referred from a private forensic psychiatrist for neuropsychological assessment. He had initiated legal action against one of his daughters for seeking to acquire a controlling interest in a large family company, of which he was the chairman. As Mr Woo and his family suspected that his ability to manage his financial affairs would be challenged in the upcoming court case, his psychiatrist was engaged to assess his mental capacity and financial matters decision-making ability.

BACKGROUND

Mr Woo was the last surviving and youngest of three siblings. He had not received any formal education and was illiterate due to poverty and the Japanese occupation. During the war he provided bicycle errand services to the Japanese Army. After the war, he began a business selling bicycle spare parts that eventually diversified into one selling motor vehicle spare parts. He got married in 1955 and had four daughters. His business steadily expanded through the years and he amassed a significant fortune (estimated to be over $200m at the time of assessment). In 1969, Mr Woo's wife was killed in a road traffic accident and he never remarried. In the ensuing period of grief and possible depression, he developed a chronic drinking problem. Following the accident, Mr Woo drank daily. Beginning early in the morning, he would proceed to consume five to eight cans of high strength beer and half a bottle of whiskey in one day. He would also smoke approximately 30 sticks of cigarettes each day. He was nonetheless in relatively good health, apart from a history of tinnitus, progressive deafness, diabetes, mild hypertension and mild renal impairment. He ate three meals a day, which were either prepared by his helper or eaten at the neighbourhood hawker centre.

Mr Woo lived in a condominium with his helper who took care of the daily chores and food preparation. He was independent and continued to drive, go on outings and manage his daily routines such as showering, dressing, and toileting without any help. He handled day-to-day monetary transactions independently and made personal financial decisions.

<table>
<tr><td colspan="2">TABLE 18.1. FIVE STATUTORY PRINCIPLES OF THE MENTAL CAPACITY ACT (SINGAPORE 2010)</td></tr>
<tr><td>1.</td><td>Assume a person has capacity unless the opposite is proven</td></tr>
<tr><td>2.</td><td>Take all practicable steps to help a person make their own decision</td></tr>
<tr><td>3.</td><td>A person has the right to make an unwise decision</td></tr>
<tr><td>4.</td><td>Always act in the person's best interests</td></tr>
<tr><td>5.</td><td>Choose the least restrictive option</td></tr>
</table>

Adapted from the Mental Capacity Act: Cap 177A, 2010 Rev Ed Sing.

ASSESSMENT

It important to keep in mind the first common law principle that every adult person has legal capacity to make his or her own decisions and is assumed to be competent until evidence is found to the contrary. Within the auspices of the Singapore Mental Capacity Act, a referring doctor must follow a two stage process to determine mental incompetence: a) the patient is suffering from an impairment or disturbance that affects the function of the brain or mind, and b) the impairment or disturbance causes inability to make a decision at a particular time. A person is deemed unable to make a decision if he or she cannot 1) understand the information presented, 2) weigh up the information, 3) remember the information, or 4) communicate the decision (Menon, 2013). As decision making is domain specific to financial abilities, and the ability to live independently, and make medical/healthcare decisions, a clear understanding of the scope of the assessment has to be outlined before the patient's abilities are tested.

In this case the goals of the assessment were 1) to determine whether Mr Woo had the cognitive capacity to understand and conduct his financial affairs, particularly in relation to personal and company financial matters; 2) to establish the manner and extent by which any cognitive impairment may have affected Mr Woo's ability to make decisions and give instructions in relation to financial matters; and 3) in the event of impaired decision making capacity, to determine whether such impairment was sufficient to prevent Mr Woo from understanding and providing clear instructions to a third party in relation to financial decisions.

Mr Woo was happy and keen to be assessed so that he could demonstrate that he "was not mad or crazy". The assessment was conducted with the assistance of a Hokkien-speaking psychologist translator. Mr Woo presented as a slightly unkempt, spirited and congenial gentleman who spoke logically and coherently. He had a tendency to wander off topic when discussing his past but was easily redirected to the task/subject. He demonstrated a good understanding of his current health status, admitting that his drinking was not healthy and probably affected his memory. While Mr Woo felt that his memory was not as good as it had been in his youth, he could give a clear account of his family background, current living situation and financial assets (*see* below). He was emotionally expressive and spoke in an animated fashion about his achievements and family. He was not depressed or anxious at the time of the assessment.

Mr Woo presented with moderate risk of injurious behaviours to self and others primarily because of his tendency to drink and drive. His drinking behaviour (despite being constant and not having caused him any trouble up till then) could compromise his cognitive functioning either temporarily or permanently, rendering driving unsafe. Mr Woo had little insight into the risks associated with drunk driving and showed no indication that he would change his behaviour. Whilst the object of the assessment was not to modify his risk, Mr Woo was adamant that drinking improved his abilities on a day-to-day basis and that he was not functionally impaired. There were no other risk issues in his mental state or day-to-day functioning.

TABLE 18.2. STRUCTURED AND SEMI-STRUCTURED COMPETENCY INSTRUMENTS

- Clinical Competency Test (Marson et al., 1995)
- Cognitive Capacity Screening Exam (Welsensee et al., 1994)
- Community Competence Scale (Searight and Hubbard, 1998)
- Competency Interview Schedule (Bean et al., 1994)
- Hopkins Competency Assessment Test (Janofsky et al., 1992)
- Incompetency Assessment Scale (Welsensee et al., 1994)
- MacArthur Competence Assessment (Grisso and Applebaum, 1995)
- Patient Competency Rating Scale (Leathem et at., 1998)
- Scale of Competency In Independent Living Skills Scale (Searight and Hubbard, 1998)
- Testament Definition Scale (Hemtk et al., 1999)

Adapted from Griffith, H.R., Belue, K., Sicola, A., Krzywanski, S., Zamrini, E., Harrell, L, & Marson, D.C.(2003). Impaired financial abilities in mild cognitive impairment: A direct assessment approach. Neurology, 60, 449–57.

A full review of his current financial situation and financial decision-making capabilities was a critical part of Mr. Woo's assessment. He began by relating a detailed summary of his current finances and the financial decisions he had made in the past decade. His business assets were divided equally amongst him and his four daughters, with each member of the family controlling 20% of the family company. His company assets included an automotive spare parts company and property investments, which were valued at over $200m. While it was not possible to independently verify these figures, a considerable level of detail was provided that matched that reported by Mr Woo's daughter in a separate interview.

One important component in evaluating mental capacity is an assessment of personal financial asset knowledge. From his personal account, Mr Woo paid himself $3,000 by GIRO each month for daily expenses. His monthly bills were taken care of by the company accountant. He reported having more than 3 million dollars in his bank account and owning a Rolls Royce and a BMW previously valued at $180,000 and $100,000 respectively. In terms of his current appreciation of monetary value, he was able to accurately estimate the price of a meal bought from a hawker centre ($5), the cost of a new pair of leather shoes ($70–80), and the approximate cost of a new shirt ($30–$40) within his tastes and preferences.

A second means of evaluating mental capacity is to assess the reasonableness and validity of a decision-making process. Mr Woo explained he was embarking on legal action against one of his daughters over an alleged financial wrongdoing, in which she had moved the company's capital and shares against his wishes. His legal action was aimed at bringing his daughter in line with his wishes. Mr Woo gave a detailed account of the financial transactions that occurred to instigate this action. He denied being influenced by any third party and maintained that he was acting on his own independent decision. Through the course of discussion Mr Woo demonstrated an in-depth understanding of the intricacies of setting up and financing a new company through contributions of paid-up capital and bank loans. He was familiar with current interest rates and was able to describe the mechanisms of distributing a company's value through shares and dividends.

When asked to weigh the pros and cons of his behaviour, Mr. Woo identified "maintaining justice" and "being fair" as positive outcomes. He believed that the best solution would be for his daughter to be realigned with the family's values of equal treatment for all. His motivation in pursuing legal action did not lie so much in teaching her a lesson but in maintaining the integrity of his entire family. He could see no disadvantages to his actions as he believed that he was in the right and would thus not lose the case. When made aware of the possibility that winning the case could in fact place further strain on family relations, he acquiesced, but was of the opinion that one family member's needs should not outweigh that of others. While his feelings towards his daughter were of concern and disappointment, his other daughters were angry with their sister and wanted her firmly rebuked through legal action. They respected their father's business acumen and achievements and could not understand why she had chosen to turn her back on the rest of the family.

Mr Woo completed a series of neuropsychological tests including tests of IQ, attention, psychomotor processing speed, memory and executive function. He demonstrated orientation to time, day, date, month, year and location. He was able to provide autobiographical information including his year and place of birth but was unable to accurately identify his date of birth as his birth certificate had been lost during World War II. His autobiographical knowledge was demonstrated in his recall of stories from his past, including memories from the second World War. He accurately recalled the year of invasion (1941) and approximate year of Singapore's independence. His knowledge of recent world events was accurate—the US elections and climate change stories were recounted accurately. He could identify the current prime minister of Singapore but not the previous one.

Apart from impediments caused by some hearing loss, Mr Woo was observed to understand questions and to answer them appropriately. He was able to follow commands on formal tests, demonstrating intact simple comprehension language skills. He could easily name drawings of common objects on the Boston Naming Test (a test whose the goal is the identification of simple line drawings of everyday objects) indicating the absence of agnosia (the inability to recognise things) which can occur in dementia. His general speech fluency was normal for his age; he was conversationally fluent and he had good comprehension. In general, there was no evidence of aphasia—an inability or impediment of speech that occurs in brain injury and dementia.

Mr Woo demonstrated moderate-to-severe impairment in visuo-spatial judgment. This was evident from his difficulty in completing visual perception tasks such as clock drawing, reading and the Hooper Test of Visual Perception, which is used to test the discrimination of complex geometric figures. He displayed moderate to severe fine motor dexterity problems on a pegboard task when compared to age-matched norms. These problems were due to his slow and tremulous responding and difficulty in guiding the actions of fine motor movements. Whilst these problems were notable, there was no gross visuo-constructional apraxia or impairment of gross motor skills. His basic attention and ability to follow conversation was intact. On formal tests of attention, Mr Woo could follow/perform basic serial tracking tasks (count 1 to 20 and list the days of the week) but it was not possible to formally assess Mr Woo's psychomotor processing speed due to his lack of education and illiteracy. Nonetheless, his immediate memory of auditory numeric sequences on a Digit Span Task was in the normal range for age. His auditory working memory was mildly impaired relative to norms. Moderate to severe impairments in tracking and repeating sequences of spatial moves on the visual span task were found. His spatial working memory was similarly impaired at the moderate to severe level relative to normative expectations for his age and education.

Mr Woo completed a formal arithmetic subtest on which he attained a scaled score in the mildly impaired range. His errors were primarily due to an inability to understand basic mathematical operations of division and multiplication and slowness in mentally processing the requirements of the questions at hand. With regards to memory, Mr Woo showed moderate to severe deficits in encoding new verbal information on tasks with a significant organisational aspect in encoding (e.g., a ten-item word list). However, deficits were not as pronounced on structured material that required less organisation of material to encode (story memory). Mr Woo could encode and immediately repeat only 33% of a word list after it was repeated three times but could discriminate between previously heard words from novel words with 70% accuracy. His initial encoding and immediate recall of the prose passages was similar and ranged from 20–40% accuracy—but after 30 minutes he could recall all that was initially encoded with up to 100% accuracy. He demonstrated average level ability in the encoding of visuo-spatial images, however, recognition and visual discrimination of previously learned complex visual material was in the moderate to severe range of impairment.

In general, people with low education perform poorly on many psychometric tests. Tests of higher cognitive function (i.e., executive function) are particularly vulnerable to education effects (Lam et al., 2013). Due to Mr Woo's illiteracy and lack of education, only limited assessment of executive function was appropriate. He demonstrated no significant problems grasping abstract concepts within normative expectations when using abstract reasoning to identifying spatial anomalies in pictures. His verbal fluency, a sensitive indicator of core executive function, was normal for age, indicating that he had the capacity to generate novel age-appropriate verbal responses.

DIAGNOSIS

Mr Woo demonstrated selective cognitive impairments that ranged from mild to severe. He had slowed fine motor dexterity, visual perception impairments, impairments in visuo-spatial and auditory working memory ("mental multi-tasking"). He demonstrated moderate to severe impairment in encoding new auditory information, particularly when the material was unstructured, and could encode such information with only 20–40% accuracy even though he could recall what he did learn with 70–100% accuracy. Similarly patchy impairments were seen in visuo-spatial new learning and recall. He demonstrated no evidence of disorientation, apraxia, agnosia or aphasia.

Under DSM-5, with the exception of delirium, the first step in the diagnostic process is to differentiate between normal neurocognitive function, mild neurocognitive disorder (mild NCD), and major neurocognitive disorder (major NCD or dementia).

Whilst Mr Woo had difficulty organising information for the purposes of encoding and recall, he possessed the ability to lay down new memories and to recognise them to some extent (albeit not within the normal range). Because of his lack of education many other tests of cognition were inappropriate. However, apart from his memory problems, there was no evidence of marked cognitive decline in the form of apraxia, agnosia or aphasia. Upon corroborative questioning with his daughter, it was found that his memory had always been poor and had not undergone progressive decline. Diagnostically, it was important that Mr Woo was independent in his daily activities. According to DSM-5 criteria, there was insufficient evidence to conclude that he was suffering from a major neurocognitive disorder.

TABLE 18.3. MODEL OF FINANCIAL CAPACITY

Basic Monetary Skills
- Naming Coins/Currency Identify specific coins and currency
- Coin/Currency relationships Indicate monetary values of coins/currency
- Counting coins/currency Accurately coont arrays of coins and currency

Financial Conceptual Knowledge
- Define financial concepts Define simple financial concepts
- Apply financial concepts Practical applications/computation using concepts

Cash Transactions
- Conduct one item transaction: verify change
- Conduct three item transaction: verify change
- Obtain change for vending machine: verify charge

Chequebook Management
- Understand checkbook Identify/explain parts of checkbook and register
- Use checkbook/register, conduct simple transaction and pay by check

Bank Statement Management
- Understand bank statement Identify/explain parts of a bank statement
- Use bank statement Identify specific transactions on bank statement
- Financial Judgement
- Detect mail fraud risk Detect/explain risks in mail fraud soliCitation
- Detect telephone fraud risk Detect/explain risks in telephone fraud solicitation

Bill Payment
- Understand bills Explain meaning and purpcse of bills
- Prioritize bills Identify overdue utility bill
- Prepare bills for mailing Prepare bills. checks. envelopes for mailing

Knowledge of Assets/Estate
- Indicate personal assets and estate arrangements

Investment Decision Making
- Understand investment options: determine returns, make and explain decision

Adapted from Griffith, et al. (2003)

Instead, Mr Woo met the criteria for mild neurocognitive disorder, as there were observable changes that impacted on his cognitive functioning; these were reported by himself and a close relative (his daughter), and were detected through objective testing.

Mr Woo's cognitive complaints were likely a result of sustained, long-term alcohol exposure and alcohol-related brain damage affecting the frontal executive component of memory functions disproportionately. This pattern of cognitive impairment was consistent with the DSM-5's substance/medication-induced NCD.

INTEGRATIVE FORMULATION

As the goals of this case involved determining Mr Woo's ability to manage his financial affairs, regardless of a diagnosis, it is important to refer to the original aims of the assessment. With regards to the first question of whether Mr Woo had the cognitive capacity to understand and conduct his financial affairs, particularly in relation to personal and company financial matters, it is necessary to keep in mind that capacity is determined by the cognitive ability to understand and appreciate context and decisions, not only the outcomes of the choices made. It was clear that Mr Woo had the ability to understand his financial affairs and to make reasonable decisions. This was because he demonstrated detailed knowledge of financial matters relating to the setting up and financial organisation of his company, as well as apparent knowledge of his company's and his own financial positions, although this was not independently verified. Furthermore, he demonstrated an understanding of the value of money in the form of current costs of living. Most importantly he demonstrated the ability to articulate reasons for making his decision to pursue legal action against his daughter, and an awareness of perceived advantages and disadvantages.

It was clear that Mr Woo was not suffering from any major impediment with regards to sensory perception. The observed impairments in fine motor dexterity did not affect his capacity to make financial decisions or conduct his financial affairs. Although testing was limited due to his lack of education, he demonstrated a relatively intact working memory and displayed some evidence of abstract reasoning ability.

Mr Woo had memory impairments that reduced the volume of new information he could encode, and compromised his ability to retrieve encoded information. However, this impairment was not severe enough to prevent Mr Woo from making a reasonable decision about his finances if information was available to him in other forms. As such, it was recommended that complex financial or legal information be explained simply to him and if necessary, repeated or written in simple statements. Provided with repetition and a written record, Mr Woo would be capable of retaining the information in his memory and have the means to revisit the finer details of his financial decisions.

Mr Woo's receptive and expressive language abilities were intact and he had the capacity to understand legal advice, when presented in a simple form, and instruct legal counsel on matters relating to his finances. He therefore could provide clear instructions in relation to his financial affairs.

TABLE 18.4. SELECTED NEUROPSYCHOLOGICAL TESTS USEFUL IN COMPETENCY ASSESSMENT

- Arithmetic (WAIS-IV)
- Matrix Reasoning (WAIS IV)
- Picture Completion (WAIS-IV)
- Repeatable Battery for the Assessment of Neuropsychological Status (RBANS)
- Similarities (WAIS-IV)
- Wide Ranging Achievement Test-4
- Brief Cognitive Status Exam (WMS-4) or MMSE/MoCA
- Colour Trail Making Test

TREATMENT

In this case, the referral question was limited in scope and goals. Whether intervention is required or desirable in this case is open to question. Mr Woo's drinking behaviour placed him and others at risk and could be the subject of an intervention program. However, from a medico-legal perspective, to begin intervention work with this patient whilst also being responsible for determining competency could be perceived in a court of law to be compromising objectivity. As such, where medico-legal questions of this nature exist, it is usually advisable that the patient be referred to an independent therapist for intervention. Mr Woo's assessment report was forwarded to the referring psychiatrist and he supported the view that Mr Woo was not demented and capable of managing his own financial affairs. Simplified versions of the views of both the psychiatrist's and neuropsychologist's opinions were entered into affidavits in evidence for court proceedings but the matter was never referred to trial, as is often the case, because an out-of-court settlement was reached between the various parties.

In reviewing the new Singapore Mental Capacity Act (2010), Menon (2013) notes that "it is a common misconception that the patient's relatives have the right to make decisions on behalf of the patient who may lack mental capacity. They have no such legal right". As such, it falls upon the courts to decide whether patients retain that capacity and, in some cases, make decisions for those who do not. In recent years, clinical psychologists, neuropsychologists and geropsychologists have been called upon by referring doctors to provide opinions relating to clients' decision-making capacity in complex issues of independence. This trend reflects recognition of the necessity to apply more standardised and comprehensive assessments to assist determinations that strike a balance between the promotion of autonomy and protection of the vulnerable (Moye, 1999). As such, there is an increasing recognition that clinically qualified psychologists, by virtue of their expertise in standardised assessment, are uniquely equipped in this respect as their assessments can enhance the accuracy and comprehensiveness of these determinations (ABA/American Psychiatric Association, 2008).

DISCUSSION

It is possible to characterise capacity as the difference between "... a person who is capable of making a decision and whose choice must therefore be respected [irrespective of the 'reasonableness' of that decision], from one who requires others to make decisions for him/her" (Wong et al., 1999). In essence, capacity is a question of independence. As previously noted, decision-making capacity is domain specific. Financial capacity refers to the ability to independently manage financial affairs in a manner consistent with self-interest and values (Marson & Hebert, 2008); it therefore involves both the ability to independently manage, but also the ability to exercise judgment on one's financial self-interest and act on values that guide financial choices (ABA/American Psychiatric Association, 2008). Marson et al. (2000) suggested that there are several levels to financial competence. The first level is the presence of *specific financial abilities* that are relevant to a particular domain of financial activity (such as paying a bill or taking out a loan, and understanding the mechanics of each). The next level refers *general financial abilities* and knowledge such as the knowledge of personal assets or the ability to perform everyday financial activities such as cash transactions, bank account management, bill payment and so on. The final level is *global financial abilities*, which refers to an overall judgment of the person's capacity to integrate information to make financial decisions that are appropriate to needs or wants.

This case highlights the importance of considering all of these aspects in order to make a comprehensive assessment of a patient's financial decision-making capability. The focus of this case was not so much the patient's ability to perform general financial judgments but more of his understanding of the financial mechanics of his company—its monetary value, how it was organized and his wishes for its future organization. Mr. Woo's legal action against his daughter was intended to safeguard the even dispersal of his assets within his family and, in doing so, he was acting in the interests of his company and his family in accordance with his values.

It would have been desirable to obtain an independent verification of Mr Woo's financial position and spending patterns. However, in the absence of this information, it was important that a report provided by his daughter corroborated his account. As there was no specific assessment tool that could address the referral question, clinical judgment was required when determining his overall level of competence in financial decision-making. This highlights a potential area of conflict between the clinical and legal definitions of competence. Clinicians often view a patient as "competent/capable", "incompetent/incapable", or "partially or marginally competent/ capable" of making decisions; whereas in the adversarial legal system, a person is simply judged to be competent or incompetent.

<table>
<tr><td colspan="2">TABLE 18.5. SIX STEP CAPACITY PROCESS</td></tr>
<tr><td>1. Trigger</td><td>There needs to be an identifiable reason to question a capacity and this should only be done if necessary.</td></tr>
<tr><td>2. Assent</td><td>The assessment of capacity is intrusive and the patient must agree to the process in order for it to be valid.</td></tr>
<tr><td>3. Information Gathering</td><td>Information relating to the person's background and the decision required (i.e., financial, testamentary, healthcare, independent living).</td></tr>
<tr><td>4. Education</td><td>Patients should have the opportunity to be educated about their decision particularly if they do not not fully understand the context of possible pros and cons.</td></tr>
<tr><td>5. Assessment</td><td>Including (but not limited to neuropsychological assessment, as a final test of the capacity to make their decision.</td></tr>
<tr><td>6. Action</td><td>Report-medico-legal or hospital. Referral to other agencies, reporting to relatives.</td></tr>
</table>

Adapted from Darzins, P., Molloy, DW., Strang D (2000) Who can decide?: The six step capacity assessment process. *Memory Australia Press, Adelaide.*

In view of the above considerations, how can a patient with a cognitive disorder be considered competent to make independent financial decisions and manage his financial affairs? Several reports have suggested that elderly patients with even mild amnestic cognitive impairment demonstrate deficits in higher-order financial abilities (as evidenced by impaired financial knowledge, bank account management and bill payment abilities; Griffith et al., 2003), while patients with mild Alzheimer's disease may exhibit diminished financial capacities across most cognitive domains (Marson et al., 2000).

Notwithstanding the association of neurocognitive impairment and impaired financial decision-making, it is important to be aware that the presence of cognitive impairment in and of itself does not necessarily preclude competence. Under common law, a patient is presumed to be competent unless clear-cut evidence of incompetence is presented. Mr Woo would not have met DSM-5 criteria for Major Neurocognitive Disorder and did not show the characteristic signs of AD—progressive decline in cognition characterised by a rapid forgetting amnesia, apraxia, aphasia or agnosia combined with functional impairment in activities of daily living. However, it was clear that he was cognitively impaired. As such, the pertinent question was whether his cognitive impairment was *severe enough* to prevent competent decision making. In this case, there was insufficient evidence to support such a view.

Cases such as these are sometimes challenging in the Singapore context due to the difficulties of psychometric testing in elderly people in Singapore. Within the local population, 65.5% of residents aged 55 and above have less than 6 years of education, whilst only 17.2% have more than 10 years of education (Department of Statistics, 2010). While general literacy rates have increased from 92.5% in 2000 to 95.9% in 2010, a significant number of older individuals have remained illiterate. Moreover, until recently there has been limited psychometric normative data available for elderly Singaporeans (although *see* Yeo et al., 1996; Lim et al., 2010; Lee et al., 2012). It has now become possible to compare the performance of low educated and aged Singaporeans using normative data from a number of different neuropsychological tests in large samples. Most recently, normative data compiled on 1,165 elderly Chinese Singaporeans aged 55–91 years from the Singapore Lifestyle and Ageing Project (SLAS) has been developed. This study, conducted at National University Hospital using the Repeatable Battery for the Assessment of Neuropsychological Status (RBANS), has led to the most comprehensive age and education stratified neuropsychological data available in Asia (Collinson et al. *In Press*). Developing local norms is critical because Asians have been shown to perform more poorly than Caucasians on some neuropsychological tests and better on others for a variety of educational, cultural and linguistic reasons (Hedden et al., 2002; Boone et al., 2007; Fuji, 2010). Consistent with most ethical codes for psychologists around the world, practitioners need to be aware of test bias, test fairness, and cultural equivalence. Singapore is no exception.

Finally, whilst the role of clinical psychologists in the assessment of capacity is increasing—and psychologists bring a high level of knowledge and expertise to this endeavour—it is worth remembering that competence is ultimately a legal determination. The psychologist's role is to provide the best possible professional opinion, even if it is nuanced or stated with caveat or qualification. Many psychologists do not wish to take on such a responsibility and/or may be confused about the definition and scope of competence and capacity. However, should psychologists be aware of ethical issues and understand the legal implications of capacity determinations, and act in good faith and according to the principles of the Mental Capacity Act to the best of current practice standards, their involvement in such cases could prove to be invaluable to the wellbeing of patients and families.

1. Why was it important for the neuropsychologist to use more than objective cognitive test scores when determining Mr Woo's cognitive capacity for financial affairs? What other assessment methods and information were useful?
2. Discuss some challenges in psychometric testing for elderly people in the Singaporean context.
3. Why do families not have the legal right to make decisions behalf of a person with diminished mental capacity?
4. What are the pros and cons of the court making decisions of capacity on a patient's behalf?
5. Why is the need to act in accordance with a patient's values important? And why is it potentially problematic?
6. Mr Woo showed some memory impairments, but they were not deemed serious enough to prevent him making reasonable decisions about his finances. In what circumstances would memory decline prohibit good financial decision-making?
7. Some people leave large sums of money to their pet/s and not their family before they die. Is this reasonable? How would we determine if this is reasonable?

CHAPTER 19

SEEING THROUGH THE CONFUSION

Dementia

PAUL FISHER AND JOY LIM

INTRODUCTION

Mr Tan, a 73-year-old Chinese male, received a diagnosis of dementia from one of the main hospitals in Singapore in 2009. In 2012, he was admitted to an inpatient ward for an assessment of his challenging behaviour at home, which was increasingly difficult to manage. His wife, who works full time, and the family's live-in domestic helper reported high levels of carer stress and were struggling to cope. The admission was initially designed to give his wife respite and allow for a more planned approach towards managing his behaviour. On the ward his continued challenging behaviours resulted in a referral by the ward's senior consultant psychiatrist to inpatient psychology services for assessment.

For the five months prior to assessment, Mr Tan had been verbally and physically aggressive towards his wife or domestic helper when they assisted him in his daily shower. On occasions he would pinch or punch them on the arms, or wring and twist their hands. He would accuse the domestic helper of trying to "rape" him when she tried to undress him for a shower. There were times when it was easier to persuade Mr Tan to shower, for example after he had soiled himself. Since admission to the ward, showering Mr Tan had become even more difficult. At times, five nurses had to attend to his personal care. He would shout vulgarities at the nurses and refuse to undress or be undressed. These incidents were significantly distressing to Mr Tan and nursing staff.

Mr Tan was also verbally aggressive and often agitated. Mrs Tan related how her husband had the habit of walking to the apartment balcony and shouting for hours when he was unable to fall asleep at night. Not only was her sleep compromised, but her stress was also increased by both the noise and the fear of disturbing the neighbours. On the ward, Mr Tan was regularly observed to be shouting and talking to someone even when no one was present. Although staff said they could cope, their response to him were varied and inconsistent. They would attempt to distract him, engage him in conversation, or ignore him.

Mr Tan's use of the toilet was also a problem. At home Mr Tan was often unaware that he needed to go to the toilet. This meant that he regularly soiled himself before his wife or domestic helper noticed any signs that he needed the toilet. When in the bathroom he appeared to not understand how to use the toilet—frequently refusing to sit down on the toilet bowl and occasionally becoming aggressive. When his domestic helper left him alone in the bathroom Mr Tan would eventually urinate and defecate outside the toilet bowl. On the ward, staff had decided that he should wear pads rather than be trained to use the toilet. From the perspective of the staff this solved the problem of his incontinence. However it was not clear if this approach would increase or decrease Mr Tan's independence post-discharge.

BACKGROUND

Mr Tan was the eldest of eight siblings. His first language was his mother's Chinese dialect; throughout his life and whilst on the ward he was always most comfortable conversing in it. He was reported to have been particularly close to his father. His parents depended on him to be a good role model for his siblings, and so had always seen himself as the person-in-charge, responsible for "moving things along". He took the initiative to engage family members and lead them to make family decisions.

Mr Tan had been married twice. His first marriage had ended in a divorce when he was in his late 30s; against his wishes he had lost contact with his three children. This was a significant loss for him and remained a point of sadness. In his early 40s, he had remarried and raised two children with his current wife. It appeared that he had a very loving relationship with his wife who, since his diagnosis of dementia in 2009, seemed a very supportive carer. According to her, he had always been a perfect gentleman who was friendly, sociable and enjoyed drinking with friends in social settings. He loved listening to "golden oldies" from the 1960s. He was reported to have no history of mental health difficulties prior to his diagnosis of dementia.

Mr Tan had previously held several jobs. He talked at length about his time in the army, where he served as an officer. This period of his life was important to him and he was proud of his military record, particularly of having mentored subordinates. Since his diagnosis of dementia in 2009 Mr Tan's occupation had been limited—he spent most of his time sitting in a chair at home. He recognised his wife's voice, and calmed down considerably whenever he heard her or when they listened to music from the 1960s together.

ASSESSMENT

The assessment of Mr Tan's case was holistic and structured around the enriched model of dementia (Kitwood, 1997). Assessment of this type attempts to understand how the following might be impacting on the current problem: the client's level of neurological impairments, his history, current lifestyle, personality, physical health and the interactions between Mr Tan and his carers. Assessment also focused on understanding the unmet psychological needs that may be communicated through his behaviours (Brooker, 2004).

Nurses on the ward completed the Challenging Behaviour Scale (Moniz-Cook, Woods, Gardiner, Silver & Agar, 2001). This provides a measure of Mr Tan's challenging behaviours—how frequently they occurred and how difficult they were to manage. Through an interview with the psychologist, Mrs Tan reported on the difficulties she experienced in managing him at home. This information was used to provide a detailed description of the behaviours Mr Tan was exhibiting.

Mr Tan's wife and others had observed changes in his cognitive functioning (e.g., becoming more forgetful), roughly a year before his diagnosis in 2009. Since then his cognition and functioning had undergone further decline. No formal neuropsychological assessment had been undertaken when he was diagnosed. Given his current agitation and high levels of confusion it was felt that a formal neuropsychological assessment would likely cause significant distress and be unlikely to produce useful findings. Instead, informal interviews were used by the psychologist to get a sense of his cognitive abilities.

Conversations with Mr Tan were conducted in his mother tongue. Mr Tan demonstrated poor eye contact, impaired processing speed and a poor attention span for visual stimulus. He was unable to recognize or name pictures of common objects or to indicate the functions of items presented. However, his verbal processing remained relatively intact. He attended well to verbal stimulus and was able to reliably follow one-step concrete instructions. He could respond to simple closed questions. He demonstrated significant word-finding difficulty in almost all sentences. For words that

Fact Box 19.1. Local epidemiological data

Recent epidemiological studies conducted estimate the age-adjusted prevalence of dementia to be between 2.4% to 5.2% (Ng, Leong, Chiam, & Kua, 2010; Sahadevan et al., 2008). Data from the National Mental Health Survey of the Elderly in Singapore suggests that the number of patients with dementia will increase from 23,000 in 2005 to a projected 53,000 in 2030 (Chiam, Ng, Tan, Ong, Ang, & Kua, 2003). Currently, an epidemiological study is being conducted by the Institute of Mental Health and updated incidence and prevalence figures for dementia will be available soon.

he could not find, Mr Tan used the word "unit" as a substitute. This appeared to be related to his army days.

Mr Tan was observed on the ward in a variety of situations. Given that the most difficult challenge for staff was giving him a shower, the decision was made, after careful consideration, to observe this interaction. This was discussed with him and his wife who agreed to the shower assessment. During the shower session it was noted that his wife's approach of talking him through each step of the shower process and checking he was comfortable appeared to calm him. While at times appearing fearful, he understood and could respond to simple, concrete verbal prompts such as, "use your left hand". Mr Tan took time to process the instructions, but when not rushed, he was able to respond accordingly.

DIAGNOSIS

Clients demonstrating behaviour like Mr Tan often receive a diagnosis of behavioural and psychological symptoms of dementia (BPSD). BPSD can be defined as "symptoms of disturbed perception, thought content, mood or behaviour that frequently occur in patients with dementia" (Hersch & Falzgraf, 2007). Cerejeira, Lagarto and Mukaetova-Ladinska (2012) provide a full review of the concept of BPSD.

BPSD can include aggression (verbal and physical), agitation, disinhibition, and hallucinations, amongst other behaviours. These behaviours can be present in many different types of dementia, such as Alzheimer's disease and vascular dementia. In the case of Mr Tan, it was not clear from available medical records if he had been diagnosed with a particular subtype of dementia. Given that his difficulties had become pronounced across many domains of functioning, establishing a subtype of dementia was no longer a priority for a psychological approach.

Similarly, coming to a diagnostic conclusion of Mr Tan's behaviours was felt to be neither necessary nor useful to either the development of a psychological understanding of the case or to the devising of an intervention plan based on non-pharmacological approaches. In contrast it was felt that a psychological formulation should be the focus of the work. This decision will be considered in the discussion.

INTEGRATIVE FORMULATION

Predisposing Factors

Mr Tan had lived a valued and meaningful life where he placed importance on being in control of both his own life and, to a lesser extent, the lives of others. He had been proud of his achievements; his time in the army, for example, had been a source of self-esteem for him. He had also placed significant value on both familial and other relationships. These experiences contributed to his sense of identity. In this way, during his adult life, his core psychological needs of attachment, identity, inclusion, occupation and comfort (Brooker, 2004) were, for the most part, met. He therefore did not experience significant psychological distress.

Precipitating Factors

The development and progression of dementia caused Mr Tan to experience significant cognitive deficits and to become increasingly confused and detached from his surroundings. His difficulties, particularly with processing information in the visual modality, caused him to experience very significant functional difficulties (e.g., to become unable to shower or use the toilet). Poor insight made it difficult for him to recognise his own difficulties.

Perpetuating Factors

As is common for persons experiencing dementia, this situation caused Mr Tan to feel confused, unsafe and uncomfortable as he struggled to make sense of his surroundings (Cheston & Bender, 1999). This was demonstrated by him accusing his domestic helper of raping him, shouting for help, resisting care and often referring to periods of his life when he felt more in control and safer (e.g., as an army officer). As can be seen Mr Tan's need for comfort was regularly unmet. This was particularly so when he received personal care, hence this being a particular trigger to his challenging behaviour.

Mr Tan's need for identity, in this case to be in control and independent, was also regularly undermined by his experience of dementia. With the decline in his cognition he regularly experienced periods of being out of control (e.g., in the shower or toilet). His response to this was to attempt to reassert himself in order to gain control and to therefore feel safer and more secure. However, with poor communication skills and a limited means of expression, his approach typically involved being physically and verbally aggressive and resisting care. Whilst his wife and domestic helper had

Fact Box 19.2. Language Use Among the Elderly

According to the 2010 Census of the Population, elderly persons (those aged 65 and above) made up 9.0% of the Singaporean population (Singapore Statistics, 2010). More than half the elderly persons surveyed (54.1%) were found to speak dialect at home. Literacy among the elderly was 75.5%, as compared to the general literacy rate of 95.9%. While most elderly persons were literate in at least one of the official languages of Singapore—English, Mandarin, Bahasa Melayu, Tamil—2.8% were found to be literate in other languages.

developed approaches to manage these behaviours (e.g., encouraging him to do as much as possible, backing off), his maladaptive behaviours were amplified on the ward, which was an unfamiliar environment with unfamiliar people. For example, being showered by nurses he did not know increased his feeling of being out of control, thereby increasing his attempts to assert himself to regain control. The nursing staff's response of increasing the number of staff during his shower time only reduced his sense of control and further exacerbated his behaviour.

Alongside this, the cognitive loss associated with Mr Tan's dementia made it increasingly difficult to meet his needs for inclusion and occupation (e.g., he was alone and under-stimulated for most of the day); this served as a further threat to his identity. The experience of dementia also heightened Mr Tan's attachment needs (Cheston and Bender, 2003). Because he felt increasingly unsafe, uncomfortable, and out of control, his needs for attachment and closeness were intensified. However it was increasingly difficult for him to get those needs met due to his cognitive difficulties, which included an inability to recognise his wife. His attachment needs were greater in the unfamiliar ward environment where he had much less access to familiar people, objects and places. The behaviours he exhibited in response to this only served to worsen the situation as they caused those close to him to feel exhausted or wary. Thus his attachment needs remained unmet. In this way the systems around Mr Tan, at home and on the ward, not only maintained his current difficulties but also pointed to ways in which he could be helped to get his needs met.

Protective Factors

In terms of protective factors, Mr Tan's psychological needs seemed to have been met in the earlier stages of his life. This would explain how, under the right conditions and with the right support he was currently able to find periods of attachment, identity, inclusion, occupation and comfort. For example, his mood was calmed by the presence of persons with whom he had developed an attachment relationship, or by objects associated with them. In addition to this, he continued to receive the support and care of his wife, who remained a dedicated carer during his admission to the ward.

PROGNOSIS

Mr Tan's prognosis was mixed. In the short term, work to meet his psychological needs and to change how he was cared for on a day-to-day basis was likely to improve his psychological well-being and reduce his levels of distress and associated challenging behaviour. A psychological approach was also likely to help those caring for Mr Tan to gain further understanding of his difficulties and to maintain or further develop empathy for him. Any progress with Mr Tan was highly dependent on working closely with those around him—providing them with information that made sense of his presentation—and acknowledging the struggles they faced. However, given the nature of dementia it was difficult to predict his prognosis in the longer term. As his cognition continued to decline, it was likely that some of his challenging behaviours would decrease, only to be replaced by other difficulties. Focusing on how Mr Tan tried to meet his basic psychological needs was likely to be useful throughout this process.

TREATMENT

For the one month of Mr Tan's admission, intervention consisted of roughly twice-weekly sessions with the ward staff team and Mrs Tan. Sessions focused on first discussing the formulation and recommendations and subsequently generating ideas for the implementation of these recommendations. Concurrent work with Mr Tan focused on understanding more about his difficulties and observing his reactions to interactions with nurses. All aspects of the intervention were designed to be consistent with a person-centred approach. They aimed to help those caring for him to find new ways to meet his psychological needs, thereby reducing his level of challenging behaviour. The intervention had three main phases, all linked to the assessment and formulation.

Mr Tan's formulation was first discussed with his wife, domestic helper and ward staff during a number of meetings. A written report was attached to his case notes for the whole multidisciplinary team to review. Mrs Tan found the formulation useful as it made sense of her husband's behaviour and absolved him of blame or being labelled "naughty". In contrast, nursing staff were initially more sceptical of the formulation and the use of psychological ideas to understand his presentation (as opposed to labeling the behaviours as BPSD) and provided limited feedback.

To help Mr Tan to orientate better to and engage more effectively with his surroundings, those around him were encouraged to use verbal cues (short, simple, concrete words) rather than visual cues. For example, rather than pointing, Mr Tan would be told that the toilet was "on [his] left". They were encouraged to avoid using the word "unit" and to substitute it with what they assumed "unit" referred to, so that his needs and intentions were clarified. As he had slowed processing speed, staff were advised to give him enough time to respond (five seconds) before providing more information or repeating something to him. This enabled him to be more engaged in communication with those around him.

To help meet Mr Tan's need for attachment and identity, it was recommended that his environment, both on the ward and at home, was filled with familiar "transitional" objects and voices. Transitional objects can provide people with a sense of attachment, safety and comfort as they remind people of their connections to important other people, such as family members (Stephens, Cheston & Gleeson, 2013). For Mr Tan, these included his daughter's old pillow and a vocal recording of his wife speaking to him, which could be played when she was away.

Letting Mr Tan listen to music was recommended to further increase his activity and stimulation. This approach, already being used by Mrs Tan, allowed her husband to stay connected to parts of his identity. Encouraging him to sing along to familiar songs helped preserve his existing skills. He was observed to be engaged and interested when familiar songs were played, and at these times rarely displayed any challenging behaviour.

To help Mr Tan feel more control over his life, and to increase his activity, he was encouraged to remain independent with people around him giving him verbal prompts and guiding his hands in tasks. For example, during meal times, he could be directed with verbal instructions to use a spoon himself instead of relying on someone to feed him. During shower times he could be encouraged to soap himself.

It was recommended that staff respected Mr Tan's wishes as far as possible when he refused personal care such as showering. Given that he was agreeable to personal care on occasion, such an approach was practical and likely to result in more positive interactions between him and the staff. This would, in turn, provide him with more comfort and a greater sense of control over his life, resulting in less distress for all. Nursing staff were advised to be vigilant for times when he was likely to be agreeable to personal care (e.g., after bowel motion). Given that showering him could take longer than other patients on the ward, they needed to consider carefully when to attend to his personal care needs as rushing this process increased his distress and agitation.

It was also recommended that the minimum number of staff required were involved when Mr Tan was being showered, or during other interactions for personal care. This was to minimise the risk of Mr Tan feeling out of control, unsafe or even violated, thereby decreasing the chances of him reacting aggressively. It was recommended that no extra staff member enter the bathroom unless the call bell had been activated and that when in the bathroom, only one staff member give guidance to him so as to avoid confusing him. This approach to personal care would enable him to use his existing skills, gently support him in the areas he found to be more challenging, while also allowing him the maximum amount of control, thus reducing his levels of distress and subsequent challenging behaviour.

Following these recommendations, small changes in the nursing staff's behaviour were noticed. A nurse, for example, brought music for Mr Tan to listen to. Nurses began attempting personal care when he was less reluctant and backing off when he was resistive. The nursing staff changed their approach to him somewhat, by being more respectful and using less infantilising language (e.g., referring to him as Mr Tan rather than using a colloquial name). Despite these modest changes, however, application of the psychologist's recommendations was not consistent.

Due to the demands already placed on the staff, no formal outcome measures for the intervention were collected. However, a reduction in Mr Tan's challenging behaviour was observed during the intervention period. He shouted less frequently. At times he resisted personal care (e.g., having his pads changed), but with a more relaxed approach from the staff, the episodes became less frequent and rarely escalated into aggression. Although his occupation levels did not significantly improve, he would listen to music quietly on the ward and began to enjoy talking with the staff.

Mrs Tan's stress levels were also reduced. The support validated much of what she was doing as her husband's carer, which she reported was helpful. It also enabled her to more fully consider both their futures. She experienced a renewed desire to care for him at home, but also began to consider the possibility that his complex needs might eventually be best managed in a nursing home environment.

Ideally the intervention was expected to have continued after Mr Tan's discharge. Unfortunately, this was not possible due to Mrs Tan's return to full-time work and inability to attend the hospital for a review. However, she seemed more capable of caring for her husband post-intervention and it was hoped that her understanding of his formulation and observation of the work carried out in the hospital would enable her to better understand and address her husband's psychological needs.

DISCUSSION

The experience of working with Mr Tan demonstrated that within dementia care the person-centred approach (Brooker, 2004; Kitwood, 1997) is often far removed from current clinical practice, which maintains its roots in the traditional "medical model" of dementia. Much of the holistic and person-centred assessment, formulation and intervention for him was very different from the ward's existing practices. However, emerging evidence from many sources demonstrates the need for a person-centred approach. From an international perspective, evidence shows that the traditional medical model of using pharmacological approaches to manage challenging behaviour has limited benefits and frequent side effects (Ballard & Waite, 2006; Kamble, Chen, Sherer, & Aparasu, 2009; Sink, Holden, & Yaffe, 2005). In contrast the person-centred formulation and intervention-based approach has been shown to be useful and cost effective (Bird, Llewellyn-Jones, & Korten, 2009; Bird, Llewellyn-Jones, Korten, & Smithers, 2007; Brodaty, Green, & Koschera, 2003).

In keeping with current worldwide trends, hospitals and other care institutions across Singapore are increasingly focused on the application of person-centred care. Person-centred care was highlighted as a philosophy of care that could be applied in dementia day programs in the 2009 Singapore National Dementia Strategy (Ministry of Health, 2009). A person-centred care steering team was also set up by the Alzheimer's Disease Association, Singapore. This steering team has focused on increasing awareness and knowledge of person-centred approaches across Singapore. This description of clinical work with Mr Tan demonstrates the practical application of the principles of person-centred care in a real-world, Singaporean, clinical setting.

Very early on, it was recognised that, because of Mr Tan's cognitive decline, Mrs Tan and the nursing staff would provide most of the relevant assessment information and would be key persons in implementing any recommendations. At the same time, it was critical to spend time with him throughout all stages of assessment and treatment, so as to maintain a clear and unbiased sense of him in mind, and to recognise that he was a unique individual struggling to make sense of his situation (Kitwood, 1997) and have his needs met (Stokes, 2000). This approach allowed for the principles of person-centred care to spill over to all aspects of the work, including those not focusing directly on Mr Tan.

One significant weakness of the work with Mr Tan was the lack of good quality outcome data to support the intervention. Although the Challenging Behaviour Scale (Moniz-Cook et al., 2001) was used as part of the assessment process, it was difficult to use as a reliable outcome measure in the hospital inpatient setting as no one member of staff could provide a consistent account of his behaviours due to staff rotating in shifts. In cases such as this the best indicator of change is the recording of clearly observable behaviours (such as shouting) in a standardised way over various time points. Dementia care mapping is one example of such a standardised approach (Brooker & Surr, 2005). Recordings could happen prior to, during the implementation of, and after the intervention phase of the work with the client. Given resource issues, this was not possible with him, but has been used before in published research of individualised formulation-based approaches to managing challenging behaviour (e.g., Bird et al., 2009). The important body of evidence on dementia care mapping shows how approaches such as those used in this case can lead to a decrease in challenging behaviour and a reduction in staff distress whilst also being cost-effective. However in terms of increasing person-centred care in a local context (e.g., the ward where Mr Tan was a patient), local data regarding the effectiveness of these approaches would be invaluable and needs to be incorporated as a standard part of casework. This will not only benefit current clients and their families—whose needs are better understood—but also future clients through better staff and organisational culture.

This case may have benefited from a broader, more systemic focus. Previous research has suggested that measures such as carers' distress are also legitimate targets for assessment and intervention (Bird et al., 2009). Examples of interventions that may have been useful to care staff could have included a reflective practice group, increasing staff's access to supervision, and focusing on building staff compassion (for both self and others). Increasing support for staff has been found to increase their psychological well-being (Cole, Scott & Skelton-Robinson, 2000); during the current work with Mr Tan a more explicit focus on staff welfare may have enabled the staff team to feel that the challenges of their role were understood and increased their openness to the psychological approach.

Mr Tan's case illustrates how very common it is for clients with challenging behaviour to be labeled as having BPSD. However a diagnosis of BPSD may not have been in his best interests as it suggested that his presentation was solely due to dementia, thus minimising other relevant factors. This diagnostic approach is generally not consistent with the person-centred approach (Kitwood, 1997) or with the concept of formulation, which is central to the work of a clinical psychologist (Bulter, 1998; Johnstone & Dallos, 2006), and it presented a significant challenge when working with Mr Tan. De-emphasising the diagnostic approach and concentrating on challenging behaviour meant taking an approach outside of the mainstream medical perspective. Along with the need to provide more support directly to staff, the difference in approach between the psychological, person-centred, perspective and the traditional medical perspective might explain why some of the nursing staff did not wholeheartedly engage in the formulation and intervention. For institutions, such as the ward where Mr Tan was a patient, staff will need additional training before they can fully engage in person-centred practice. Training would focus on the principles of person-centred care and, in particular, aim to support and supervise the application of person-centred care principles while maintaining an appropriate focus on the medical aspects of a client's presentation.

The person-centred approach aims to make sense of the experiences and challenging behaviours of clients with dementia in a way that is both respectful and builds on the psychological evidence base. Working with Mr Tan required the building of a meaningful relationship with him and required those around him to make small but important changes to his care and environment to enable his basic human needs to be met. This case study highlights the need for good outcome data, even in routine clinical practice, to demonstrate the value of applying person-centred principles. Further, this case illustrates the need to consider the system around the client when trying to make any changes to their care. Using person-centred principles enables clinicians to see through the confusion that these cases can generate and allows them to connect with the person beneath.

DISCUSSION QUESTIONS

1. The broad and detailed assessment undertaken in this case was structured around the need to gather information regarding the client's level of neurological impairments, his history, current lifestyle, personality, physical health and the interactions between him and his carers. Which of these was most important in the development of a formulation?

2. How do you think Mr Tan feels when he is taken into the bathroom? Rather than writing a list, write a paragraph or two from Mr Tan's perspective as he struggles to make sense of what is happening.

3. If you were to find yourself in a very confused and disoriented state one day, possibly due to dementia, write a list of how you would want your life to be and how you would want others to treat you so that you felt safe, content and valued. When you have finished your list consider how well the items can fit under the following headings: attachment, identity, inclusion, occupation and comfort.

4. If instead of developing the formulation, the psychologist, and other professionals in the team had diagnosed the client as experiencing BPSD, how would the proposed intervention have been different?

CHAPTER 20.

THE MIND-BODY-GUT CONNECTION

Irritable Bowel Syndrome

NENNA NDUKWE

INTRODUCTION

Madam Choo was a 68-year-old Chinese Singaporean lady who was referred for psychological assessment by her doctor, a consultant gastroenterologist. Madam Choo had been diagnosed with Irritable Bowel Syndrome (IBS), a functional gastrointestinal disorder in which individuals often report distressing symptoms including abdominal pain, bloating, diarrhoea and constipation (Gerson et al., 2006). The referral stated that Madam Choo struggled to effectively manage her IBS and this had resulted in a flare up of the typical symptoms of IBS. As a consequence, Madam Choo was feeling low and was worried her symptoms would worsen. She was also embarrassed by her symptoms and had withdrawn from social activities, such as dining out with friends and volunteering in church. Moreover, she had difficulty choosing and adhering to an appropriate dietary plan to aid her IBS.

BACKGROUND

Madam Choo was a retired bank administrator who had been married to her husband for 32 years. She had three children, two of whom lived in Singapore while the youngest studied in the United Kingdom. Madam Choo had experienced frequent complaints of stomachache, nausea and diarrhoea for many years. Over the past year, she had felt increasingly anxious and low in mood as she had been unable to control the flare up of these symptoms.

Following periods of being symptom-free, she would often assume that her symptoms would eventually improve. While she suspected that stress and her diet played a significant role in triggering these symptoms, she remained unclear about their pattern and not entirely certain of her actual triggers, leading her to feel, on the whole, helpless and pessimistic about her condition improving.

Initially preoccupied by the thought that she might have bowel cancer, Madam Choo spent a lot of time seeking opinions about her symptoms from her physician, friends, family, and the internet. Mr Choo was concerned about his wife's level of discomfort and her concerns. He encouraged her to approach her GP for help. He also suggested that she try using Chinese medicine to alleviate her symptoms. However, Madam Choo was reluctant to do so and did not feel that it would benefit her much. Her eventual consultation with her GP led to a prescription of pain-relieving medication and a referral to a specialist gastroenterology (GI) clinic; it was here that she was formally diagnosed with irritable bowel syndrome (IBS), and referred to a specialist clinical psychologist. While reluctant to consult psychological services at first, she decided to seek help six months later.

Madam Choo acknowledged that she had always been an anxious person. She recounted feeling easily affected by "too much pressure" and significant changes in her life. She reflected that her anxiety was triggered during stressful periods, such as when she felt incapable of meeting increasing demands at work. One episode occurred when her husband had been ill for a protracted period of time and she had to struggle to single-handedly manage household matters. Madam Choo noticed that during periods of heightened anxiety she often experienced headaches, difficulty sleeping and stomachaches. In terms of coping, she had always been unable to balance demands and had a tendency to internalize her feelings rather than voice them.

Prior to her referral, Madam Choo had experienced two episodes of depression. The first occurred in 2000 when her husband became ill with heart problems and she feared that he might die. She was prescribed Prozac by her physician to reduce her depressive symptoms and she eventually stopped taking medication a year later. In 2006, she experienced a second episode of depression following work stress. Her work environment had become too demanding, yet she feared losing her job if she complained. Once again, she was able to reduce her depressive symptoms by taking medication and allowing herself time to process the triggering events. Madam Choo had no previous involvement with psychology and counselling services.

ASSESSMENT

Given the nature of Madam Choo's presenting problems (emotional distress, reduced activity, negative thinking and physical complaints) a cognitive behavioural framework was used to structure and gather assessment data (White, 2001). The first session was spent clarifying Madam Choo's understanding of why she had been referred, and what her main concerns were. Madam Choo was initially sceptical about what could be achieved as her primary goal was symptom relief for her IBS condition. She also worried about the stigma associated with seeking help from a psychologist. She was immediately defensive: "What are you going to do to me today?", "I'm not mental, so not sure why am I here?" Her fear was that she would be sent to the mental health hospital. Accordingly, she had a tendency to minimize her concerns and repeatedly enquire how psychology services could help her. The clinical psychologist was able to help Madam Choo to understand what would take place in the sessions and answer her questions. Spending time building rapport and allowing Madam Choo to ask questions about the assessment and treatment plan was essential.

The assessment revealed that Madam Choo's physical symptoms, low mood and anxiety became more prevalent following a one-year period of increased stress characterized by financial difficulties and various life and work transitions. She also viewed herself as the problem solver of the family, and tended to take on too much and not ask for help.

Madam Choo attributed her complaints of abdominal pain, nausea and diarrhoea to her IBS being out of her control. Her thoughts included "I do not understand IBS", "It's too hard to manage and I've tried everything", "I want to be able to enjoy my life but I can't as I'm in pain" and ongoing fears of possible bowel cancer. She reported feelings of sadness and anxiety due to uncertainty about the cause of her IBS. She also remained fearful of her prognosis and uncertain on how to manage her condition. On top of feeling easily fatigued and nauseous due to her condition, Madam Choo's poor management of IBS meant that she also experienced regular bloating, abdominal pain and diarrhoea. These symptoms had caused her to withdraw from social activities such as eating out, mixing with friends and regular outings. She felt that these symptoms were an inconvenience and disruption to her quality of life. She chose to isolate herself rather than be a burden to others. Furthermore, she exhibited low self-efficacy with regards to coping. For example, she often discontinued her IBS medication and sought various remedies such as using painkillers, drinking herbal tea and making changes to her diet to alleviate her concerns, but to no avail.

Madam Choo was a devout Christian who attended church regularly. She enjoyed the support of this community, in addition to the company of her husband, family and friends. Madam Choo's faith seemed to help her in remaining hopeful that her health would improve once she understood the cause of her IBS and meaning of her symptoms. Her supportive family and social network reduced her feelings of isolation and occasionally helped in her to have a positive outlook.

The IBS-Symptom Severity Scale (IBS-SSS; Francis, Morris & Whorell, 1997), was used to gauge the severity of Madam Choo's physical symptoms. The IBS-SSS categorizes IBS symptoms as mild, moderate or severe. Madam Choo's scores classed her as having severe symptoms. A baseline measure of her symptoms was taken using the Hospital Anxiety and Depression Scale (HADS), developed by Zigmond & Snaith (1983). The HADS consists of a 14-item scale (seven for anxiety and seven for depression) marked out of a total score of 21. It was used to assess Madam Choo's emotional state and levels as a baseline measure of anxiety and depression. Madam Choo endorsed scores for anxiety (16 out of 21) and depression (17 out of 21) in the severe range, indicating marked distress. After being told what these scores meant, she confirmed that these were an accurate reflection of the impact of living with IBS.

Madam Choo was not found to be at risk of suicidal ideation, and she did not pose any risk to herself or others.

Madam Choo was diagnosed with IBS by her gastroenterologist. Diagnosis of IBS is achieved using a system known as the Rome III Criteria (Longstreth et al., 2006), which is used to classify functional gastrointestinal disorders. The criteria for a diagnosis of IBS includes recurrent abdominal pain or discomfort and change in bowel habit for at least six months. Symptoms have to be experienced on at least three days per month in the last three months, with at least two of the following criteria: 1) pain relieved by bowel movement; 2) onset of pain is related to a change in frequency of stool; 3) onset of pain is related to a change in the appearance of stool.

Madam Choo exhibited IBS-specific anxiety and low mood. Psychological factors and somatisation have been strongly associated with IBS (Choung, 2009). Madam Choo's anxiety was characterised by worry about physical symptoms and hypervigilance. She experienced physical complaints linked to her psychological symptoms, and avoided situations that might be associated with or trigger her physical symptoms. According to the DSM-5, Madam Choo met the criteria for Anxiety Related to a Medical Condition in addition to her meeting the criteria for Somatic Symptom Disorder as a differential diagnosis. She did not meet the criteria for any of the anxiety or depressive disorders as per the DSM-5.

INTEGRATIVE FORMULATION

A psychological formulation of Madam Choo's IBS and associated anxiety and low mood was conducted during session three. This formulation was shared with her and she was encouraged to contribute to the process.

Predisposing Factors

Madam Choo's history of unresolved gastrointestinal (GI) complaints had led to fixed beliefs of her incapacity to manage, or to be in control of her physical symptoms. These experiences predisposed her to having an external locus of control and a pessimistic outlook with regards to symptom management. Madam Choo's history of depression and anxiety further predisposed her to feeling vulnerable and prone to marked periods of distress and negative thinking when events were perceived to be out of her control.

Precipitating Factors

While there are multiple causes for GI complaints, acute periods of stress in Madam Choo's life appear to have been a precipitating factor to GI difficulties as well as to heightened periods of emotional distress she experienced.

Perpetuating Factors

Madam Choo's GI symptoms were perpetuated by ongoing stress, poor adherence to medication, and a lack of knowledge about her IBS condition and ways to successfully manage it. This increased her sense of helplessness and produced feelings of anxiety and low mood. In addition, Madam Choo's tendency to focus on her GI symptoms resulted in her hypersensitivity to flare ups, which she was unable to manage. Madam Choo's anxiety and low mood were maintained by her negative thoughts, in which she believed her condition to be out of her control, catastrophic thoughts of her symptoms pointing to ovarian cancer, and feared that she would be sent to a mental hospital. In addition, she perceived herself to be a burden to others, which led to a withdrawal from social and pleasurable activities. This increased her sense of isolation and further contributed to her low mood and anxiety.

Protective Factors

Important protective factors that encouraged positive outcomes included Madam Choo's religious faith, supportive family, social network and her willingness to seek help from health care services once she realised that she could not cope on her own.

PROGNOSIS

The prognosis for people living with IBS can be positive once there is a good understanding of the condition, and an adherence to an appropriate diet and certain lifestyle changes. Adherence to medication and psychological therapy are also beneficial. While Madam Choo was initially sceptical, her increasing engagement over the first few sessions illustrated an important resolve to gain and apply knowledge and skills from therapy. Psychological treatments such as cognitive behavioural treatment (CBT) have been shown to be effective in treating individuals living with IBS (Tang, Lin & Zhang, 2013). Therefore, it was expected that Madam Choo would develop useful strategies to help with managing her anxiety, low mood and GI symptoms.

Madam Choo's struggles adjusting to her condition and emotional management were factors that could impede her progress if not managed appropriately. There was a possibility that Madam Choo could become overwhelmed by the challenges of therapy. Therefore, it would be important to be mindful of discussing and addressing this issue with Madam Choo during therapy.

TREATMENT

Madam Choo worked with the psychologist to compile concrete goals for therapy. These included learning more about IBS and using this knowledge to reduce symptoms, develop strategies to improve her low mood and anxiety, resume normal levels of activity, such as dining out regularly with family and friends, volunteering in church, and socialising with friends. Therapy was conducted over seven structured sessions across a three-month period. Madam Choo attended these weekly sessions and was always punctual for her appointments.

The treatment plan included familiarising Madam Choo with the CBT model. She was given information to aid her in understanding of CBT as a form of collaborative and problem-solving based therapy. Figure 20.1 illustrates the focus of CBT on the behaviours, thoughts, and feelings impacting Madam Choo's IBS symptoms. She was introduced to the concept of "CBT homework", in which she would learn new skills during the week and monitor her own progress. Madam Choo had initially hoped that CBT could eliminate her GI symptoms. It was explained that CBT could not remove IBS, but could help her manage its symptoms, which could significantly improve her quality of life.

Madam Choo revealed that, at the time of her diagnosis, there had been too much new information to remember about IBS and too little time to pursue symptom management in depth. Her curiosity and questioning nature provided a positive forum for education on the nature of IBS and how to manage it—an essential component of therapy. She was told how IBS can affect the digestive system, received confirmation that abdominal pain, bloating, nausea, diarrhoea and fatigue are typical symptoms of IBS, and how these symptoms could be aggravated by diet, stress and poor compliance to her medical regime. She was surprised to hear that many people become frustrated, moody and anxious because they have to deal with uncomfortable symptoms. This insight made her "feel normal" and helped to allay her initial fears of going mad and the embarrassment of seeing a psychologist. She was encouraged to keep a record of her questions concerning IBS and to seek opportunities to consult with her physician in order to gain another perspective on the cause and management of IBS.

Madam Choo agreed to keep a diary of her GI symptoms, which would help her to identify triggers to GI flare ups and track patterns of setbacks and progress in symptom management. She found that this increased her confidence in the self-management of IBS. Madam Choo was taught to be more proactive in managing her health and diet and encouraged to gradually increase the time she spent on pastimes and leisure activities with the support of her loved ones. She gradually increased her outings and experimented with different foods without encountering any challenges. Eventually, Madam Choo began to feel a greater sense of control over her condition and less of a failure. Positive affirmation from the psychologist at each consultation helped her to remain optimistic, validated her efforts and reinforced the good feedback she was receiving from her family and friends regarding self-management.

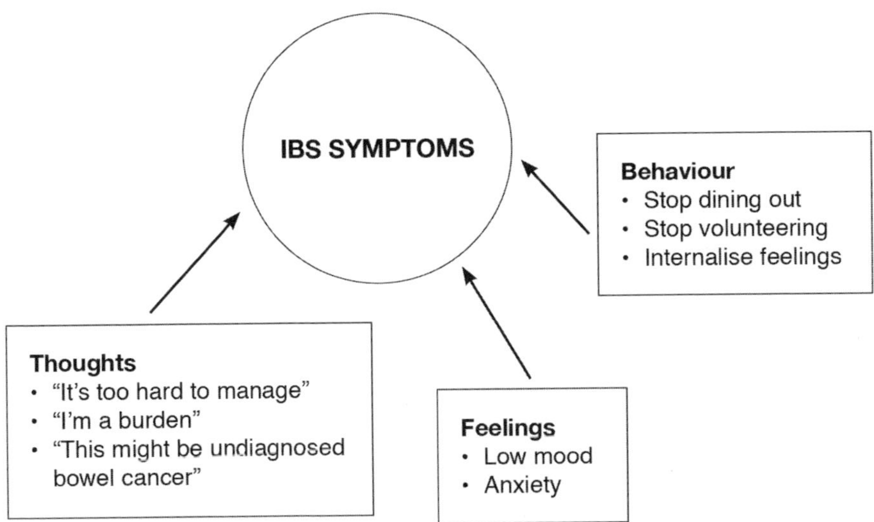

Through therapy, Madam Choo was able to learn that thoughts such as "I'm a burden", "I have ovarian cancer", "I can't cope", "I will end up in a mental hospital", "I need to see a doctor to tell me what is really wrong" contributed to feelings of anxiety, low mood and diminished effectiveness in managing her GI symptoms. She was thus taught to monitor negative or unhelpful thoughts using another diary and encouraged to evaluate their validity. Madam Choo decided to begin by examining the statement "I'm a burden to others", which she believed to be true. IBS caused her to feel dependent on others and she assumed that people viewed her as a sickly person. Asking her husband and close friends what they thought of her was a challenge as she felt embarrassed about "losing face" and appearing weak and sickly. With gentle encouragement, she was able to gather mixed feedback from her family and friends.

From her husband, she found out that while not perceived to be a burden, she sometimes spoke too much about her condition. This made him feel hopeless at times, yet it made him aware that Madam Choo was really struggling to cope. He subsequently encouraged her to seek support and to talk more openly about her IBS. Furthermore, Madam Choo's close friends gave her affirmation that she was loved. They encouraged her to ask for help and readily availed themselves to support her. Through this homework exercise Madam Choo's perception of herself was changed. Rather than a burden, she saw herself as loved and valued. She made a commitment to consider how she could reach out to her family and friends for support.

Madam Choo also worked hard to improve her ability to ask for help. She practiced expressing her needs (e.g., asking a friend for support and encouragement when her symptoms felt unmanageable), during role play within and outside of sessions. Madam Choo was able to express her needs well in sessions, but felt that she needed more practice before she could feel at ease and not anxious when doing so.

During therapy sessions Madam Choo was encouraged to explore her other negative thoughts. She progressed from the belief that IBS was destroying her life to feeling more empowered: "I will not be defeated by IBS", "I deserve to enjoy myself and be happy", "I will have days were I feel defeated but I can try again tomorrow". Madam Choo also realised that continuously seeking help from medical services fueled her worries about having a more serious diagnosis. To minimise her tendency to catastrophize, Madam Choo learnt to challenge her negative thoughts, to practice behavioural strategies (diaphragmatic breathing, guided imagery, progressive muscle relaxation) and to divert her attention to more positive activities (watching television or going for a short walk).

Madam Choo also found relaxation helpful in managing stressful situations. For example, she used to avoid social outings and dining out. This was because certain foods would aggravate her symptoms and she was fearful of bloating and frequent trips to the bathroom in the presence of others. With relaxation techniques, she felt calm enough to set herself small targets such as making better food choices, sharing her concerns rather than hiding them, and quelling her agitation rather than resorting to panicking, feeling helpless and embarrassed.

In terms of relapse prevention Madam Choo learnt that because IBS symptoms wax and wane it was important for self-management to be a normal part of her life. She was pleased with her progress in therapy and received positive feedback about management of her symptoms from her gastroenterologist.

When HADS was administered at the end of therapy, Madam Choo's scores placed in the mild range. This was compared to her initial assessment profile, which was in the severe range for anxiety and depression. Madam Choo attributed her progress to a combination of several factors such as her uptake of medication for symptom management, her positive response to therapy and her receipt of family and social support. She had been able to gather new information through therapy, attain her goals, and observe improvement in her overall well-being, and she felt her IBS symptoms were much more manageable. Madam Choo had also gained more confidence and reported feeling happier. Madam Choo recognized the importance of maintaining her progress and planned to join an existing hospital-based IBS support group in the hospital and to offer her support to others. In addition Madam Choo noted that she would continue to practice the strategies learnt during therapy.

DISCUSSION

IBS arises from an interplay of biological and psychosocial factors (Longstreth, et al., 2006). It is prevalent in both Asian and Western countries (Talley, 2008), and is known to affect 5–11% of the population (Spiller et al., 2007). In Singapore, a community survey showed 8.6% of respondents fulfilled the diagnostic criteria for IBS (Gwee, Lu & Ghoshal, 2009). Indeed, incident rates in Asia have been comparable to Europe (9.6%) and Australia (6.9%), although not as high as Canada and the UK (12%), (Gwee et al. 2009).

Although IBS is not a life-threatening condition, the impact of symptoms on individuals is significant. It is normal for people like Madam Choo to ask why they have been diagnosed with IBS and to seek symptom relief. In addition they may experience a range of emotions connected to their diagnosis such as anxiety, low mood, despair and helplessness. Therefore, it is critical that people living with IBS are equipped with adequate knowledge of IBS and the practical skills to effectively manage their condition and to seek appropriate help (Halpert et al. 2007).

Despite being provided with information about IBS during her diagnosis, Madam Choo felt insufficiently prepared to deal with it. The responsibility for communicating with the client at the point of diagnosis should be with the treating physician or gastroenterologist. For example, the role of medication in reducing symptoms could be explained by the treating physician. Information about condition management could also be reinforced at follow-up visits. Additionally, psychologists working within functional gastrointestinal disorder clinics should possess knowledge of IBS, the digestive system, and the role of various biopsychosocial factors such as diet, stress and their relationship to GI symptoms. Such knowledge would be helpful in understanding clients' experiences and the unique challenges associated with IBS.

Many people living with IBS, such as Madam Choo, will require help in understanding misconceptions regarding their health. When IBS symptoms are severe and chronic, these persons may fear underlying diseases such as cancer. Misunderstanding their symptoms can cause clients anxiety and increase their level of distress. They may also display low mood, frustration, poor self-efficacy and have

---

Fact Box 20.1. The role of clinical psychologists in IBS settings

1. Psycho-education regarding IBS and links to thoughts, feelings and behaviour
2. Undertaking of assessments
3. Client-centred formulation
4. Therapeutic interventions
5. Multidisciplinary team working
6. Research, teaching, training of interns in physical health and other allied professionals

problems coping with IBS because of overwhelming demands. In addition, many clients may struggle to manage perceived losses, changes to their quality of life and an acceptance of IBS. Given these challenges clinicians and therapists play an important role in listening actively to their clients, encouraging them to share their experiences and concerns, and enabling them to feel that their concerns are valid and taken seriously (Azpiroz & Whorwell, 2009).

Seeking appropriate help from psychological services in addition to medical services can be beneficial for people living with IBS. However, help-seeking might be hampered by fear and stigmatisation of mental health. For example, Madam Choo was initially anxious about seeing a psychologist, because she was embarrassed about seeing a "doctor of the mind", did not want to risk losing face and was worried about how she would be perceived by those closest to her. In cases like this, it is especially important that psychologists are aware of and understand their client's cultural beliefs concerning psychological distress, mental health, physical symptoms and help-seeking behaviours, and when explaining their role to clients, ensure their explanations fit with their client's beliefs and frames of reference (Kramer et al. 2002).

The role of psychologists in GI services in Singapore is noteworthy because there has been an absence of such specialist services. This could be partly attributed to the fact that clinical psychology in medical settings within Singapore is still a developing profession, with few specialist clinical psychologists working in physical health. One of the recent developments in Singapore for people living with IBS was a Functional Gastrointestinal Disorder (FGID) psychology service that was established at the National University Hospital Singapore in 2010. Given the initiation of a FGID psychology unit in Singapore, continued investment in the service should be a priority. Attention should be given to understanding help-seeking behaviour among Singaporeans living with IBS, their perceptions and explanations for their GI symptoms and any cultural beliefs regarding their condition. Singapore should also continue to raise the profile and value of clinical psychology in medical settings (Castelnuovo, 2010). As awareness already exists amongst professionals of the significance of addressing the psychological aspect of disease management, it is hoped that the same benefits will be apparent to the recipients of psychological and IBS medical services.

DISCUSSION QUESTIONS

1. Madam Choo was initially reluctant to receive psychological input as she was unsure about what this would entail. She was also sceptical about the relevance of clinical psychology to her. How could education about clinical psychology in Singaporean medical settings be promoted?

2. Historically there has been an absence of specialist clinical health psychology services in Singapore for clients with IBS or other chronic physical health conditions. Discuss some of the benefits of including a clinical psychologist in the IBS services within the Singapore healthcare setting.

3. IBS is a functional gastrointestinal disorder that can lead to a variety of distressing symptoms. As a psychologist you have been asked to design a self-help book for people living with IBS. What important components should be included?

4. Research has suggested that people in different cultural contexts perceive and respond to their IBS condition differently. How might a psychologist respond to the needs of Singaporeans living with IBS? What cultural factors would need to be considered? How could the psychologist work sensitively with this population in Singapore?

5. Draw a diagram illustrating the cognitive, behavioural, emotional, physical, and systemic factors that exacerbated Madam Choo's IBS symptoms. For each factor, identify one or more specific treatment strategies that could be addressed in therapy with her.

REFERENCES

INTRODUCTION

Ang, R. P., Lim, K. M. & Tan A-G. (2004). Effects of gender and sex role orientation on help-seeking attitudes. *Current Psychology*, *23*(3), 203–14.

Bernal, G., & Sáez-Santiago, E. (2006). Culturally centered psychosocial interventions. *Journal of Community Psychology*, *34*, 121–32.

Coleman, H. L. K., Wampold, B. E., & Casali, S. L. (1995). Ethnic minorities' ratings of ethnically similar and European American counselors: A meta-analysis. *Journal of Counseling Psychology*, *42*(1), 55–64.

Chong, S-A. (2007). Mental health in Singapore: A quiet revolution? *ANNALS Academy of Medicine*, *36*(10), 795–6.

Chong, S-A., Mythily, S. & Verma, S. (2005). Reducing the duration of untreated psychosis and changing help-seeking behaviour in Singapore. *Social Psychiatry and Psychiatry Epidemiol*, *40*, 619–21.

Chong, R., Tan, W-M., Wong, L-M. & Cheah, J. (2012). Integrating mental health: The last frontier? *International Journal of Integrated Care*. ISSN 1568–4156. Available at: <http://www.ijic.org/index.php/ijic/article/view/1058/1902>.

Chong, S. A. et al. (2012). A population-based survey of mental disorders in Singapore. *ANNALS Academy of Medicine Singapore*, *41*, 24–66.

———. (2012). Prevalence and impact of mental and physical comorbidity in the adult Singapore population. *ANNALS Academy of Medicine Singapore*, *41*, 105–14.

Collinson S. L., Fang S. H., Lim M. L., Feng L., Ng T. P. (2014) Normative Data for the Repeatable Battery for the Assessment of Neuropsychological Status (RBANS) in Elderly Chinese. *Archives of Clinical Neuropsychology*, *29*(5), 442–55

Fassberg, M. M., van Orden, K. A., Duberstein, P., Erlangsen, A., Lapierre, S., et al. (2012). A systematic review of social factors and suicidal behaviour in older adults. *International Journal of Environmental Research and Public Health*, *9*, 722–45.

Foo, K. H., Merrick, P. L. & Kazantzis, N. (2006). Counseling/psychotherapy with Chinese Singaporean clients. *Asian Journal of Counselling*, *13*(2), 271–93.

Kessler, R. C., Pethuhova, M., Sampson, N. A., Zaslavsky, A. M. & Wittchen, H-U. (2012).

Twelve-month and lifetime prevalence and lifetime morbid risk of anxiety and mood disorders in the United States. *International Journal of Methods in Psychiatric Research, 21*(3), 169–84.

Merikangas, K. R., Jin, R., He, J-P., Kessler, R. C., Lee, S., et al. (2012). Prevalence and correlates of bipolar spectrum disorder in the World Mental Health Survey. *Archives of General Psychiatry, 68*(3), 241–51.

Ministry of Health. (2007). MediShield Scheme. Retrieved from: http://www.pqms.moh.gov.sg

Phua, H. P., Chua, A. V., Ma, S., Heng, D. & Chew, S. K. (2004). Singapore's burden of disease and injury. *Singapore Medical Journal,50*, 468–78.

Smith, T. B., Rodriguez, M. M. D., & Bernal, G. (2011). Culture. In Norcross, J. C. (Ed.) *Psychotherapy relationships that work: Evidence-based responsiveness.* New York, NY: Oxford University Press.

Tan, H-Y., Choo, W-C., Doshi, S., Lim, L. E. C. & Kua, E-H. (2004). A community study of the health-related quality of life of schizophrenia and general practice outpatients in Singapore. *Social Psychiatry and Psychiatric Epidemiology, 39*, 106–12.

Tiong, W. W., Yap, P., Huat Koh, G. C., Phoon Fong, N., & Luo, N. (2013). Prevalence and risk factors of depression in the elderly nursing home residents in Singapore. *Aging & Mental Health, 17*(6), 724–31. DOI:10.1080/13607863.2013.775638

Woo, B.S.C., et al. (2007). Emotional and behavioural in Singaporean children based on parent, teacher and child reports. *Singapore Medical Journal, 48*(12), 1100–6.

World Health Organization. First report on suicide prevention. Available online: http://www.who.int/mediacentre/news/releases/2014/suicide-prevention-report/en/ (accessed 5 Sept 2014).

CHAPTER 1. EATING DISORDER (ANOREXIA NERVOSA)

American Psychiatric Association. (2013). Diagnostic and statistical manual of mental disorders (5th ed.). Arlington, VA: American Psychiatric Publishing.

Baello, J., & Mori, L. (2007). Asian values adherence and psychological help-seeking attitudes of Filipino Americans. *Journal of Multicultural, Gender and Minority Studies, 1*(1), 1–14.

Borzekowski, D. L. G., Schenk, S., Wilson, J. L., & Peebles, R. (2010). E-Ana and e-Mia: A content analysis of pro-eating disorder websites. *American Journal of Public Health, 100*(8), 1526–34.

Chen, A., Mond, J. M., & Kumar, R. (2010). Eating disorders mental health literacy in Singapore: Beliefs of young adult women concerning treatment and outcome of bulimia nervosa. *Early Intervention in Psychiatry, 4,* 39–46.

Crow, S., & Swigart, S. (2005). Medical Assessment. In J.E.Mitchell & C.B.Peterson (Eds.), *Assessment of eating disorders* (pp. 120–8). New York, NY: Guilford Press.

Eisler, I., Lock, J., & Le Grange, D. (2010). Family-based treatments for adolescents with anorexia nervosa: Single-family and multifamily approaches. In C. M. Grilo & J. E. Mitchell (Eds.), *The treatment of eating disorders* (pp. 150–74). New York, NY: Guildford Press.

Fairburn, C. G., & Beglin, S. (2008). Eating disorder examination questionnaire (EDE-Q 6.0). In

C. G. Fariburn (Ed.), *Cognitive behaviour therapy and eating disorders* (pp. 265–308). New York, NY: Guilford Press.

Garner, D. M., Olmstead, M. P., Bohr, Y. & Garfinkel, P. E. (1982). The eating attitudes test: Psychometric features and clinical correlates. *Psychological Medicine, 12*, 871–8.

Haines, J. & Neumark-Sztainer, D. (2006). Prevention of obesity and eating disorders: A consideration of shared risk factors. *Health Education Research, 21(6)*, 770–82.

Health Promotion Board. (2002). BMI-for-age for boys and girls. Available at: http://www.hpb.gov.sg/HOPPortal/health-article/632

Ho, T. F. (2010). Prevention and management of obesity in children and adolescents—the Singapore experience. In J. A. O'Dea & M. Eriksen (Eds.), *Childhood obesity prevention: International research, controversies, and interventions* (pp. 240–9). Oxford, UK: Oxford University Press.

Ho, T. F., Tai, B. C., Lee, E. L., Cheng, S., Liow, P. H. (2006). Prevalence and profile of females at risk of eating disorders in Singapore. *Singapore Medical Journal, 47*, 499–503.

Johnson, J. G., Cohen, P., Kasen, S., Brook, J. S. (2002). Eating disorders during adolescence and the risk for physical and mental disorders during early adulthood. *Archives of General Psychiatry, 59(6)*, 545–52.

Kok, L. P., & Tian, C. S. (1994) Susceptibility of Singapore Chinese schoolgirls to anorexia nervosa—Part 1 (Psychological factors). *Singapore Medical Journal, 35*, 481–85.

Le Grange, D. & Lock, J. (2007). *Treating bulimia in adolescents: A family-based approach.* New York, NY: Guildford Press.

Lee, H. Y., Lee, E. L., Pathy, P., Chan, Y.H. (2005). Anorexia nervosa in Singapore: An eight-year retrospective study. *Singapore Medical Journal, 46*, 275–81.

Leong, F. T. L., & Lau, A. S. L. (2001). Barriers to providing effective mental health services to Asian Americans. *Mental Health Services Research, 3,* 201–14.

Lin, K. M., & Cheung, F. (1999). Mental health issues in Asian Americans. *Psychiatric Services, 50,* 774–80.

Lock, J., Le Grange, D., Agras, W. S., & Dare, C. (2001). *Treatment manual for anorexia nervosa: A family-based approach.* New York, NY: Guildford Press.

Maine, M. & Bunnell, D. W. (2010). A perfect biopsychosocial storm: Gender, culture, and eating disorders. In M. Maine, B. Hartman McGilley, & D. W. Bunnell (Eds.), *Treatment of eating disorders: Bridging the research-practice gap* (pp. 3–16). London, UK: Academic Press Elsevier.

Mond, J. M., Chen, A., Kumar, R. (2010). Eating-disordered behaviour in Australian and Singaporean women: A comparative study. *International Journal of Eating Disorders, 43,* 717–23.

Mueller, M., & Pekarik, G. (2000). Treatment duration prediction: Client accuracy and its relationship to dropout. *Psychotherapy: Theory, Research, Practice, Training, 37,* 117–23.

National Institute for Health and Clinical Excellence. (2004). *Core interventions in the treatment and management of anorexia nervosa, bulimia nervosa and related disorders.* Available at: http://publications.nice.org.uk/eating-disorders-cg9.

Rieger, E., Touyz, S., Schotte, D., Beumont, P., Russell, J., Clarke, S., Kohn, M., Griffiths, R. (2000). Development of an instrument to assess readiness to recover in anorexia nervosa. *International Journal of Eating Disorders, 28,* 387–96.

Sansone, R. A., & Levitt, J. L. (2004). The prevalence of self-harm behaviour among those with eating disorders. In J. L. Levitt, R. A. Sansone, & L. Chon (Eds.), *Self-harm behaviour and eating disorders: Dynamics, assessment and treatment* (pp. 3–13). New York, NY: Brunner-Routledge.

Sansone, R. A., Levitt, J. L., & Sansone, L. A. (2004). An overview of psychotherapy strategies for the management of self-harm behaviour. In J. L. Levitt, R. A. Sansone, & L. Chon (Eds.), *Self-harm behaviour and eating disorders: Dynamics, assessment and treatment* (pp. 121–34). New York, NY: Brunner-Routledge.

Saunders, S. M. (2000). Examining the relationship between the therapeutic bond and the phases of treatment outcome. *Psychotherapy, 37,* 206–18.

Soh, N. L., Touyz, S., Dobbins, T. A., Surgenor, L. J., Clarke, S., Kohn, M. R., Lee, E. L., Leow, V., Rieger, E., Ung, K. E., Walter, G. (2007). Restraint and eating concern in North European and East Asian women with and without eating disorders in Australia and Singapore. *Australia and New Zealand Journal of Psychiatry, 41,* 536–45.

Stice, E., & Shaw, H. (2004). Eating disorder prevention programs: A meta-analytic review. *Psychological Bulletin, 130,* 207–27.

Stice, E., Shaw, H., Marti, C. N. (2007). A meta-analytic review of eating disorder prevention programs: Encouraging findings. *Annual Review of Clinical Psychology, 3,* 233–57.

The National Bureau of Asian Research Center for Health and Aging (2008). Obesity prevention and control efforts in Singapore: 2008 case study. Available at: http://www.nbr.org/publications/issue.aspx?id=174#/h.

Wang, M. C., Ho, T. F., Anderson, J. N., Sabry, Z. I. (1999). Preference for thinness in Singapore, a newly industrialised society. *Singapore Medical Journal, 40,* 502–7.

Wilson, J. L., Peebles, R., Hardy, K. K., & Litt, I. F. (2006). Surfing for thinness: A pilot study of pro-eating disorder website usage in adolescents with eating disorders. *Pediatrics, 118,* 1635–43.

CHAPTER 2. ENCEPHALITIS AND CHALLENGING BEHAVIOURS

Beck, A. (2006). Addressing the mental health needs of looked after children who move placement frequently. *Adoption & Fostering, 30,* 60–5. DOI: 10.1177/030857590603000308.

Golding, K. S. (2010). Multi-agency and specialist working to meet the mental health needs of children in care and adopted. *Clinical Child Psychology and Psychiatry, 15*(4), 573–87. DOI: 10.1177/1359104510375933.

Manara, R., Franzoi, M., Cogo, P., & Battistella, P, A. (2006). Acute necrotising encephalopathy: combined therapy and favourable outcome in a new case. *Child's Nervous System, 22,* 1231–36. DOI: 10.1007/s00381–006–0076–9.

McAuley, C., & Davis, T. (2009). Emotional well-being and mental health of looked after children in England. *Child & Family Social Work, 14*(2), 147–55. DOI: 10.1111/j.1365–2206.2009.006.19.

Mizuguchi, M., Abe, J., Mikkaichi, K., Noma, S., Yoshida, K., Yamanaka, T., & Kamoshita, S. (1995). Acute necrotising encephalopathy of childhood: A new syndrome presenting with multifocal, symmetric brain lesions. *Journal of Neurology, Neurosurgery, and Psychiatry, 58,* 555–61.

Mizuguchi, M., Yamanouchi, H., Ichiyama, T., & Shiomi, M. (2007). Acute encephalopathy associated with influenza and other viral infections. *Acta Neurologica Scandinavica, 115,* 45–56

CHAPTER 3. ADHD AND OPPOSITIONAL DEFIANT DISORDER

Achenbach, T. M., & Rescorla, L. A. (2001). *Manual for the ASEBA School-Age Forms and Profiles.* Burlington, VT: University of Vermont, Research Center for Children, Youth, and Families

———. (2007). *Multicultural supplement to the manual for the ASEBA school-age forms and profiles.* University of Vermont, Research Centre for Children, Youth, and Families, Burlington.

American Psychiatric Association (2013). *Diagnostic and Statistical Manual of Mental Disorders* (5th ed.). Arlington, VA: American Psychiatric Publishing.

Ang, R., Rescorla, L., Achenbach, T., Yoon, P., Fung, D. & Woo, B. (2012). Examining the Criterion Validity of CBCL and TRF Problem Scales and Items in a Large Singapore Sample. *Child Psychiatry Human Development, 43,* 70–86.

Bardo, M. Fishbein, D & Milch (2011). *Inhibitory control and drug abuse prevention: from research to translation.* New York, NY: Springer.

Barkley, R. & Murphy, K. (2006). *Attention-deficit hyperactivity disorder: A clinical workbook* (3rd ed.). New York, NY: Guilford Press.

Brassett-Harknett A. & Butler, N. (2007). Attention-deficit/hyperactivity disorder: An overview of the etiology and a review of the literature relating to the correlates and life course outcomes for men and women. *Clinical Psychology Review, 27,* 188–210.

Greenberger & Padesky. (1995). *Mind over Mood: Changing how you feel by changing the way you think.* New York, NY: Guilford Press.

Institute of Mental Health. (2012). *Child Guidance Clinic Research Unit.* Available at: http://www.imh.com.sg/research/page.aspx?id=343 (accessed 2 May 2013).

Kapalka, G., (2010) *Counselling boys and men with ADHD.* New York, NY: Routledge.

National Institute for Health and Care Excellence. (2013). *Attention deficit hyperactivity disorder (ADHD): NICE guideline. CG72.* London, UK: National Institute for Health and Care Excellence.

Patterson, G. R. (1982). *Coercive family process. Cognitive-behavioural therapy for anger in children and adolescents: A meta-analysis.* Eugene, OR: Castalia Publishing.

Polanczyk, G., Silva de Lima, M., Horta, B., Biederman, J. & Rohde, L. (2007). The worldwide prevalence of adhd: a systematic review and metaregression analysis, *American Journal of Psychiatry, 164*, 942–8.

Solanto, M. Marks, D., Mitchell, K., Wasserstein, J. & Kofman, M. (2008). Development of a New Psychosocial Treatment for Adult ADHD, *Journal of Attention Disorders, 11*(6), 728–36.

Verhulst F.C., Prince J., Vervuurt-Poot C. & de Jong J.B. (1989). Mental health in Dutch children: (IV) self-reported problems for ages 11–18. *Acta Psychiatric Scandanavia, 80*(356), 1–48.

Woo, B., Ng, T., Fung, D., Chan, Y., Lee, Y., Koh, J. & Cai, Y. (2007). Emotional and behavioural problems in Singaporean children based on parent, teacher and child reports. *Singapore Medical Journal, 48*(12), 1100 .

CHAPTER 4. ANXIETY AND AUTISM SPECTRUM DISORDER

American Psychiatric Association. (2000). *Diagnostic and statistical manual of mental disorders (4th ed., text rev.).* doi:10.1176/appi.books.9780890423349.

American Psychiatric Association. (2013). Diagnostic and statistical manual of mental disorders (5th ed.). Arlington, VA: American Psychiatric Publishing.

Bernard-Opitz, V., Kwook, K.-W., & Sapuan, S. (2001). Epidemiology of autism in Singapore: Findings of the first autism survey. *International Journal of Rehabilitation Research, 24*, 1–6.

Cardaciotto, L., & Herbert, J. D. (2004). Cognitive behavior therapy for social anxiety disorder in the context of Asperger's syndrome: A single-subject report. *Cognitive and Behavioral Practice, 11*, 75–81.

Committee on Educational Interventions for Children with Autism, Board on Behavioral, Cognitive, and Sensory Sciences, Board on children, Youth and Families, Division of Behavioral and Social Sciences and Education, & National Research Council. (2001). *Educating children with autism.* Washington, DC: National Academy Press.

Elsabbagh, M., Divan, G., Koh, Y.J., Kim, Y.S., Kauchali, S., Marcín, C., Montiel-Nava, C., Patel, V., Paula, C.S., Wang, C., Yasamy, M.T., & Fombonne, E. (2012). *Global Prevalence of Autism and Other Pervasive Developmental Disorders. Autism Research,* 160–79. http://onlinelibrary.wiley.com/doi/10.1002/aur.239/pdf

Fombonne, E., Heavey, L., Smeeth, L., Rodrigues, L.C., Cook, C., Smith, P.G., Meng, L., & Hall, A.J. (2004). Validation of the diagnosis of autism in general practitioner records. *BMC Public Health 4*(5). doi:10.1186/1471-2458-4-5.

Garretson, H., Fein, D., & Waterhouse, L. (1990). Sustained attention in children with autism. *Journal of Autism and Developmental Disorders, 20*, 101–14.

Geschwind, D. H., & Levitt, P. (2007). Autism spectrum disorders: Developmental disconnection syndromes. *Current Opinion in Neurobiology, 17*(1), 103–11.

Gould, J., & Ashton-Smith, J. (2011). Missed diagnosis or misdiagnosis? Girls and women on the autism spectrum. *Good Autism Practice, 12*(1), 34–41.

Gray, C. (2010). What are Social Stories? In the Gray Center. Retrieved from http://www.thegraycenter.org/social-stories/what-are-social-stories.

Hare, D. J. (1997). The use of cognitive-behavioral therapy with people with Asperger syndrome: A case study. *Autism, 1*, 215–225.

Harpaz-Rotem, I., & Rosenheck, R.A. (2004) Changes in outpatient psychiatric diagnosis in privately insured children and adolescents from 1995 to 2000. *Child Psychiatry Human Development, 34*, 329–40.

Helverschou, S.B., Bakken, T.L., & Martinsen, H. (2011). Psychiatric disorders in people with autism spectrum disorders: Phenomenology and recognition. In J. L. Matson & P. Sturmey (Eds.), *International handbook of autism and pervasive developmental disorders* (pp. 53–74). New York: Springer. ISBN 9781441980649. OCLC 746203105.

Joseph, R. M., Tager-Flusberg, H., & Lord, C. (2002). Cognitive profiles and social-communicative functioning in children with autism spectrum disorder. *Journal of Child Psychology and Psychiatry, and Allied Disciplines, 43*(6), 807–21.

Knickmeyer, R. C., Wheelwright, S., & Baron-Cohen, S. B. (2008). Sex-typical play: Masculinization/defeminization in girls with an autism spectrum condition. *Journal of Autism and Developmental Disorders, 38*(6), 1028–35.

Leyfer, O., Folstein, S., Bacalman, S., Davis, N., Dinh, E., Morgan, J., et al. (2006). Comorbid psychiatric disorders in children with autism: Interview development and rates of disorders. *Journal of Autism and Developmental Disorders, 36*, 849–61.

Lian, W. B., & Ho, S. K. (2012). Profile of children diagnosed with autistic spectrum disorder managed at a tertiary child development unit. *Singapore Medical Journal, 53*(12), 794–800.

Lord, C., Rutter, M., DiLavore, P. C., & Risi, S. (2000). *Autism Diagnostic Observation Schedule (ADOS)*. Los Angeles, CA: Western Psychological Services.

Lord, C., Rutter, M., DiLavore, P. C., Risi, S., Gotham, K., Bishop, S. L. B (2012), *Autism Diagnostic Observation Schedule, second edition (ADOS-2) manual (part 1): Modules 1–4*. Torrance, CA: Western Psychological Services.

Mesibov, G., Shea, V., & Schopler, E. (2005). *The TEACCH approach to autism spectrum disorders*. New York: Plenum Press.

Ooi, Y.P., Tan, Z.J., Lim, C.X., Goh, T.J., & Sung, M. (2011). Prevalence of behavioural and emotional problems in children with high-functioning autism spectrum disorders. *Australian and New Zealand Journal of Psychiatry, 45*(5), 370–5. doi: 10.3109/00048674.2010.534071

Rutter, M., Le Couteur, A., Lord, C. (2003), *Autism Diagnostic Interview-Revised (ADI-R) manual*. Los Angeles: Western Psychological Services.

Schopler, E. (1994). Behavioral priorities for autism and related developmental disorders. In E. Schopler & G.B. Mesibov (Eds.), *Behavioral issues in autism* (pp. 557–5). New York: Plenum Press.

Skokauskas, N., & Gallagher, L. (2010). Psychosis, affective disorders and anxiety in autistic spectrum disorder: Prevalence and nosological considerations. *Psychopathology*, 8–16.

Towbin, K. E., Pradella, A., Gorrindo, T., Pine, D.S., & Leibenluft, E. (2005). Autism spectrum traits in children with mood and anxiety disorders. *Journal of Child and Adolescent Psychopharmacology, 5*(3), 452–64. doi:10.1089/cap.2005.15.452.

Tsakanikos, E., Underwood, L., Kravariti, E., Bouras, N., & McCarthy, J. (2011). Gender differences in co-morbid psychopathology and clinical management in adults with autism spectrum disorders. *Research in Autism Spectrum Disorders, 5*(2): 803–8. doi:10.1016/ j.rasd.2010.09.009. ISSN 1750-9467.

Weiss, J. A., & Lunsky, Y. (2010). Group cognitive behaviour therapy for adults with Asperger syndrome and anxiety or mood disorder: A case series. *Clinical Psychology and Psychotherapy, 17*, 438–46.

Whiteley, P., Todd, L., Carr, K., & Shattock, P. (2010). Gender ratios in autism, Asperger syndrome and autism spectrum disorder. *Autism Insights*, 2, 17–24.

CHAPTER 5. SELECTIVE MUTISM

American Psychiatric Association. (2000). *Diagnostic and statistical manual of mental disorders (4th ed., text rev.)*. Washington, DC: Author.

American Psychiatric Association. (2013). *Diagnostic and statistical manual of mental disorders (5th ed.)*. Arlington, VA: American Psychiatric Publishing.

Bergman, R. L., Keller, M. L., Piacentini, J., & Bergman, A. J. (2008). The development and psychometric properties of the selective mutism questionnaire. *Journal of Clinical Child and Adolescent Psychology, 37*(2), 456–64.

Birmaher, B., Khetarpal. S., Cully, M., Brent, D., & McKenzie, S. (1995). *Screen for child anxiety related disorders (SCARED)*. Western Psychiatric Institute and Clinic, University of Pittsburgh.

Bögels, S.M., Alden, L., Beidel, D. C., Clark, L. A., Pine, D. S., Stein, M. B., Voncken, M. (2010). Social anxiety disorder: Questions and answers for the DSM-V. *Depression and Anxiety. 27*, 168–189.

Chavira, D. A., Shipon-Blum, E., Hitchcock, C., Cohan, S., & Stein, M. B. (2007). Selective mutism and social anxiety disorder: All in the family? *Journal of the American Academy of Child and Adolescent Psychiatry, 46*, 1464–1472.

Dickstein, S. G. (2013). Can my child have both autism and selective mutism, and be treated for both? Retrieved from http://www.childmind.org/en/posts/ask-an-expert/2013-7-16-can-child-have-both-autism-and-selective-mutism-an

Elizur, Y., & Perednik, R. (2003). Prevalence and description of selective mutism in immigrant and native families: A controlled study. *Journal of the American Academy of Child & Adolescent Psychiatry, 42*, 1451–1459.

Fung, D., Kenny, A., & Mendlowitz, S. (2000). *Meeky Mouse: A cognitive behavioral treatment program for children with selective mutism*. Unpublished manuscript.

Goodman, R. (1997). The Strengths and Difficulties Questionnaire: A research note. *Journal of Child Psychology and Psychiatry, 38*, 581–6.

Kee, C., H. Y., Fung, D. S S., & Ang, L-K. (2001). An electronic communication device for selective mutism. *Journal of the American Academy of Child & Adolescent Psychiatry, 40*, 389.

Kendall, P. C. (1992). *The Coping Cat workbook*. Ardmore, PA: Workbook Publishing.

Kopp, S., & Gillberg, C. (1997) Selective mutism: A population-based study: a research note. *Journal of Child Psychology and Psychiatry, 38* (2), 2576–2.

Kristensen, H. (2000). Selective mutism and comorbidity with developmental disorder delay, anxiety disorder, and elimination disorder. *Journal of the American Academy of Child & Adolescent Psychiatry, 39,* 249–56.

Kristensen, H., & Oerbeck, B. (2006). Is selective mutism associated with deficits in memory span and visual memory?: An exploratory case–control study. *Depression and Anxiety, 23,* 71–76.

Kwan, C. (2013). *Online portal for treatment of children with Selective Mutism.* Oral presentation at the Serious Games & Social Connect Conference, Singapore.

Kwan, C., Sung, S. C., Ooi, Y. P., Wong, Z. J., Tan, Y. R. & Fung, D. (2014). *Virtual Reality Exposure Therapy for Children with Selective Mutism: A Case Series.* Poster presentation at the International Association for Child and Adolescent Psychiatry (IACAPAP) Congress.

Malini, R. (2011). *Understanding selective mutism from maternal and childhood characteristics* Unpublished Master of Psychology (Clinical) dissertation, School of Psychology at James Cook University, Singapore.

Mendlowitz, S., Manassis, K., Bradley, S., Scapiliato, D., Miezitis, S., Shaw, B. F. (1999). Cognitive-behavioral group treatments in childhood anxiety disorders. *Journal of the American Academy of Child and Adolescent Psychiatry, 38,* 1223–9.

Ng, J. J., & Lee, A. (2013). Schools making small strides in shifting focus from academics. Retrieved from http://www.todayonline.com/singapore/schools-making-small-strides-shifting-focus-academics.

Ooi, Y. P., Raja, M., Sung, S. C., Fung, D. S. S. (2012). Application of a web-based cognitive-behvaioural therapy programme for the treatment of selective mutism in Singapore: a case series study. *Singapore Medical Journal, 53*(7), 446–50.

Remschmidt, H., Poller, M., Herpertz-Dahlmann, B., Hennighausen, K., & Gutenbrunner, C. (2001). A follow-up study of 45 patients with elective mutism. *European Archives of Psychiatry and Clinical Neuroscience, 251,* 284–296.

Roid, G. H., & Miller, L. J. (1997). *Leiter International Performance Scale-Revised.* Wood Dale, IL: Stoelting Co.

Rutter, M., Le Couteur, A., & Lord, C. (2003). *Autism Diagnostic Interview- Revised (ADI-R).* Los Angeles: Western Psychological Services.

Shipon-Blum, E. (2007). When the words just won't come out: Understanding selective mutism. Retrieved from http://www.selectivemutism.org/resources/library/SM%20General%20Information/When%20the%20Words%20Just%20Wont%20Come%20Out.pdf

Shipon-Blum, E. (2012). Selective Mutism Anxiety Research and Treatment Center. Retrieved from www.selectivemutismcenter.org

Steinhausen, H-C., Wachter, M., Laimbock, K., & Metzke, C. W. (2006). A long-term outcome study of selective mutism in childhood. *Journal of Child Psychology and Psychiatry, 47*(7), 751–6.

Tan, J., & Gopinathan, S. (2000). Education reform in Singapore: Towards greater creativity and innovation? *NIRA Review, 7*(3), 5–10.

Viana, A. G., Beidel, D. C., & Rabian, B. (2009). Selective mutism: A review and integration of the last 15 years. *Clinical Psychology Review, 29*, 57–67.

CHAPTER 6. GENERALIZED ANXIETY DISORDER

Allen, J. L., Rapee, R. M., & Sandberg, S. (2008). Severe life events and chronic adversities as antecedents to anxiety in children: A matched control study. *International Society for Research in Child and Adolescent Psychopathology, 36*, 1047–56.

American Psychiatric Association. (2013). *Diagnostic and statistical manual of mental disorders* (5th ed.). Arlington, VA.

Barrett, P. M., Duffy, A. I., Dadds, M. R., & Rapee, R. M. (2001). Cognitive-behavioural treatments of anxiety disorders in children. Long-term (6-year) follow-up. *Journal of Consulting and Clinical Psychology, 69*, 135–41.

Birmaher, B., Axelson, D. A., Monk, K., Kalas, C., Clark, D. B., Ehmann, M., Bridge, J., Heo, J., & Brent, D. A. (2003). Fluxetine for the treatment of childhood anxiety disorders. *Journal of the American Academy of Child & Adolescent Psychiatry, 42*, 415–23.

Bittner, A., Egger, H. L., Erkanli, A., Costello, E. J., Foley, D. L., & Angold, A. (2007). What do childhood anxiety disorders predict? *Journal of Child Psychology and Psychiatry, 48*, 1174–83.

Chambless, D. L., & Ollendick, T. H. (2001). Empirically supported psychological interventions: Controversies and evidence. *Annual Review of Psychology, 52*, 685–716.

Chong, S. A., Vaingankar, J. A., Sherbourne, C., Yap, M., Lim, Y. W., Wong, H. B., Ghosh-Dastidar, B., Kwok, K. W., & Subramaniam, M. (2012). A population-based survey of mental disorders in Singapore. *Annals of the Academy of Medicine Singapore, 41*, 49–66.

Dubow, E. F., Tisak, J., Causey, D., Hryshko, A., & Reid, G. (1991). A two-year longitudinal study of stressful life events, social support and social problem-solving skills: Contributions to children's behavioural and academic adjustment. *Child Development, 62*, 583–99.

D'Zurilla, T. J., & Goldfried, M. R. (1971). Problem-solving and behaviour modification. *Journal of Abnormal Psychology, 78*, 107–126.

Grych, J. H., & Fincham, F. D. (1992). Interventions for children of divorce: Toward greater integration of research and action. *Psychological Bulletin, 111*, 434–54.

Hidalgo, R. B., Tupler, L. A., & Davidson, J. R. T. (2007). An effect-size analysis of pharmacologic treatments for generalized anxiety disorder. *Journal of Psychopharmacology, 21*, 864–72.

Hirshfeld-Becker, D. R., Biederman, J. & Rosenbaum, J. F. (2004). Behavioural Inhibition. In T. L. Morris & March, J.S (Eds.). *Anxiety disorders in children and adolescents* (2nd ed.) (pp. 27–58). New York, NY: Guilford Press.

Kagan, J., Reznick, J. S., Clarke, C., Snidman, N., & Garcia-Coll, C. (1984). Behavioural inhibition to the unfamiliar. *Child Development, 55*, 2212–25.

Kagan, J., Reznick, J. S., & Gibbons, J. (1989). Inhibited and uninhibited types of children. *Child Development, 60*, 838–45.

Kazdin, A. E., Siegel, T. C., Bass, D. (1992). Cognitive problem-solving skills training and parent management training in the treatment of antisocial behaviour in children. *Journal of Consulting and Clinical Psychology, 60*, 733–47.

Kendall, P. C. (Ed). (2006). *Child and adolescent therapy: Cognitive-behavioural procedures* (3rd ed.) New York, NY: Guilford Press.

Kendall, P. C., & Southam-Gerow, M. A. (1996). Long-term follow-up of a cognitive-behavioural therapy for anxiety-disordered youth. *Journal of Consulting and Clinical Psychology, 64*, 724–30.

Kessler, R. C., Berglund, P., Demler, O., Jin, R., Merikangas, K. R., & Walters, E. E. (2005). Lifetime prevalence and age-of-onset distributions of DSM-IV disorders in the National Comorbidity Survey Replication. *Archives of General Psychiatry, 62*, 593–602.

Kleiner, L., Marshall, W. L., & Spevack, M. (1987). Training in problem-solving and exposure treatment for agoraphobics with panic attacks. *Journal of Anxiety Disorder, 1*, 219–38.

Leitenberg, H., & Callahan, E. J. (1973). Reinforced practice and reduction of different kinds of fears in adults and children. *Behaviour Research and Therapy, 11*, 19–30.

Masi, G., Millepiedi, S., Poli, P., Bertini, N. & Milantoni, L. (2004). Generalized anxiety disorder in referred children and adolescents. *Journal of the American Academy of Child and Adolescent Psychiatry, 43*, 752–60.

Michael, K. D., Payne, L. O., & Albright, A. E. (2012). An adaptation of the coping cat program: The successful treatment of a 6-year-old boy with generalized anxiety disorder. *Clinical Case Studies, 11*, 426–40.

Moore, M. & Carr, A. (2000). Anxiety disorder. In A. Carr (Ed.), *What works with children and adolescents? A critical review of psychological interventions with children* (pp. 178–202). Florence, KY: Taylor & Francis/Routledge.

Nordahl, H. M., Wells, A., Olsson, C. A., & Bjerkeset, O. (2010). Association between abnormal psychosocial situations in childhood, generalized anxiety disorder and oppositional defiance disorder. *Australian and New Zealand Journal of Psychiatry, 44*, 852–8.

Ollendick, T. H., & King, N. J. (2000). Empirically supported treatments for children and adolescents. In P. C. Kendall (Ed.), *Child and adolescent therapy: Cognitive behavioural procedures* (2nd edn, pp. 386–425). New York: Guilford Press.

Ossterlaan, J. (2001). Behavioural inhibition and development of childhood anxiety disorders. In W. K. Silverman & P. O. S Treffers (Eds.). *Anxiety disorders in children and adolescents: Research, assessment and intervention* (pp. 45–71). New York, NY: Cambridge University Press.

Patel, G. P., & Fancher, T. L. (2013). Generalized Anxiety Disorder. *Annals of Internal Medicine, 159*, 1–11.

Rubin, L. (Ed.). (2006). *Using superheroes in counseling and play therapy.* New York, NY: Springer.

Rynn, M. A., Siqueland, L., & Rickels, K. (2001). placebo-controlled trial of sertraline in the treatment of children with generalized anxiety disorder. *American Journal of Psychiatry, 158,* 2008–14.

Sanders, M. R. (1999). Triple P—positive parenting program: Towards an empirically validated multilevel parenting and family support strategy for the prevention of behaviour and emotional problems in children. *Clinical Child and Family Psychology Review, 2,* 71–90.

Sheslow, D. V., Bondy, A. S., & Nelson, R. O. (1982). A comparison of graduated exposure, verbal coping skills, and their combination in the treatment of children's fear of the dark. *Child and Family Behaviour Therapy, 4,* 33–45.

Silverman, W. K., & Kurtines, W. M. (2005). Progress in developing an exposure-based transfer-of-control approach to treating internalizing disorders in youth. In E. D. Hibbs, & P. S. Jensen (Eds.), *Psychosocial treatments for child and adolescent disorders* (2nd ed., pp. 97–119). Washington, DC: American Psychological Association.

Silverman, W. K., Pina, A. A., & Viswesvaran, C. (2008). Evidence-based psychosocial treatments for phobic and anxiety disorders in children and adolescents: A review and meta-analyses. *Journal of Clinical Child & Adolescent Psychology, 37,* 105–30.

Spence, S. H. (1997). The structure of anxiety symptoms among children: A confirmatory factor analytic study. *Journal of Abnormal Psychology, 106,* 280–97.

Webster-Stratton, C., Reid, J., & Hammond, M. (2001). Social skills and problem-solving training for children with early-onset conduct problem: Who benefits? *Journal of Child Psychology and Psychiatry, 42,* 943–52.

Whitton, S. W., Luiselli, J. K., & Donaldson, D. L. (2006). Cognitive-behavioural treatment of generalized anxiety disorder and vomiting phobia in a elementary-age child. *Clinical Case Studies, 5,* 477–87.

Wolchik, S. A., West, S. G., Westover, S., Sandler, I. N., Martin, A., Lustig, J., Tein, J-Y., Fisher, J. (1993). The children of divorce parenting intervention: outcome evaluation of an empirically based program. *American Journal of Community Psychology, 21,* 293–331.

CHAPTER 7. FRONTAL LOBE EPILEPSY

Braakman, H. M. H., Vaessen, M. J., Hofman, P. A. M., Debij-van Hall, M. H., Backes, W. H., Vles, J. S. H., & Aldenkamp, A. P. (2011). Cognitive and behavioural complications of frontal lobe epilepsy in children: A review of the literature. *Epilepsia, 52*(5), 849–56.

Dixon, L. Q. (2011). The role of home and school factors in predicting English vocabulary among bilingual kindergarten children in Singapore. *Applied Psycholinguistics, 32*(1), 141–68.

Fosi, T., Lax-Pericall, M. T., Scott, R. C., Neville, B. G., & Aylett, S. E. (2013). Methylphenidate treatment of attention deficit hyperactivity disorder in young people with learning difficulty and difficult-to-treat epilepsy: Evidence of clinical benefit. *Epilepsia, 54*(12), 2071–81.

Hale, J. B., Reddy, L. A., Semrud-Clikeman, M., Hain, L. A., Whitaker, J, Morley, J., Lawrence, K., Smith, A., & Jones, N. (2011). Executive impairment determines ADHD medication response: Implications for academic achievement. *Journal of Learning Disabilities, 44*(2), 196–212.

Harpin, V. A. (2005). The effect of ADHD on the life of an individual, their family and community from preschool to adult life. *Archives of disease in childhood.* 90(Suppl I):i2–i7. DOI: 10.1136/adc.2004.059006.

Hermann, B., Jones, J., Dabbs, C. A., Allen, Sheth, R., Fine, J., McMillan, A., & Seidenberg, M. (2007). The frequency, complications and aetiology of ADHD in new onset paediatric epilepsy. *Brain, 130,* 3135–48.

Jones-Gotman, M., Smith, M. l., Risse, G. L., Westerveld, M., Swanson, S. J., Giovagnoli, A, R., Lee, T., Mader-Joaquim, M. J. & Piazzini. (2010). The contribution of neuropsychology to diagnostic assessment in epilepsy. *Epilepsy and Behaviour, 18,* 3–12.

Kanner, A. (2011). Depression and Epilepsy: A bidirectional relationship. *Epilepsia, 52* (Suppl 1), 21–7.

MacAllister, W. S., Vasserman, M., Vekarla, P., Miles-mason, E., Hochsztein, N., & Bender, H. A. (2012). Neuropsychological endophenotypes in ADHD with and without epilepsy. *Applied Neuropsychology: Child, 1*(2), 121–8.

Rugg-Gunn, F. J. & Sander, J. W. (2012). Management of chronic epilepsy. *British Medical Journal*, 345, e4576, DOI: 10.1136/bmj.e4576.

Shaw, M., Hodgkins, P., Caci, H., Young, S., Kahle, J., Woods A. G. & Arnold, L. E. (2012). A systematic review and analysis of long-term outcomes in attention deficit hyperactivitiy disorder: effects of treatment and non-treatment. *BMC Medicine, 10*(99), DOI: 10.1186/ 1741–7015–10–99.

Sherman, E. M. S., Brooks, B. L., Akday, S., Connolly, M. B., & Wiebe, S. (2010). Parents report more ADHD symptoms than to teachers in children with epilepsy. *Epilepsy and Behaviour, 19,* 428–35.

Stoeckel, R. E., Colligan, R. C., Barbaresi, W. J., Weaver, A. L., Killian, J. M., Katusic, S. (2013). Early speech-language impairment and risk for written language disorder: A population-based study. *Journal of Developmental & Behavioural Pediatrics, 34*(1), 38–44.

Van Bogaert, P., Urbain, C., Galer, S., Ligot, N., Peigneus, P., & De Tiege, X. (2011). Impact of focal interictal epileptiform discharges on behaviour and cognition in children. *Clinical Neurophysiology, 42,* 53–8.

VanStraten, A . F. & Ng, Y-T. (2012). What is the worst part about having epilepsy? A children's and parent's perspective. *Pediatric Neurology, 47,* 431–5.

Wechsler, D. (2004). The Wechsler intelligence scale for children (4th ed.). London, UK: Pearson Assessment.

Westerveld, M. (2010). Childhood epilepsy. In K. O. Yeates, M. D., Ris, H. G. Taylor, & B. F. Pennington (Eds), *Pediatric Neuropsychology: Research theory and practice* (pp 71–91). New York, NY: Guilford Press.

Wei, X., Yu, J. W. & Shaver, D. (2014). Longitudinal effects of ADHD in children with learning disabilities or emotional disturbances. *Exceptional Children, 80*(2), 205–19.

Yap J. A. P., Hoh S-Y., Lim E. L. S., Cox, C. A., Kao, M. I. M., Teo, M. P. W., Lee, S. K., & Chan D. W. S (2014). Concerns and needs of parents of children with epilepsy: Singapore local needs assessment. Unpublished data.

Zhang, D-Q., Li, F-H., Zhu, Z-B, & Sun R-P. (2014). Clinical observations on attention deficit hyperactivity disorder (ADHD) in children with frontal lobe epilepsy. *Journal of Child Neurology, 29*(1), 54–7.

CHAPTER 8. PHYSICAL ABUSE AND POST-TRAUMATIC STRESS DISORDER

American Academy of Child & Adolescent Psychiatry (2010). Practice parameter for the assessment and treatment of children and adolescents with posttraumatic stress disorder. *Journal of the American Academy of Child & Adolescent Psychiatry, 49*(4), 414–30.

American Psychiatric Association. (2013). *Diagnositc and statistical manual of mental disorders, (5th edition)*. Washington, DC: Author.

Bene, E., & Anthony, E. (1957). *Manual for the Family Relationship Test.* Windsor, UK, NFER-Nelson.

Cary, C.E. & McMillen, C. (2012). The data behind the dissemination: A systematic review of trauma-focused cognitive behavioural therapy for use with children and youth. *Children and Youth Services Review, 34*, 748–57.

Cohen, J.A., Mannarino, A.P. & Deblinger, E. (2012).*Trauma-focused CBT for children and Adolescents: Treatment Applications*. New York, NY: Guilford Press.

Cohen, J.A., Deblinger, E., Mannarino, A.P., & Steer, R. (2004). A multi-site, randomized controlled trial for children with abuse-related PTSD symptoms. *Journal of the American Academy of Child & Adolescent Psychiatry, 43*(4), 393–402.

Cohen, J.A., Mannarino, A.P., & Deblinger, E. (Eds.). (2006). *Treating trauma and traumatic grief in children and adolescents*. New York, NY: Guilford Press.

Cohen, J.A., Mannarino, A.P., Kliethermes, M., & Murray, L.A. (2012). Trauma-focused CBT for youth with complex trauma. *Child Abuse and Neglect, 36*, 528–41.

Cohen, J.A., Mannarino, A.P. (1997). A treatment study of sexually abused preschool children: Outcome during one year follow-up. *Journal of the American Academy of Child & Adolescent Psychiatry, 36*(9), 1228–35.

Cohen, J.A., Mannarino, A.P. (2008). Trauma-focused cognitive behavioural therapy for children and parents. *Child and Adolescent Mental Health, 13*(4), 158–62.

Cohen, J.A., Mannarino, A.P. & Staron, V.R. (2006). A pilot study of modified cognitive-behavioral therapy for childhood traumatic grief. *Journal of the American Academy of Child and Adolescent Psychiatry, 45*(12), 1465–73.

Deblinger E., Lippmann J. & Steer R. (1996). Sexually abused children suffering posttraumatic stress symptoms: Initial treatment outcome findings. *Child Maltreatment, 1*, 310–21.

Dorsey, S., Briggs, E.C., & Woods, B.A. (2011). Cognitive-behavioral treatment for posttraumatic stress disorder in children and adolescents. *Child and Adolescent Psychiatric Clinics of North America, 20*(2), 255–69.

Foa, E., Keane, T., Friedman, M., & Cohen, J. (2009). *Effective treatments for PTSD, second edition*. New York: Guilford Publications.

Ford, J. & Courtois, C. (Eds.). (2013). *Treating complex traumatic stress disorders in children and adolescents: Scientific foundations and therapeutic models.* New York, NY: Guilford Press.

Goodman, R. (1997) The Strengths and Difficulties Questionnaire: A research note. *Journal of Child Psychology and Psychiatry, 38*, 581–6.

Jaycox, L.H., Cohen, J.A., Mannarino, A.P., Walker, D.W., Langley, A.K., Gegenheimer, K.L., & Schonlau, M., (2010). *Children's mental health care following Hurricane Katrina: A field trial of trauma-focused psychotherapies. Journal of Traumatic Stress, 23*(2), 223–31.

Kauffman Best Practices Project (2004). *Closing the quality chasm in child abuse treatment: Identifying and disseminating best practices. The findings of the Kauffman best practices project to help children heal from child abuse.* National Crime Victims Research and Treatment Center.

Kovacs, M. (1992). *Children's Depression Inventory, 2nd edition.* Toronto, Canada: Multi-Health Systems.

Murray, L.K., Dorsey, S., Skavenski, S., Kasoma, M., Imasiku, M., Bolton, P., Bass, J., & Cohen, J.A. (2013). Identification, modification, and implementation of an evidence-based psychotherapy for children in a low income country: The use of TF-CBT in Zambia. *International Journal of Mental Health Systems, 7*, 24.

SAMHSA (2008). Review of trauma-focused cognitive behavioural therapy. Retrieved from www.nrepp.samhsa.gov

Piers, E.V., Harris, D.B., & Herzberg, D.S. (2002). *The Piers-Harris Children's Self Concept Scale-2nd edition.* Los Angeles, CA: Western Psychological Services.

Pynoos, R., Rodriguez, N., Steinberg, A., Stuber, M., & Frederick, C. (1998). *UCLA PTSD index for DSM-IV.*

CHAPTER 9. OPPOSITIONAL DEFIANT DISORDER

Achenbach, T. M., & Rescorla, L. (2001). *ASEBA school-age forms & profiles.* Aseba., P International.

Bandura, A., Walters, R. H., & Sears, R. R. (1959). Adolescent aggression: a study of the influence of child-training practices and family interrelationships. *American Sociological Review, 25*(3), 438. doi:10.2307/2092109.

Bronfenbrenner, U. (1986). Ecology of the family as a context for human development: Research perspectives. *Developmental Psychology, 22*(6), 723.

Carr, A. (2006). *The handbook of child and adolescent clinical psychology: A contextual approach.* London, UK: Routledge.

Chan, J.S., Chow, Y., & Elliott, J.M. (2000). *Professional and public perceptions of physical child abuse and neglect in Singapore.* Singapore: Singapore Children's Society.

Crick, N. R., & Dodge, K. A. (1994). A review and reformulation of social information-processing mechanisms in children's social adjustment. *Psychological Bulletin, 115*(1), 74.

Fergusson, D. M., Lynskey, M. T., & Horwood, L. J. (1996). Factors associated with continuity and changes in disruptive behavior patterns between childhood and adolescence. *Journal of Abnormal Child Psychology 24*: 533–53.

French, R. (2001). A guide to keeping cool: A group program for aggression control. *Centre for Clinical Interventions*. Retrieved from http://www.cci.health.wa.gov.au/

Fung, D. S. S., & Cai Y. (2005). A guide to child and adolescent psychiatry. Unpublished manuscript.

Hill, J. (2002). Biological, psychological and social processes in the conduct disorders. *Journal of Child Psychology and Psychiatry, 43*(1), 133–64.

Johnson, T. P., & Van de Vijver, F. J. (2003). Social desirability in cross-cultural research. *Cross-cultural survey methods,* 195–204.

Lau, A.S., Garland, A.F., Yeh, M., McCabe, K.M., Wood, P.A., & Hough, R. (2004). Race/ethnicity and informant discrepancies in assessing adolescent psychopathology. *Journal of Emotional and Behavioral Disorders. 12*, 145–56.

Leung P.W., Hung S.F., Ho T.P., Lee, Liu, Tang & Kwong (2008). Prevalence of DSM-IV disorders in Chinese adolescents and the effects of an impairment criterion: A pilot community study in Hong Kong. *European Child and Adolescent Psychiatry, 17*(7), 452–61.

Maxwell, S. R. A. (2001). A focus on familial strain: Antisocial behavior and delinquency in Filipino society. *Sociological Enquiry, 3*, 256–92.

Novaco, R.W. (1975). *Anger control: The development and evaluation of an experimental treatment*. Massachusetts: Lexington Books.

Ooi, Y. P., Ang, R., Fung, D., Wong, G., & Cai, Y. (2007). Effects of CBT on children with disruptive behaviour disorders: Findings from a Singapore study. *ASEAN Journal of Psychiatry, 8*(2), 71–81.

Pevalin, D. J., Wade, T. J., & Brannigan, A. (2003). Precursors, consequences and implications for stability and change in pre-adolescent antisocial behaviors. *Prevention Science, 4*(2), 123–36.

Spivack, G., & Shure, M. B. (1982). The cognition of social adjustment: Interpersonal cognitive problem-solving thinking. In B. B. Lahey, (Eds.), *Advances in clinical child psychology* (pp. 323–72). New York, NY: Plenum Press.

Tong, C.K., Elliott, J.M. and Tan, P.M.E.H. (1996). *Public perceptions of child abuse and neglect in Singapore*. Singapore: Singapore Children's Society.

CHAPTER 10. PYROMANIA

Andrews, D. A., & Bonta, J. (2010). *The psychology of criminal conduct* (5th ed.). Cincinnati, OH: Anderson Publishing.

Andrews, D. A., Bonta, J., & Wormith, J. S. (2004). *The level of service/case management inventory (LS/CMI)*. Toronto, Ontario: Multi-Health Systems.

Andrews, D. A., & Dowden, C. (2005). Managing correctional treatment for reduced recidivism: A meta-analytic review of program integrity. *Legal and Criminological Psychology, 10*, 173–87.

Bennett, W. M., & Hess, K. M. (1984). *The arsonist: A closer look*. Springfield, IL: Charles C Thomas.

Bishop, S. R., Lau, M., Shapiro, S., Carlson, L., Anderson, N. D., Carmody, J., Segal, Z. V.,

Abbey, S., et al. (2004). Mindfulness: A proposed operational definition. *Clinical Psychology: Science & Practice, 11*, 230–41.

Bourget, D., & Bradford, J. M. (1989). Female arsonists: A clinical study. *Bulletin of the American Academy of Psychiatry and the Law, 17*, 293–300.

Bradford, J. M. (1982). Arson: A clinical study. *Canadian Journal of Psychiatry, 27*, 188–93.

Bryant, C. (2008). Understanding bushfire: trends in deliberate vegetation fires in Australia *Technical and background paper series no. 27.* Canberra, AU: Australian Institute of Criminology.

Butcher, J. N., Dahlstrom, W. G., Graham, J. R., Tellegen, A. M., & Kreammer, B. (1989). *The Minnesota Multiphasic Personality Inventory-2 (MMPI-2): Manual for administration and scoring.* Minneapolis, MN: University of Minneapolis Press.

Canter, D., & Fritzon, K. (1998). Differentiating arsonists: A model of fire setting actions and characteristics. *Legal and Criminological Psychology, 3*, 73–96.

Chu, C. M., Ward, T., & Willis, G. (2014). Practicing the Good Lives Model. In F. McNeill & I. Durnescu (Eds.), *Understanding penal practice* (pp. 206–22). London, United Kingdom: Routledge.

Clare, I. C. H., Murphy, G. H., Cox, D., & Chaplin, E. H. (1992). Assessment and treatment of fire-setting: A single case investigation using a cognitive-behavioural model. *Criminal Behaviour and Mental Health, 2*, 253–68.

Emmons, R. A. (1999). *The psychology of ultimate concerns.* New York, NY: Guilford Press.

Fineman, K. R. (1980). Fire setting in childhood and adolescence. *Psychiatric Clinics of North America, 3*, 483–99.

Gannon, T. A., Ó Ciardha, C., Doley, R. M., & Alleyne, E. (2012). The multi-trajectory theory of adult fire setting (M-TTAF). *Aggression and Violent Behaviour, 17*, 107–21.

Gannon, T. A., & Pina, A. (2010). Fire setting: Psychopathology, theory and treatment. *Aggression and Violent Behaviour, 15*, 224–38.

Grant, J. E., & Kim, S. W. (2007). Clinical characteristics and psychiatric comorbidity of pyromania. *Journal of Clinical Psychiatry, 68*, 1717–22.

Hall, J. R., Jr. (2007). *Intentional fires and arson.* Quinsey, MA: Fire Analysis and Research Division, National Fire Protection Association.

Heath, G. A., Hardesty, V. A., Goldfine, P. E., & Walker, A. M. (1983). Diagnosis and childhood fire setting. *Journal of Clinical Psychology, 41*, 571–5.

Hill, R. W., Langevin, R., Paitich, D., Handy, L., Russon, A., & Wilkinson, L. (1982). Is arson an aggressive act or a property offense? A controlled study of psychiatric referrals. *Canadian Journal of Psychiatry, 27*, 648–54.

Jackson, H., Glass, C., & Hope, S. (1987a). Why are arsonists not violent offenders? *International Journal of Offender Therapy and Comparative Criminology, 31*, 143–51.

———. (1987b). A functional analysis of recidivistic arson. *British Journal of Clinical Psychology, 26*, 175–85.

McCarty, C. A., & McMahon, R. J. (2005). Domains of risk in the developmental continuity of fire setting. *Behaviour Therapy, 36*, 185–95.

Moore, J. M., Jr., Thompson-Pope, S. K., & Whited, R. M. (1996). MMPI-A profiles of adolescent boys with a history of fire setting. *Journal of Personality Assessment, 67*, 116–26.

Muckley, A. (1997). *Fire setting: Addressing offending behaviour. A resource and training manual.* Redcar and Cleveland, UK: Redcar and Cleveland Psychological Service.

Murphy, G. H., & Clare, I. C. H. (1996). Analysis of motivation in people with mild learning disabilities (mental handicap) who set fires. *Psychology, Crime and Law, 2*, 153–64.

Novaco, R. W. (2003). *The Novaco Anger Scale and Provocation Inventory (NAS-PI).* Los Angeles, CA: Western Psychological Services.

Palmer, E. J., Hollin, C. R., Hatcher, R. M. & Ayres, T. C. (2010). Arson. In F. Brookman, M. Maguire, H. Pierpoint, & T. Bennett (Eds.), *Handbook of crime* (pp. 380–92). Cullompton, UK: Willan Publishing.

Paulhus, D. L. (1984). Two-component models of socially desirable responding. *Journal of Personality and Social Psychology, 46*, 598–609.

Plaud, J., & Gaither, G. (1997). A clinical investigation of the possible effects of long-term habituation of sexual arousal in assisted covert sensitization. *Journal of Behaviour Therapy and Experimental Psychiatry, 28*, 281–90.

Paunonen, S. V, & LeBel, E. P. (2012). "Socially desirable responding and its elusive effects on the validity of personality assessments". *Journal of Personality and Social Psychology 103* (1), 158–75. doi:10.1037/a0028165

Räsänen, P., Puumalainen, T., Janhonen, S., & Väisänen, E. (1996). Fire setting from the viewpoint of an arsonist. *Journal of Psychosocial Nursing and Mental Health Services, 34*, 16–21.

Rice, M. E., & Chaplin, T. (1979). Social skills training for hospitalized male arsonists. *Journal of Behaviour Therapy and Experimental Psychiatry, 10*, 105–8.

Rice, M. E., & Harris, G. T. (1996). Predicting the recidivism of mentally disordered firesetters. *Journal of Interpersonal Violence, 11*, 364–75.

———. (2008). Arson. In V. N. Parrillo (Ed.), *The encyclopedia of social problems* (pp. 57–58). Thousand Oaks, CA: Sage.

Rix, K. J. B. (1994). A psychiatric study of adult arsonists. *Medicine Science and Law, 34*, 21–34.

Royer, F. L., Flynn, W. F., & Osadca, B. S. (1971). Case history: Aversion therapy for fire setting by a deteriorated schizophrenic. *Behavior Therapy, 2*, 229–32.

Showers, J., & Pickrell, E. (1987). Child firesetters: A study of three populations. *Hospital and Community Psychiatry, 38*, 495–501.

Soothill, K., Ackerley, E., & Francis, B. (2004). The criminal careers of arsonists. *Medicine Science and the Law, 44*, 27–40.

Stewart, L. A. (1993). Profile of female firesetters: Implications for treatment. *British Journal of Psychiatry, 163*, 248–256.

Swaffer, T., Haggett, M., & Oxley, T. (2001). Mentally disordered firesetters: A structured intervention programme. *Clinical Psychology and Psychotherapy, 8*, 468–75.

Taylor, J. L., Thorne, I., Robertson, A., & Avery, G. (2002). Evaluation of a group intervention for convicted arsonists with mild and borderline intellectual disabilities. *Criminal Behaviour and Mental Health, 12,* 282–93.

Taylor, J. L., Thorne, I., & Slavkin, M. L. (2004). Treatment of fire setting behaviour. In W. Lindsay, J. Taylor, & P. Sturmey (Eds.), *Offenders with developmental disabilities* (pp. 221–41). Chichester, UK: Wiley.

Vaughn, M. G., Fu, Q., DeLisi, M., Wright, J. P., Beaver, K. M., Perron, B., E., & Howard, B., E. (2010). Prevalence and correlates of fire-setting in the United States: Results from the National Epidemiological Survey on Alcohol and Related Conditions. *Comprehensive Psychiatry, 51,* 217–23.

Ward, T. (2002). Good lives and the rehabilitation of offenders: Promises and problems. *Aggression and Violent Behavior, 7,* 513–28.

Ward, T., & Gannon, T. A. (2006). Rehabilitation, etiology, and self-regulation: The comprehensive good lives model of treatment for sexual offenders. *Aggression and Violent Behavior, 11,* 77–94.

Ward, T., & Stewart, C. A. (2003). The treatment of sex offenders: Risk management and good lives. *Professional Psychology: Research and Practice, 34,* 353–60.

Williams, D. (2005). *Understanding the arsonist: From assessment to confession.* Tucson, AZ: Lawyers and Judges Publishing.

Yates, P. M., & Ward, T. (2008). Good lives, self-regulation, and risk management: An integrated model of sexual offender assessment and treatment. *Sexual Abuse in Australia and New Zealand: An Interdisciplinary Journal, 1,* 3–20.

CHAPTER 11. BORDERLINE PERSONALITY DISORDER

Adams, H. E., Bernat, J. A., and Luscher, K. A. (2001). Borderline personality disorder: An overview. In P. B. Sutker and H. E. Adams (Eds.), *Comprehensive Handbook of Psychopathology.* New York, NY: Kluweer Academic/Plenum Press.

American Psychiatric Association. (2013). Diagnostic and Statistical Manual of Mental Disorders (5th ed.). Arlington, VA: American Psychiatric Association.

Beck, A. T., Freeman, A., and Davis, D. D. (2004). Cognitive Therapy of Personality Disorders (2nd ed.). New York, NY: Guildford Press.

Beck A. T., Steer R. A., and Brown G. K. (1996). Manual for Beck Depression Inventory II (BDI-II). San Antonio, TX: Psychology Corporation

Bornovalova, M. A. and Daughters, S. B. (2007). How does dialectical behaviour therapy facilitate treatment retention among individuals with comorbid borderline personality disorder and substance use disorders? *Clinical Psychology Review, 27,* 923–43.

Briere, J. (2000). *Inventory of altered self-capacities—Professional manual.* Tallahassee, FL: Psychological Assessment Resources Inc.

Buss, A. H., and Warren, W. L. (2000). Aggression Questionnaire: Manual. Los Angeles, CA: Western Psychological Services

Carver, C. S. (1997). You want to measure coping but your protocol's too long: Consider the Brief COPE. *International Journal of Behavioural Medicine, 4*(1), 92–100.

Chatziandreou, M., Tsani, H., Lamnidis, N., Synodinou, C., and Vaslamatzis, G. (2005). Psychoanalytic psychotherapy for severely disturbed borderline patients: Observations on the supervision group of psychotherapists. *American Journal of Psychoanalysis, 65*, 135–47.

Dimeff, L., and Linehan, M. M. (2001). Dialectical behaviour therapy in a nutshell. *The California Psychologist, 34*, 10–13.

Linehan, M. M. (1993a). *Cognitive Behavioural Treatment for Borderline Personality Disorder.* New York, NY: Guildford Press.

Linehan, M. M. (1993b). *Skills Training Manual for Treating Borderline Personality Disorder.* New York, NY: Guildford Press.

———. (1996) *Reasons for Living Scale.* Behavioural Research and Therapy Clinics. Seattle, WA: University of Washington.

Linehan, M. M., Comtois, K. A., Murray, A. M., Brown, M. Z., et al. (2006). Two-year randomized controlled trial and follow-up of dialectical behaviour therapy vs therapy by experts for suicidal behaviours and borderline personality disorder. *Archives of General Psychiatry, 63*, 757–66.

Livesley, W. J. (2007). A framework for integrating dimensional and categorical classifications of personality disorder. *Journal of Personality Disorders, 21*, 199–224.

Nee, C. and Farman, S. (2005). Female prisoners with borderline personality disorder: some promising treatment development. *Criminal Behaviour and Mental Health, 15*, 2–16.

———.. (2007). Dialectical behaviour therapy as a treatment for borderline personality disorder in prisons: Three illustrative case studies. *Journal of Forensic Psychiatry and Psychology, 18*, 160–180.

Paris, J. (1993). The treatment of borderline personality disorder in light of research on its long term outcome. *Canadian Journal of Psychiatry, 38*, S28-S34.

———. (2005). Borderline personality disorder. *Canadian Medical Association Journal, 172*, 1579–83.

Paris, J. and Zweig-Frank, H. (2001). A 27-year follow-up of patients with borderline personality disorder. *Comprehensive Psychiatry, 42*, 482–7.

Perseius, K. I., Kaver, A., Ekdahl, S., Asberg, M. and Samuelsson, M. (2007). Stress and burnout in psychiatric professionals when starting to use dialectical behavioural therapy in the work with young self-harming women showing borderline personality symptoms. *Journal of Psychiatric and Mental Health Nursing, 14*, 635–43.

Russell, J. J., Moskowitz, D. S., Zuroff, D.C., Sookman, D., and Paris, J. (2007). Stability and variability of affective experience and interpersonal behaviour in borderline personality disorder. *Journal of Abnormal Psychology, 116*, 578–88.

Singleton, N., Meitzer, H., Gatward, R., Coid, J., and Deasy, D. (1998). *Psychiatric morbidity among prisoners in England and Wales: A survey carried out in 1997 by the Social Survey Dimension of ONS on behalf of the Department of Health.* London, HMSO.

Skodol, A., Buckley, P., and Charles, E. (1983). Is there a characteristic pattern to the treatment history of clinical outpatients with borderline personality disorder? *Journal of Mental and Nervous Disease, 171*, 405–10.

Skodal, A. E., Gunderson, J. G., Pfohl, B., Widiger, T. A., Livesley, W. J., and Siever, L. J. (2002). The borderline diagnosis: Psychopathology, comorbidity, and personality structure. *Biological Psychiatry, 51,* 936–50.

Spielberger, C. D. (1983). *Manual for the State-Trait Anxiety Inventory (STAI).* Palo Alto, CA: Consulting Psychologists Press.

Swartz, M., Blazer, D, George, L., Winfield, I. (1990). Estimating the prevalence of borderline personality disorder in the community. *Journalof Personality Disorders, 4,* 257–72.

Watson D., Clark L. A., and Tellegen A. (1988). Development and validation of brief measures of positive and negative affect: The PANAS scales. *Journal of Personality and Social Psychology, 54,* 1063–70.

Zeigler-Hill V., and Abraham, J. (2006). Borderline personality features: Instability of self-esteem and affect. *Journal of Social and Clinical Psychology, 25,* 668–87.

CHAPTER 12. AUTISM SPECTRUM DISORDER

American Psychiatric Association. (2000). *Diagnostic and statistical manual of mental disorders* (4th ed., text rev.). Washington, DC: American Psychiatric Publishing.

———. (2013). *Diagnostic and statistical manual of mental disorders* (5th ed.). Arlington, VA: American Psychiatric Publishing.

Andersson, G., Gillberg, C., & Miniscalco, C. (2013). Pre-school children with suspected autism spectrum disorders: Do girls and boys have the same profiles? *Research in Developmental Disabilities, 34,* 413–22.

Attwood, T. (2006). The pattern of abilities and development of girls with Asperger's syndrome. In *Asperger's and girls* (pp. 1–7). Arlington, TX: Future Horizons.

———. (2007). *The complete guide to Asperger's syndrome.* London, UK: Jessica Kingsley Publishers.

Baron-Cohen, S., Wheelwright, S., Skinner, R., Martin, J., & Clubley, E. (2001). The autism spectrum quotient (AQ): Evidence from asperger syndrome/high functioning autism, males and females, scientists and mathematicians. *Journal of Autism and Developmental Disorders, 31,* 5–17.

Dworzynski, K., Ronald, A., Bolton, P., & Happé, F. (2012). How different are girls and boys above and below the diagnostic threshold for autism spectrum disorders? *Journal of the American Academy of Child and Adolescent Psychiatry, 51*(8), 788–97.

First, M. B., Gibbon, M., Spitzer, R. L., Williams, J. B. W., & Benjamin, L. S. (1997). *Structured clinical interview for DSM-IV axis II personality disorders, (SCID-II).* Washington, DC: American Psychiatric Press.

Fombonne, E. (2005). Epidemiological studies of pervasive developmental disorder. In Volkmar, F., Paul, R., Klin, A., & Cohen, D., (Eds). *Handbook of autism and pervasive developmental disorders* (pp. 42–69). Hoboken, NJ: Wiley.

Freeth, M., Sheppard, E., Ramachandran, R., & Milne, E. (2013). A cross-cultural comparison of autistic traits in the UK, India and Malaysia. *Journal of Autism and Developmental Disorders, 43*(11), 2569–2583.

Gaus, V. L. (2007). *Cognitive-behavioural therapy for adult asperger syndrome.* New York, NY: Guilford Press.

Gillberg, C. & Coleman, M. (2000). *The biology of autistic syndromes* (3rd ed.). London, UK: Mac Keith Press.

Gould, J., & Ashton-Smith, J. (2011). Missed diagnosis or misdiagnosis? Girls and women on the autism spectrum. *Good Autism Practice, 12*(1), 34–41.

Head, A., McGillivray, J., & Stokes, M. (2012). *The female profile of autism: An examination of friendships.* Paper presented at the First Scientific Meeting of the Australasian Society for Autism Research (ASfAR), Sydney.

Jones, L., Goddard, L., Hill, E.L., Henry, L.A., & Crane, L. (2014). Experiences of receiving a diagnosis of Autism Spectrum Disorder: A survey of adults in the United Kingdom. *Journal of Autism and Developmental Disorders*, DOI : 10.1007/s10803–014–2161–3.

Jones et al., 2014; National Autistic Society UK. http://www.autism.org.uk/About-autism/All-about-diagnosis/Diagnosis-information-for-adults.aspx

Kirkovski, M., Enticott, P., & Fitzgerald, P. (2013). A review of the role of female gender in autism spectrum disorders. *Journal of Autism and Developmental Disorders*, 43(11), 2584–603.

Knickmeyer, R. C., Wheelwright, S., & Baron-Cohen, S. B. (2008). Sex-typical play: Masculinization/defeminization in girls with an autism spectrum condition. *Journal of Autism and Developmental Disorders, 38*(6), 1028–35.

Lai, M-C, Lombardo, M. V., Pasco, G., Ruigrok, A. N. V., Wheelwright, S. J., et al. (2011). A behavioural comparison of male and female adults with high functioning autism spectrum conditions. *PLoS ONE, 6*(6): e20835. DOI:10.1371/journal.pone.0020835

Lord, C., Rutter, M., DiLavore, P., Risi, S., Gotham, K., & Bishop, S. L. (2012). Autism Diagnostic Observation Schedule (2nd ed.) (ADOS-2) Manual (Part I): Modules 1–4, Torrance, CA: Western Psychological Services.

Lovibond, S. H., & Lovibond, P. F. (1995). *Manual for the Depression Anxiety Stress Scales* (2nd ed.). Sydney: Psychology Foundation.

National Institute for Health and Care Excellence. (2012). *The NICE guideline on recognition, referral, diagnosis and management of adults on the autism spectrum.* London, UK: The British Psychological Society and The Royal College of Psychiatrists.

Petalas, M. A., Hastings, R. P., Nash, S., Hall, L. M., Joannidi, H., & Dowey, A. (2012). Psychological adjustment and sibling relationships in siblings of children with autism spectrum disorders: Environmental stressors and the broad autism phenotype. *Research in Autism Spectrum Disorders, 6*(1), 546–55.

Rosenberg, R. E., Kaufman, W. E., Law, J. K., & Law, P. A. (2011). Parent report of community psychiatric comorbid diagnoses in Autism Spectrum Disorders. Autism Research and Treatment. OPEN ACCESS, available at: http://www.hindawi.com/journals/aurt/2011/405849/

van Steensel, F. J., Bögels, S. M., & Perrin, S. (2011). Anxiety disorders in children and adolescents with adolescents with autistic spectrum disorders: A meta-analysis. *Clinical Child and Family Psychology Review, 14*(3), 302–17. DOI: 10.1007/s10567–011–0097–0.

Wagner, S. (2006). Educating the female student with Asperger's. In T. Attwood, T. Grandin, C. Faherty, et al. (Eds.) *Asperger's andgirls: World-renowned experts join those with Asperger's syndrome to resolve issues that girls and women face every day!* (pp. 15–32). Arlington, TX: Future Horizons.

Willey, L. H. (1999). *Pretending to be normal: Living with Asperger's syndrome.* London, UK: Jessica Kingsley Publishers.

Wu, D. Y. H. (1996). Chinese childhood socialization. In M. H. Bond (Ed.), *The handbook of Chinese Psychology* (p. 143–54). Hong Kong, HK: Oxford University Press.

Xu, Y. Y., & Farver, J. A. M. (2008). What makes you shy? Understanding situations elicitors of shyness in Chinese children. *International Journal of Behavioural Development, 33*(2), 97–104.

CHAPTER 13. DEVIANT SEXUAL BEHAVIOUR

American Psychiatric Association. (2013). *Diagnostic and Statistical Manual of Mental Disorders* (5th ed.). Washington, DC: American Psychiatric Publishing.

Andrews, D. A., & Bonta, J. (2010). *The Psychology of Criminal Conduct* (5th ed.). Cincinnati, OH: Anderson Publishing.

Baratta, A., Javelot, J., Morali, A., Halleguen, O., & Weiner , L. (2012). The role of anti-depressants in treating sex offenders. *Sexologies, 21*(3), 106–8.

Darcangelo, S. (2007). Fetishism. In Laws, R., & O'Donohue, W. T., *Sexual Deviance: Theory, Assessment and Treatment* (2nd ed.). New York, NY: Guildford Press.

Food and Drug Administration. (May, 2007). FDA proposes new warnings about suicidal thinking, behaviour in young adults who take antidepressant medications. Available at: http://www.fda.gov/NewsEvents/Newsroom/PressAnnouncements/2007/   ucm108905.htm (accessed 12 June 2014).

Garcia, F. D., Delavenne, H. G., Assumpção Ade, F., Thibaut, F. (2013). Pharmacologic Treatment of Sex Offenders with Paraphilic Disorder. *Current Psychiatry Reports*, 15(5), 356.

Koh, K. G. W. W., Lee, J., Phang, S., & Goh, J. (2013). The mandatory treatment order—The first year in Singapore. *ASEAN Journal of Psychiatry, 14*(2), 103–8.

Nichols, H. R., & Molinder, I. (2010). *The multiphasic sex inventory—II.* Nichols and Molinder Assessments, Inc.

Ward, T., Melzer, J., & Yates, P. (2007). Reconstructing the Risk Need Responsibility model: A theoretical elaboration and evaluation. *Aggression and Violent Behaviour*, 12, 208–28.

CHAPTER 14. MAJOR DEPRESSION AND PARANOID PERSONALITY DISORDER

American Psychiatric Association. (2013). *Diagnostic and Statistical Manual of Mental Disorders* (5th ed.). Arlington, VA: American Psychiatric Association.

Berman, A. L. (2006). Risk management with suicidal patients. *Journal of Clinical Psychology, 62,* 171-84.

Bongar, B. (2002). *The suicidal patient: Clinical and legal standards of car* (2nd Ed). Washington, DC: American Psychiatric Association.

Chia, B. H. & Chia, A. (2010). Suicide in Singapore: The Singapore family. *Physicia, 36,* 26–9.

———. (2012). Prevention of suicide in Singapore. *Annals Academy of Medicine,41*(9), 375–6.

Comtois, K. A. & Linehan, M. M. (2006). Psychosocial treatments of suicidal behaviours: A practice-friendly review. *Journal of Clinical Psychology, 62*(2), 161–70.

Gormley, B. (2004). Application of adult attachment theory to the treatment of chronically suicidal, traumatised women. *Psychotherapy: Theory, Research, Practice, Training, 41*(2), 136–43.

Hazan, C. & Shaver, P. (1987). Romantic Love conceptualized as an attachment process. Journal of Personality and Social Psychology, 52(3), 511–24.

Hesse, E. (1999). The Adult Attachment Interview: Historical and current perspectives. In J. Cassidy & P. R. Shaver (Eds.), *Handbook of attachment: Theory, research, and clinical applications* (pp. 395–433). New York, NY: Guilford Press.

Jobes, D. A. (2000). Collaborating to prevent suicide: A clinician-research perspective. *Suicide and Life Threatening Behaviour, 30*(1), 8–17.

Main, M., & Goldwyn, R. (1998). *Adult attachment scoring and classification system.* Unpublished manuscript, Department of Psychology, University of California

Matthews, J. D. (2012). *Cognitive behavioural therapy approach for suicidal thinking and behaviours in depression.* Available at: http://dx.doi.org/10.5772/52418.

Meichenbaum, D. (2005). 35 years of working with suicidal patients: Lessons learned. *Canadian Psychology, 46*(2), 64–72.

Millon, T. (1999). *Personality guided therapy.* Hoboken, NJ: Wiley.

Morey, L. C. (1991). The Personality Assessment Inventory professional manual. Odessa, FL: Psychological Assessment Resources.

Rudd, M. D. (2000). The suicide mode: A cognitive-behavioural model of suicidality. *Suicide and Life Threatening Behaviour, 30*(1), 18–33.

Ruiz, M. & Ochshorn, E. (2010). Clinical applications of the PAI in criminal justice settings. In Blais, M.A., Baity, M.R., & Hopwood, C. J. (Eds.) *Clinical applications of the Personality Assessment Inventory* (pp. 113–34). New York, NY: Routledge.

Samaritans of Singapore (2013). *National Suicide Statistics.* Available at: www.samaritans.org.sg

Scroufe, L. A., Carlson, E. A., Levy, A. K., & Egeland, B. (1999). Implications of attachment theory for developmental psychopathology. *Development and Psychopathology, 11,* 1–13.

Singapore Prison Service. (2004). *Suicide Risk Assessment Questionnaire.*

Strack, S. (1999). Essentials of MCMI-III Assessment in *Essentials of Millon Inventories Assessment* (pp. 1–52). Hoboken, NJ: Wiley.

Thong, J. Y., Su, A. H., Chan, Y. H., & Chia, B. H. (2008). Suicide in psychiatric patients: case control study in Singapore. *Australia New Zealand Journal of Psychiatry, 42*(6), 509–19. DOI: 10.1080/0048670802050553

Worden, J. W. (2001). *Grief counselling and grief therapy: A handbook for the mental health professional.* New York, NY: Springer.

CHAPTER 15. GAMBLING DISORDER

Abbott, M.W. & McKenna, B.G. (2005). Gambling and problem gambling among recently sentenced women in New Zealand prisons. *Journal of Gambling Studies. 21*(4), 559–81.

Blaszczynski, A. (2000). Pathways to Pathological Gambling: Identifying Typologies. *Journal of Gambling Issues, 1.* doi: 10.4309/jgi.2000.1.1

Blaszczynski, A., & Nower, L. (2002). A pathways model of problem and pathological gambling. *Addiction, 97*, 487–99.

Dowling, N., Smith, D. & Thomas, T. (2006). Treatment of female pathological gambling: the efficacy of a cognitive behavioural approach. *Journal of Gambling Studies, 22*(4), 355–72.

Dowling, N., Smith, D. & Thomas, T. (2009). A preliminary investigation of abstinence and controlled gambling as self-selected goals of treatment for female pathological gambling. *Journal of Gambling Studies, 25*(2), 201–14.

George, S. & Murali, V. (2005). Pathological gambling: an overview of assessment and treatment. *Advances in Psychiatric Treatment, 11*, 450–6.

Holdsworth, L., Nuske, E. & Breen, H. (2013). All mixed up together: Women's experiences of problem gambling, comorbidity and co-occurring complex needs. *International Journal of Mental Health and Addiction, 11*, 315–28.

Lesieur, H.R. & Blume, S.B. (1991). When lady luck loses: women and compulsive gambling. In *Feminist Perspectives on Addictions*, ed. Nan van Den Bergh, pp.181–97. New York: Springer Publishing Co.

Lim P.L. (2009). Casino Control Act. *Singapore Infopedia.* Retrieved from http://eresources.nlb.gov.sg/infopedia/articles/SIP_1615_2009-11-30.html

Loo, J.M.Y., Raylu, N. & Ooi, T.P.S. (2008) Gambling among the Chinese: a comprehensive review. *Clinical Psychology Review, 28*, 1152–66.

Manning, V., Gomez, B., Guo, S., Low Y.D., Koh, P.K. and Wong, K.E. (2012). An exploration of quality of life and its predictors in patients with addictive disorders: Gambling, alcohol and drugs. *International Journal of Mental Health and Addiction, 10*(4), 551–62.

Prochaska, J.O. & DiClemente, C.C. (1982). Transtheoretical therapy: Toward a more integrative model of change. *Psychotherapy 19*, 276–88.

Rosenthal, R.J. & Lorenz, V.C. (1992). The pathological gambler as criminal offender. Comments on evaluation and treatment. *Psychiatric Clinics of North America 15*(3), 647–60.

Tang, C.S.K., Wu, A.M.S. & Tang, J.Y.C. (2007). Gender differences in characteristics of Chinese treatment-seeking problem gamblers. *Journal of Gambling Studies, 23*, 145–56.

Teo, P., Mythily, S., Anantha, S. & Winslow, M. (2007) Demographic and Clinical Features of 150 Pathological Gamblers Referred to a Community Addictions Programme. *Annals, Academy of Medicine, Singapore, 36,*165–8.

Wong, J. & Tse, S. (2003) The face of Chinese migrants' gambling: A perspective from New Zealand. *Electronic Journal of Gambling Issues, 9*, 1–11.

CHAPTER 16. PANIC DISORDER

American Psychiatric Association. (2013). *Diagnostic and Statistical Manual of Mental Disorders* (5th ed.) (DSM-5). Arlington, VA: American Psychiatric Publishing.

American Psychiatric Association. (2000). *Diagnostic and Statistical Manual of Mental Disorders* (4th ed. Text Revision) (DSM-IV-TR). Washington, DC: American Psychiatric Association.

Ayuso-Mateos, J. L. (2012). *Global Burden of panic disorder in the year 2000: Version 1 Estimates*. GBD 2000 Working Paper. Geneva, CH: WHO.

Ballenger, J. C. & Fyer, A. J. (1996). Panic disorder and agoraphobia. In T. A. Widiger, A. J. Frances, H. A., Pincus, R. Ross, M. B. First & W. W. Davis (Eds.), *DSM-IV sourcebook* (Vol. 2, pp. 411–71). Washington, DC: American Psychiatric Association.

Bourne, E. J. (2000). *The anxiety and phobia workbook* (3rd ed.). Oakland, CA: New Harbinger Publications.

Chambless, D. L., Caputo, G. C., Bright, P., & Gallagher, R. (1984). Assessment of fear of fear in agoraphobics: The body sensations questionnaire and the agoraphobic cognitions questionnaire. *Journal of Consulting and Clinical Psychology, 52*, 1090–7.

Chong, S. A., Abdin, E., Vaingankar, J. A., Heng, D., Sherbourne, C., Yap, M., Lim, Y. W., Wong, H. B., Ghosh-Dastidar, B., Kwok, K. W., Subramaniam, M. (2012). A population-based survey of mental disorders in Singapore. *Annals Academy of Medicine Singapore,41*, 49–66.

Clark, D. M. (1986). A cognitive approach to panic. *Behaviour Research and Therapy, 24*, 461—70.

Craske, M. G. & Barlow, D. H. (2000). *Master your anxiety and panic: Client work-book* (3rd ed.). New York, NY: Graywind.

Lewis-Fernandez, R., Hinton, D. E., Laria, A. J., Patterson, E. H., Hofmann, S. G., Craske, M. G., Stein, D. J., Asnaani, A., & Liao, B. (2011). Culture and the anxiety disorders: Recommendations for DSM-5. *Focus, 9*(3), 351–68.

Lovibond, S. H. & Lovibond, P. F. (1995). *Manual for the Depression anxiety StressScales* (2nd ed.). Sydney, AU: Psychology Foundation.

Soh, K.C. & Lee, C. (2010). Panic Attack and its Correlation with Acute Coronary Syndrome—More Than Just a Diagnosis of Exclusion, *Annals Academy of Medicine Singapore, 39*(3): 197–202.

Taylor, S. (2000). *Understanding and treating panic disorder. Cognitive-behavioural approaches.* New York, NY: Wiley.

Taylor, S. (2001). Breathing retraining in the treatment of panic disorder: Efficacy, caveats and indications. *Scandinavian Journal of Behavior Therapy, 30*, 1–8.

Weissman, M. M., Bland, R. C., Canino, G. J., Faravelli, C., Greenwald, S., Hai-Gwo, H., Joyce, P. R., Karam, E. G., Lee, C. K., Lellouch, J.Lepine, J. P., Newman, S. C., Oakley-Browne,M.

A., Rubio-Stipec,M., Wells, J. E., Wickramarante, P. J., Wittchen, H. U., & Yeh, E. K. (1997). The cross-national epidemiology of panic disorder. *Archives of General Psychiatry, 54*, 305–9.

Wittchen, H. U., Reed, V. & Kessler, R. C. (1998). The relationship of agoraphobia and panic in a community sample of adolescents and young adults. *Archives of General Psychiatry, 55*, 1017–24.

Wood, M. M., Brendtro, L. K., Fecser, F. A., & Nichols, P. (1999). *Psycho-education: An idea whose time has come.* Reston, VA: Council for Children with Behavioral Disorders.

CHAPTER 17. OBSESSIVE-COMPULSIVE DISORDER

Abramowitz, J. S., Franklin, M. E., & Foa, E. B. (2002). Empirical status of cognitive-behavioral therapy for obsessive-compulsive disorder: A meta-analytic review. *Romanian Journal of Cognitive and Behavioral Psychotherapies, 2,* 89–104.

American Psychiatric Association. (2013). Diagnostic and statistical manual of mental disorders (5th ed.). Arlington, VA: American Psychiatric Association.

Chong, S. A., Abdin, E., Vaingankar, J. A., Subramaniam, M. (2012). A population survey of mental disorders in Singapore. *Annals Academy of Medicine Singapore, 41,* 49—66.

Clark, D. A., & Beck, A. T. (2010). *Cognitive therapy of anxiety disorders: Science and practice.* New York, NY: Guilford Press.

Davey, G. C. L., Field, A. P., & Startup, H. M. (2003). Repetitive and iterative thinking in psychopathology: Anxiety-inducing consequences and a mood-as-input mechanism. In R. G., Menzies & P. Silva (Eds.), *Obsessive-compulsive disorder: Theory, research and treatment* (pp. 79–100). London, UK: Wiley.

Foa, E. B., Kozak, M. J., Salkovskis, P. M., Coles, M. E., & Amir, N. (1998). The validation of a new obsessive-compulsive disorder scale: The obsessive-compulsive inventory. *Psychological Assessment, 10,* 206–14.

Foo, K., Merrick, P. L., & Kazantis, N. (2006). Counseling/psychotherapy with Chinese Singaporean clients. *Asian Journal of Counselling, 13,* 271—93.

Goodman, W. K., Price, L. H., Rasmussen, S. A., Mazure, C. Fleischmann, R. L. Hill, C. L., Heninger, G. R., & Charney, D. S. (1989). The Yale–Brown Obsessive-Compulsive Scale. I. Development, use, and reliability. *Archives of General Psychiatry, 46,* 1006—11.

Hatch, M. L., & Friedman, S. (1996). Behavioral treatment of obsessive-compulsive disorder in African Americans. *Cognitive and Behavioral Practice, 3,* 303–15.

Jones, D. W. (2002). *Myths, Madness and the Family: The Impact of Mental Illness on the Family.* United Kingdom: Palgrave.Karno, M., Golding, J. M., Sorenson, S. B., & Burnam, M. A. (1988). The epidemiology of obsessive compulsive disorder in five US communities. *Archive of General Psychiatry, 45,* 1094–9.

Kobak, K. A., Greist, J. H., Jefferson, J. W., Katzelnick, D. J., & Henk, H. J. (1998). Behavioral versus pharmacological treatments of obsessive compulsive disorder: A meta-analysis. *Psychopharmacology, 136,* 205–16.

Kuhajda, M. C., Thorn, B. E., Gaskins, M. W., Day M. A., & Cabbil, C. M. (2011). Literacy and cultural adaptations for cognitive behavioral therapy in a rural pain population. *Translational Behavioral Medicine, 1,* 216–23.

March, J. S., Frances, A., Kahn, D. A., & Carpenter, D. (Eds.). (1997). The expert consensus guidelines: Treatment of obsessive-compulsive disorder. *Journal of Clinical Psychiatry, 58* (Suppl. 4), 1–72.

National Institute for Health and Clinical Excellence, (2005). Obsessive-compulsive disorder: Core interventions in the treatment of obsessive-compulsive disorder and body dysmorphic disorder. Available at: http://www.nice.org.uk/CG031.

Riccardi, C. J., Timpano, K. R., & Schmidt, N. B. (2010). A case study perspective on the importance of motivation in the treatment of obsessive compulsive disorder. *Clinical Case Studies, 9,* 273–84.

Salkovskis, P. M. (2007). Psychological treatment of obsessive-compulsive disorder. *Psychiatry, 6,* 229–33.

Salkovskis, P. M., Wroe, A. L., Morrison, E. F., Richards, C., Reynolds, M., & Thorpe, S. (2000). Responsibility attitudes and interpretations are characteristic of obsessive-compulsive disorder. *Behaviour Research and Therapy, 38,* 347–72.

Teo, P., Graham, E., Yeoh, B. S. A., & Levy, S. (2003). Values, change and inter-generationalties between two generations of women in Singapore. *Ageing and society, 23,* 327–47.

CHAPTER 18. NEUROPSYCHOLOGICAL ASSESSMENT OF FINANCIAL DECISION MAKING

Adapted from Griffith, H.R., Belue, K., Sicola, A., Krzywanski, S., Zamrini, E., Harrell, L, & Marson, D.C.(2003). Impaired financial abilities in mild cognitive impairment: A direct assessment approach. Neurology, 60, 449–457.

Bean, G., Nishisato, S., Rector, N. A., and Glancy, G. (1994). The psychometric properties of the Competency Interview Schedule. *Canadian Journal of Psychiatry—Revue Canadienne de Psychiatrie 39*(8): 368–76.

Boone, K. B., Victor, T. L., Wen, J., Razani, J., & Pontón, M. (2007). The association between neuropsychological scores and ethnicity, language, and acculturation variables in a large patient population. *Archives of Clinical Neuropsychology, 22*(3), 355–65.

Collinson S. L., Fang S. H., Lim M. L., Feng L., Ng T. P. (2014) Normative Data for the Repeatable Battery for the Assessment of Neuropsychological Status (RBANS) in Elderly Chinese. *Archives of Clinical Neuropsychology.* In Press.

Darzins, P., Molloy, D. W., Strang D. (2000) Who can decide? : The six step capacity assessment process. Adelaide, AU: Memory Australia Press.

Department of Statistics, Singapore Population: Census 2010. Available at: http://www.singstat.gov.sg/publications/publications_and_papers/cop2010/cop2010_sr1.html

Fuji, D. E. M. (2010). *The neuropsychology of Asian-Americans.* London, UK: Psychology Press.

Griffith, H. R., Belue, K., Sicola, A., Krzywanski, S., Zamrini, E., Harrell, L, & Marson, D.

C. (2003). Impaired financial abilities in mild cognitive impairment: A direct assessment approach. *Neurology, 60,* 449–57.

Grisso, T., and Appelbaum, P. S. (1995). MacArthur treatment competence study. *Journal of the American Psychiatric Nurses Association 1*(4): 125–7.

Hedden, T., Park, D. C., Nisbett, R., Ji, L. J., Jing, Q., & Jiao, S. (2002). Cultural variation in verbal versus spatial neuropsychological function across the life span. *Neuropsychology, 16*(1), 65–73.

Heinik, J., Werner, P., & Lin, R. (1999). How do cognitively impaired elderly patients define "testament": Reliability and validity of the testament definition scale. *Israeli Journal of Psychiatry and Related Sciences, 36*(1), 23–8.

Janofsky, J. S., McCarthy, R. J., & Folstein,M. F. (1992). The Hopkins Competency Assessment Test: A brief method for evaluating patients' capacity to give informed consent. *Hospital and Community Psychiatry, 43,* 132–6.

Lam, M, Eng., G. K., Rapisarda, A., Kraus, M., Subramaniam, M., Keefe, R. S. E., Collinson, S. L. (2013). Formulation of the age-education index: Accounting for age and education effects in neuropsychological performance. *Psychological Assessment, 25,* 61–70.

Leathem, J. M., Murphy, L. J., and Flett, R. A. (1998). Self- and informant-ratings on the patient competency rating scale in patients with traumatic brain injury. *Journal of Clinical and Experimental Neuropsycholology, 20*(5): 694–705.

Lee K. Y. C., Collinson, S. L., Feng, L., Ng, T. P. (2012). Normative Neuropsychological Data for an Elderly Chinese Population. *Clinical Neuropsychologist, 26,* 321–34.

Marson, D. C., Ingram, K. K., Cody, H. A., and Harrell, L. E. (1995). Assessing the competency of patients with Alzheimer's disease under different legal standards: A prototype instrument. *Archives of Neurology, 52,* 949–54.

Marson, D. C., Sawrie, S., McInturff, B., Snyder, S., Chatterjee, A., Stalvey, T., Boothe, A. & Harrell, L. (2000). Assessing financial capacity in patients with Alzheimer's disease: A conceptual model and prototype instrument. *Archives of Neurology, 57,* 877–84.

Marson, D. C., & Hebert, T. (2008a). Financial capacity. In B. L. Cutler (Ed.), *Encyclopedia of psychology and the law* (Vol. 1, pp. 313–16). Thousand Oaks, CA: Sage.

Martin, R., Griffith, R., Belue, K., Harrell, L., Zamrini, E., Anderson, B., Bartolucci, A., & Marson, D. (2008). Declining financial capacity in patients with mild Alzheimer's disease: A one-year longitudinal study. *American Journal of Geriatric Psychiatry, 16,* 209–19.

Mental Capacity Act: Cap 177A, 2010. Rev Ed Sing.

Menon, S. (2013). The Mental Capacity Act: Implications for Patients and Doctors Faced with Difficult Choices. *Annals of the Academy of Medicine Singapore, 42,* 200–2.

Moye, J., & Karel, M. J. (1999). Evaluating decisional capacities in older adults: Results of two clinical studies. *Advances in Medical Psychology, 10,* 71–84.

Searight, H. R., and Hubbard, S. L. (1998). Evaluating patient capacity for medical decision making: Individual and interpersonal dimensions. *Family, Systems and Health, 16,* 41–53.

Weisensee, M. G., Kjervik, D. K., and Anderson, J. B. (1994). Impairment of short-term memory as a criterion for determination of incompetency. *Geriatric Nursing, 15*(1), 35–40.

Wong, J. G., Clare, C. H., Gunn, M. J., and Holland, A. J. (1999). Capacity to make health care decisions: Its importance in clinical practice. *Psychological Medicine, 29*, 437–46.

Yeo, D., Gabriel, C., Chen, C., Lee, S. H., Loenneker, T., & Wong, M. C. (1997). Pilot validation of a customized neuropsychological battery in elderly Singaporeans. *Neurological Journal of South East Asia, 2*, 123–7.

CHAPTER 19. DEMENTIA

Ballard, C., & Waite, J. (2006). The effectiveness of atypical antipsychotics for the treatment of aggression and psychosis in Alzheimer's disease. *Cochrane DatTanase Systematic Review*(1), CD003476. DOI: 10.1002/14651858.CD003476.pub2

Bird, M., Llewellyn-Jones, R. H., & Korten, A. (2009). An evaluation of the effectiveness of a case-specific approach to challenging behaviour associated with dementia. *Aging & Mental Health, 13*(1), 73–83.

Bird, M., Llewellyn-Jones, R. H., Korten, A. & Smithers, H. (2007). A controlled trial of a predominantly psychosocial approach to BPSD: Treating causality. *International Psychogeriatrics, 19*(5), 874–891

Brodaty, H., Green, A., & Koschera, A. (2003). Meta-analysis of psychosocial interventions for caregivers of people with dementia. *Journal of the American Geriatric Society, 51*(5), 657–64.

Brooker, D. (2004). What is person-centred care in dementia? *Reviews in Clinical Gerontology, 13*, 215–22.

Brooker, D., & Surr, C. (Eds.). (2005). *Dementia care mapping: Principles and practice.* University of Bradford, UK: Bradford Dementia Group, Division of dementia studies.

Butler, G. (1998). Clincal formulation. In A. S. Bellack & M. Hersen (Eds). *Comprehensive clinical psychology*. Oxford: Pergamon

Cerejeira, J., Lagarto, L. & Mukaetova-Ladinska (2012). Behavioural and psychological symptoms of dementia. frontiers in neurology, 3, 1–21.

Chiam, P. C., Ng, T. P., Tan, L. L., Ong, P.S., Ang, A. & Kua, E. H. (2004). Prevalence of dementia in Singapore—results of the national mental health survey of the elderly 2003. *Annuls of the Academy of Medicine, Singapore, 33*(5 Suppl), *S14–15*.

Cole, R.P., Scott, S., & Skelton-Robinson, M. (2000). The effect of challenging behaviour, and staff support, on the psychological wellbeing of staff working wit older adults. *Aging and Mental Health, 4*(4), 359–65

Hersch, E. C., & Falzgraf, S. (2007). Management of the behavioural and psychological symptoms of dementia. *Clinical Interventions in Aging, 2*(4), 611–21

Johnstone, L., & Dallos, R. (2006). Introduction to formulation. In Johnstone, L. & Dallos, R. (Eds.), *Formulation in psychology and psychotherapy* (pp. 1–16). New York, NY: Routledge.

Kamble, P., Chen, H., Sherer, J. T., & Aparasu, R. R. (2009). Use of antipsychotics among elderly nursing home residents with dementia in the US: an analysis of National Survey Data. *Drugs & Aging, 26*(6), 483–92. DOI: 10.2165/00002512-200926060-00005

Kitwood, T. (1997). *Dementia reconsidered: The person comes first*. Maidenhead, UK: Open University Press.

Moniz-Cook, E., Woods, R., Gardiner, E., Silver, M., & Agar. (2001). The Challenging Behaviour Scale (CBS): Development of a scale for staff caring for older people in residential and nursing homes. *British Journal of Clinical Psychology, 40*(3), 309–22.

Ministry of Health. (2009). *Report of the National Dementia Strategy.* Singapore, SG: Ministry of Health.

Ng, T. P., Leong, T., Chiam, P. C., & Kua, E. H. (2010). Ethnic variations in dementia: the contributions of cardiovascular, psychosocial and neuropsychological factors. *Dementia and Geriatric Cognitive Disorders, 29*(2), 131–138. DOI: 10.1159/000275668

Public Guardian Singapore. (2008). Code of practice, Singapore Mental Capacity Act. Singapore, SG: Ministry of Health.

Sahadevan, S., Saw, S. M., Gao, W., Tan, L. C., Chin, J. J., Hong, C. Y., & Venketasubramanian, N. (2008). Ethnic differences in Singapore's dementia prevalence: the stroke, Parkinson's disease, epilepsy, and dementia in Singapore study. *Journal of the American Geriatrics Society, 56*(11), 2061–8. DOI: 10.1111/j.1532–5415.2008.01992.

Sink, K. M., Holden, K. F., & Yaffe, K. (2005). Pharmacological treatment of neuropsychiatric symptoms of dementia: a review of the evidence. *Journal of the American Medical Association, 293*(5), 596–608. DOI: 10.1001/jama.293.5.596.

Stokes, G. (2000). *Challenging behaviour in dementia: A person centred approach.* Bicester, UK: Speechmark.

Stephens, A., Cheston, R. and Gleeson, K. (2013). An exploration into the relationships people with dementia have with physical objects: An ethnographic study. *Dementia, 12* (6), 697–712. ISSN 1471–3012.

CHAPTER 20. IRRITABLE BOWEL SYNDROME

American Psychiatric Association. (2013). *Diagnostic and statistical manual of mental disorders* (5th ed). Arlington, VA: American Psychiatric Publishing.

Azpiroz, F. & Whorwell, P. J. (2009). The challenge of developing new therapies for irritable bowel syndrome. *Therapeutic advances in gastroenterology, 2*(4), 201–3.

Castelnuovo, G. (2010). No medicine without psychology: The key role of psychological contribution in clinical settings. *Frontiers in Psychology,* 1(4).

Choung, R. S., Locke, G. R. the Third, Schleck, C. D., Zinsmeister, A. R. & Talley, N. J. (2009). Psychosocial distress and somatic symptoms in community subjects with irritable bowel syndrome: a psychological component is the rule. *American Journal of Gastroenterology, 104*(7), 1722–9.

Drossman, D. A. (1996). Gastrointestinal illness and the biopsychosocial model. *Journal of Clinical Gastroenterology,* 22, 252–4.

Fones, C. S., Kua, E. H., Ng, T. P. & Ko, S. M. (1998). Studying the mental health of a nation: A preliminary report on a population survey in Singapore. *Singapore Medical Journal, 39*(6), 251–5.

Foo, K. H., Merritt, P. L., & Kazantzis, N. (2006). Counselling/psychotherapy with Chinese Singaporean clients. *Asian Journal of Counselling, 3*(2), 271–93.

Francis, C. Y., Morris, J. & Whorell, P. J (1997). The irritable bowel severity scoring system: A simple method of monitoring irritable bowel syndrome and its progress. *Ailmentary Pharmacology & Therapeutics, 11*(2), 395–402.

Gerson, M-J., Gerson, C. D., Awad, R. A., Dancey, C., Poitras, P., Porcelli, P. & Sperber, A. D. (2006). An international study of irritable bowel syndrome and mind-body attributions. *Social Science and Medicine, 62*, 2838–47.

Gwee, K. A., Lu, C. L., Ghoshal, U. C. (2009). Epidemiology of irritable bowel syndrome in Asia: Something old, something new, something borrowed. *Journal of Gastroenterology and Hepatology, 24*, 1601–7.

Halpert, A. et al. (2007). What patients know about irritable bowel syndrome (IBS) and what they would like to know. National survey on patient eductaional needs in IBS and development and validation of the patient educational. *American Journal ofGastroenterology, 102*(9), 1972–82.

Huang, S., & Spurgeon, A. (2006). The mental health of Chinese immigrants in Birmingham, UK. *Ethnicity & Health, 11*, 365–87.

Kanazawa, M., Hongo, M., & Fukudo, S. (2011). Visceral hypersensitivity in irritable bowel syndrome. *Journal of Gastroenterology & Hepatology, 26*(3), 119–1021.

Kramer, E. J., Kwong, K., Lee, E. & Chung, H. (2002). Cross cultural factors influencing the mental health of Asian Americans. *Western Journal of Medicine, 176*(4), 227–31.

Leong, F. T. L. & Lau, A. S. L. (2001). Barriers to providing effective mental health services to Asian Americans. *Mental Health Services Research. 3*(4), 201–14.

Levy, R. L., Olden, K. W., Naliboff, B. D., Bradley, L. A., Francisconi, C., Drossman, D. A. & Creed, F. (2006). Psychosocial aspects of functional gastrointestinal disorders. *Gastroenterology, 130,* 1447–14458.

Longstreth, G. F., Thompson, W. G., Chey, W. D., Houghton, L. A., Mearin, F. & Spiller, R. C. (2006). *Gastroenterology, 131*(2), 688.

Quigley, E.M. (2012). Probiotics in the management of functional bowel disorders; promise fulfilled? *Gastroenterology Clinics North America, 41*(4), 805–19.

Spiller, R., Aziz, Q., Creed, F., Emmanuel, A., Houghton, L., Hungin, P., Jones, R. Kumar, D. & Rubin, G. (2007). Guidelines on irritable bowel syndrome: Mechanisms and practical management. *Gut, 56*(12), 1770–98.

Tang, Q-L., Lin, G-Y., & Zhang, M-Q. (2013). Cognitive-behavioural therapy for the management of irritable bowel syndrome. *World Journal of Gastroenterology, 19*(46), 8605–10.

Wang, Y. T., Lim, H. Y., Tai, D., Krishnamoorthy, T. L., Tan, T., Barbier, S. & Thumboo, J. (2012). The impact of irritable bowel syndrome on health related quality of life: A Singapore perspective. *BMC Gastroenterology, 12*, 104.

White, C. A. (2001). *Cognitive behaviour therapy for chronic medical problems. A guide to assessment and treatment in practice.* Hoboken, NJ: Wiley.

Zigmond, A. S., & Snaith, R. P. (1983). The hospital anxiety and depression scale. *Acta Psychiatrica Scandinavia, 67*(6), 361–70.

LIST OF CONTRIBUTORS

EDITORS

Dr. Gregor Lange, B.A. (Hons)., M. Sc., D. Psych. Sc.

Senior Lecturer, National University of Singapore
Consultant Clinical Psychologist and Supervisor, Private Practice

Gregor is a German-born, Irish- and American-trained clinical psychologist. His work experiences include working in public health care services (Ireland), private clinics (Ireland, USA, Vietnam), and lecturing at Universities (Ireland & Singapore). He has also worked as an independent consultant, researcher, and author. Gregor has been working with families, couples and individual adults with a variety of problems for more than 10 years. His work includes helping diverse people deal with difficult emotions, family and relationship problems, stress, and other psychological or behavioural difficulties. He is a registered with the Psychological Society of Ireland (PSI) and a member of the Singapore Psychological Society. Gregor is particularly interested in mindfulness-based interventions for mental health problems.

Dr. John Davison, B.Sc. (Hons)., D. Clin. Psy.

Senior Clinical Psychologist, AT&R Unit, Middlemore Hospital, New Zealand

John is a clinical psychologist with experience in both clinical and academic positions in Singapore, New Zealand and Australia. In Singapore, he worked as a lecturer in the Psychology Department of the National University of Singapore. John was a council member for the Singapore Psychological Society and was actively involved in the Singapore Neuropsychology Discussion Group. He has recently returned to NZ, where he provides psychological and neuropsychological assessment, treatment and rehabilitation for adults, older adults and families adjusting to medical and neurological disorders, as well as staff consultation and training. John is registered with the Australian Psychological Society College of Clinical Psychologists and the

NZ Psychology Board, and is a member of the APS Ageing Interest Group and the New Zealand Psychologists for Older People. John completed his Doctorate of Clinical Psychology at the University of Auckland, in collaboration with Harvard University/Mass General Hospital.

SUB-EDITOR

Deborah Amanda Goh, B.Sc. (Hons).

Research Assistant, Department of Psychology, National University of Singapore
Child Protection Officer, Rehabilitative and Protective Branch, Ministry of Social and Family Development

Deborah majored in Life Sciences (Biomedical Science) and Psychology at the National University of Singapore. Through research, she has worked with older adults to study the impact of Type II diabetes on cognition, and with children and their caregivers to determine how various child, maternal and family factors affect the reporting of autistic traits in preschoolers. Her current work in child protection services is motivated by her passion for the welfare of children and the integrity of families in Singapore.

CONTRIBUTORS

Ms Charis Qian Ru CHEW, B.A. (Hons).

Psychologist, Ministry of Social and Family Development

Charis is a Psychologist for the Ministry of Social and Family Development (MSF), where she has been working for five years with children, youth and families with experiences of trauma. Her work includes providing assessments and evidence-based individual and group interventions, as well as providing consultations to children's homes. Charis is currently pursuing her postgraduate studies in clinical psychology in the University of Queensland and is researching mindfulness-based interventions for enhancing parent and child emotional regulation. She also has experience in the Triple P parenting program and in the area of psycho-oncology.

Desiree CHOO, B. Soc. Sci. (Hons)., M. Psych (Clinical).

Clinical Psychologist, Institute of Mental Health

Desiree completed her training at the National University of Singapore and began her practice at the Child Guidance Clinic in 2010. Her experience includes working with survivors of childhood emotional, physical and sexual abuse, juvenile offenders, at-risk youth, as well as children and adolescents with a variety of other psychological or behavioural difficulties. Desiree also has a particular interest in journeying with children and adolescents coping with parental divorce.

Dr. CHU Chi Meng, B.A., B. Soc. Sci. (Hons)., D. Psych (Clinical).

Principal Clinical and Forensic Psychologist, Ministry of Social and Family Development
Adjunct Assistant Professor, National University of Singapore

Chi Meng obtained his Doctor of Psychology in Clinical Forensic Psychology from Australia, and has worked extensively with offenders with mental illnesses during his clinical forensic psychology internship at the Victorian Institute of Forensic Mental Health in Melbourne. He currently heads the Centre for Research on Rehabilitation and Protection at the Ministry of Social and Family Development (MSF) as a Senior Assistant Director. In addition, Chi Meng is concurrently the Principal Clinical and Forensic Psychologist at the Clinical and Forensic Psychology Branch (MSF), where he has previously headed a forensic health service that specialises in the assessment and treatment of offending behaviours.

Dr. Simon COLLINSON, B.Sc. (Hons)., M. Sc., D. Phil.

Associate Professor & Deputy Director, Clinical Psychology Programmes, National University of Singapore

Simon trained in Clinical Neuropsychology at Macquarie University, Sydney, Australia and holds a Doctorate in Clinical Medicine (Psychiatry) from the University of Oxford. He has previously held research posts in Australia and the UK, including the Mental Health Research Institute of Victoria (MHRI), Departments of Psychiatry at Oxford, Charing Cross/Imperial College Medical School London. He is the author of more than 50 scientific papers and texts in the field of neuropsychology. Simon has worked as a Senior Clinical Neuropsychologist in Neurosurgery at the Alfred and Cedar Court Rehabilitation Hospitals in Melbourne, Australia and the Department of Psychological Medicine, National University Hospital, Singapore. In addition to his research and teaching, he is in private practice and sees clients with neuropsychological disorders from all over Southeast Asia.

Dr. Catherine COX, D. Psy (Clin Neuropsy).

Clinical Neuropsychologist, KK Women's and Children's Hospital

Catherine Cox completed her Doctorate in Clinical Neuropsychology at Melbourne's La Trobe University in 2001. She worked in Australia in adult and geriatric settings until her family's relocation to Singapore in 2008. While Catherine was keen to continue to work as a neuropsychologist in Singapore, she realised that her grasp of Chinese and dialects is very poor. Working with Singapore's mostly English-speaking children presented the best option for her. She began working at KK Women's and Children's Hospital in March 2008, and was the first neuropsychologist employed by the hospital. The bulk of her work has been with children with epilepsy, as the hospital was establishing an epilepsy program at the time. She also sees children with other neurodevelopmental and acquired brain disorders receiving the bulk of her referrals from neurology and neurosurgery.

Dr. Paul FISHER, D. Clin. Psy.

Lecturer in Clinical Psychology, University of East Anglia

Paul has worked clinically and as an academic within the UK and Singapore. He gained his qualification from the Bristol Doctorate in Clinical Psychology training course in 2007. He is a passionate advocate for the role of individualised and person-centred formulations to the work of clinical psychologists. He has significant experience working with people with a diagnosis of dementia, including those who are labelled as having 'challenging behaviour'. His enthusiasm for working with this client group is evident across his clinical work, his research interests and his teaching and supervision of psychologists in training. Having worked across hospital, community and residential settings, Paul has developed knowledge and skills to work alongside complex staff teams in varied settings. During his time in Singapore he collaborated closely with the Community Psychogeriatric Programme (CPGP) based out of Changi General Hospital. This allowed him to experience a Singaporean approach to supporting persons with a diagnosis of dementia.

Dr. GWEE Kenji, B.A. (Hons)., D. Clin. Psych (Clin Forensic).

Senior Clinical Forensic Psychologist, Institute of Mental Health
Adjunct Lecturer, National University of Singapore

As a clinical forensic psychologist, Kenji performs both forensic as well as clinical roles. He conducts a variety of forensic assessments, including risk assessments, mental state at the time of offense, fitness to plead, and capacity assessments. His work includes providing consultation to lawyers and courts on forensic matters such as false confessions, malingering, intellectual functioning and alleged memory loss. Kenji is also engaged in treatment and works therapeutically with offenders on their psychiatric challenges as well as offending behavior. When playing a non-forensic role, he provides psychological assessment and treatment to non-offending adult clients with a range of emotional and psychiatric difficulties. Kenji has a keen practical and research interest in psychological assessments.

HO Wei Tshen, B. Soc. Sci., M.A. App. Psy (Counselling).

Senior Psychologist, Clinical and Forensic Psychology Branch, Ministry of Social and Family Development

Wei Tshen has been working with adolescents and their families for more than 15 years. Her work experience ranges from community- and school-based work with at-risk youth to institutional juvenile offender rehabilitation. She is currently involved in the assessment and treatment of adolescent and adult offenders with psychological difficulties and offending issues, particularly sexual offending.

Jade JANG Leong Yeok, , B.A., B. Soc. Sci. (Hons)., M.A. App. Psy (Educational Psychology).

Senior Educational Psychologist, Institute of Mental Health

At the Child Guidance Clinic (CGC), Jade has been working with children and adolescents with various mental health conditions, such as Mood and Anxiety Disorders, as well as Autism Spectrum Disorders. Her clinical duties include conducting diagnostic, cognitive, educational and adaptive behavioural assessments, as well as delivering individual and group therapy. She also provides psycho-education and support for their parents and caregivers to help them manage their child's behaviours, as well as understand and cope with their child's diagnosis. She believes in conducting research to better understand mental health issues as well as to guide clinical practice, and has several publications. She is also passionate about sharing knowledge through conducting trainings and providing supervision.

Dr. Jasmin KAUR, B.Sc., D. Psych.

Senior Assistant Director, Singapore Prison Service

Jasmin is a senior psychologist with Singapore Prison Service. She conducts research on offending patterns, forensic risk assessment tools, and offending behavior. In addition to her research portfolio, Jasmin has been a practicing clinician for more than 10 years, and sees clients with a variety of behavioural difficulties and mental health issues. Her work has included group interventions for personality-disordered and violent offenders. Jasmin provides professional supervision to other psychologists in Singapore Prison Service. Jasmin completed her Bachelor of Social Sciences (Honours) from National University of Singapore and holds a Doctorate in Clinical Psychology from James Cook University, Australia. She is a member of the Australian Psychological Society and the Singapore Psychological Society.

Clare H. M. KWAN, M.A. Clin. Psych.

Senior Clinical Psychologist

Clare has been working in an outpatient tertiary psychiatric hospital setting for the last five years, providing psychological intervention to children, adolescents and their families. She has extensive clinical experience in treatment of mood and anxiety psychiatric issues as well as treatment of teenagers engaging in sexualized behaviours, trauma relating to physical/sexual abuse and neglect. Clare has been providing evidenced-based treatment in a range of treatment modalities such as Cognitive Behavioural Therapy (CBT), Dialectical Behavioural Therapy (DBT), Child-Centred Play Therapy, Trama Focus-CBT (TF-CBT), and Eye Movement Desensitisation Reprocessing (EMDR). Clare is also an active researcher and presents at conferences locally and internationally. She is a member of the Singapore Psychological Society and the Australian Psychological Society.

Dr Julia CY LAM, B. Soc. Sc. (Hons)., M. Phil., M.Sc., D. Psych (Forensic).

Forensic Psychologist and Director of Forensic Psych Services, Winslow Clinic, Promises Healthcare Pte Ltd

Julia is a Forensic Psychologist who specializes in assessment and report-writing for Court purposes in the criminal, civil and family law contexts. A scientist-practitioner, her work experiences include working in universities, hospitals, prisons and correction services, gambling treatment facilities and private clinics. She has expertise in Impulse-Control Disorders, Problem Gambling, Atypical Theft Offending and Addictions, and their respective offending. Her research and lecturing experiences span across three countries (Hong Kong, Australia and Singapore) over two decades which include training medical, nursing, psychology and social work students, as well as mental health professionals and addiction counsellors. She currently teaches addiction counselling of a master program at a local university in Singapore. She is a registered psychologist in Hong Kong, Australia and Singapore. She was a Council Member (Newsletter Editor) of the Singapore Psychological Society from 2009 to 2015.

Joy LIM, B.Sc. (Hons).

Psychologist, Changi General Hospital

Joy has participated actively in clinical research in older adults since 1996, and has
published several papers on the validation of psychometric batteries and screening
tests for the assessment of dementia, and depression in older Singaporean adults,
in international peer reviewed journals. As a psychologist with the Community
Psychogeriatric Programme (CPGP) at Changi General Hospital, Joy was involved
in providing training and support for common mental health problems in older
adults for eldercare staff, and empowering care partners with the necessary skill
sets to promote good quality of life particularly in people with dementia in the
community. Her clinical work includes conducting assessments and intervention
using a formulation-led approach to understanding 'challenging behaviour' of people
diagnosed with dementia. Joy has attained an Advanced User status in Dementia
Care Mapping (DCM) and is using the tool to support quality care in eldercare staff.
She is currently a candidate for the Doctorate in Clinical Psychology program at
James Cook University.

Dr. Joy LOW, B.Sc. (Hons). Psy., D. Clin. Psych & Clin Neuropsych.

Senior Clinical Psychologist & Clinical Neuropsychologist, Clinical & Forensic
Psychology Branch (CFPB), Ministry of Social and Family Development (MSF)

Joy is interested in trauma and its impact on the developing brain. She conducts
assessment and therapy for children, youth and families who have experienced
trauma from intrafamilial abuse and neglect. She supervises clinical psychologists
within CFPB, heads operations of its sexual abuse intervention team, facilitates
community training of CID officers and counsellors, and is involved in consultation
projects for multi-agency workgroups. She is also part of the National CARE
network, which is trained to respond to national and international crises or
emergencies. Joy's undergraduate studies at the University of York, England, were
fully sponsored by MSF. She subsequently completed her Doctorate of Clinical
Psychology and Clinical Neuropsychology at the University of Queensland in
Brisbane, Australia. During her postgraduate studies, Joy specialised in paediatric
brain injury and adult substance abuse and was registered as a provisional
psychologist under the Australian Health Practitioner Regulation Agency (AHPRA).
She is currently registered as a full member of the Singapore Psychological Society.

Dr. Iliana MAGIATI, B.Sc., M.Sc., PhD., D. Clin. Psy.

Assistant Professor, National University of Singapore

Iliana is a chartered clinical psychologist. She completed her doctoral training in clinical psychology at the Institute of Psychiatry, King's College London and her Ph.D. on early intervention in autism at St. George's Hospital Medical School. She has worked in both academic and research settings, and as a clinical psychologist within multidisciplinary child development and psychology teams in the UK National Health Service. She has specific knowledge of and experience in the assessment, diagnosis and intervention of children and young people with ASD and other developmental and learning difficulties and in working with children and families. Her research and clinical interests include screening and diagnosis of ASD, anxiety difficulties in people with ASD, and long term outcomes in individuals with ASD. She supervises clinical interns in their clinical placements and is also an ADOS trainer.

Dr. Nenna NDUKWE, D. Clin. Psy., M. Sci., B. Sci. (Hons)., C. Psychol., C. Sci., AFBPsS.

Consultant Clinical Psychologist/Regional Director of Operations California Counselling Pte Ltd Singapore

Nenna holds a Doctorate in Clinical Psychology, Master of Science Degree in Forensic & Legal Psychology and a Bachelor of Science Degree in Psychology. She has more than 10 years of clinical experience working with children, adolescents and their families; couples and adults. Her experience in mental and physical health spans a wide range of settings, including hospitals, private practice, corporate organizations, education and correctional settings. She has also worked as an academic in universities teaching psychology and conducting psychological-based research.Nenna's clinical experience includes providing clinical supervision, consultation, and working with clients experiencing anxiety, depression, stress, self-harm, trauma, eating and feeding difficulties, grief and loss, relationship conflicts, and adjustment issues. She also has a special interest in working with clients who experience somatic complaints (relating to chronic fatigue, irritable bowel syndrome, chronic pain and other medically unexplained symptoms). Working overseas with various diverse cultures has meant that Nenna is familiar with and able to offer support to clients experiencing difficulties relating to expatriation. She is trained in the use of cognitive behavioural therapy, child and family systemic therapy, psychodynamic therapy and psychometric testing.Nenna completed her training in psychology in the UK and is certified as a Chartered Psychologist and Full Member of the British Psychological Society's Division of Clinical Psychology.

Dr. Adaline NG, D. Clin. Psy.

Senior Assistant Director, Psychological Services, Singapore Prison Service

Adaline oversees the provision of psychological services to offenders and staff, such as risk assessments, offender interventions, and staff counselling. She has worked at Singapore Prison Service for the past 13 years. She has assumed various portfolios during her time there and pioneered program evaluation initiatives.A clinical psychologist by training, her clinical experience includes assessing the risk of re-offending in areas such as domestic and sexual violence. She has also delivered group-based interventions for young male offenders with violence antecedents, and worked with personality-disordered offenders. Adaline's main areas of clinical interest include personality disorders, addictions, and violence. She also provides clinical supervision to psychologists at Singapore Prison Service, as well as postgraduate clinical psychology students. In addition, she co-teaches a Correctional Psychology module at the National University of Singapore.

Jeffrey ONG, MA. Clin. Psy.

Senior Clinical Psychologist, Institute of Mental Health

Jeffrey obtained his Masters degree in Clinical Psychology from the National University of Singapore. He has been working with the Institute of Mental Health since 2009, at the outpatient clinic of the Child Guidance Clinic (CGC). He is currently part of the REACH (Response, Early intervention and Assessment in Community mental Health for students) team. Jeffrey works primarily with children and adolescents in relation to clinical issues such as developmental disorders, anxiety, depression, addictions and anger management. His clinical experience includes conducting diagnostic and psychometric assessments, provision of individual and group therapy, and conducting training for school counsellors.

Elaine Li-Ying SUM, B. Soc. Sc. (Hons)., M. Psych (Clinical).

Clinical Psychologist, Institute of Mental Health

Elaine completed her Masters in Psychology (Clinical) in a joint Masters program from University of Melbourne and National University of Singapore and also received her Bachelor of Social Science in Psychology (Hons) from National University of Singapore. Elaine is currently working at the Institute of Mental Health (Singapore) with the adult general psychiatric population. She does psychological therapy, both in the individual and group formats, and also provides psychological, neuropsychological and forensic assessments.

TAN Li Jen, B. Soc. Sci. (Hons)., M. Clin. Psych.

Senior Principal Clinical Psychologist and Senior Assistant Director, Clinical & Forensic Psychology Branch, Ministry of Social & Family Development

Li Jen has been a practicing clinical psychologist for over 15 years. She currently oversees the provision of clinical services for child abuse and sexual abuse victims and their families, and the implementation of evidence-based programs for trauma, parenting and associated problems in child welfare settings. Li Jen has also worked in adult and pediatric hospital settings with patients across the lifespan who presented with a wide range of mental disorders. Li Jen has special interests in trauma, anxiety and stress, and is also involved in crisis intervention and disaster mental health work. She believes in the importance of integrating trauma informed care and evidence based treatments within a systems approach in providing effective interventions for clients and families.

TAY Sze Yan, B.A., B. Soc. Sci. (Hons)., M. Soc. Sci., M. Clin. Psy.

Senior Psychologist, Singapore General Hospital (SGH)

Sze Yan is a Clinical Psychologist at the Department of Neurology, SGH. She has more than 10 years of experience working with patients with neurological issues, and is also experienced in working with individuals with a variety of psychological and behavioral issues. Her roles have included conducting neuropsychological evaluation for patients with neurological disorders (specifically memory problems in elderly patients), helping patients manage their moods, adjustment issues, stress, caregiving issues and cognitive difficulties, and facilitating support groups for patients with dementia. Sze Yan is actively involved in clinical research related to the areas of Neuropsychology and Neurology, and had presented at a number of local and international conferences. She has also contributed her research findings to a range of peer-reviewed journals. She completed her Masters in Clinical Psychology at the National University of Singapore and is a member of the Singapore Psychological Society.

Nishta Geetha THEVARAJA, B.A., M. Psych (Clinical).

Clinical Psychologist, REACH (Response, Early intervention and Assessment in Community Mental Health), Institute of Mental Health

Nishta is experienced in working with individuals with mild intellectual disability and with children and adolescents with mental health conditions in Singapore. She is a member of Silver Ribbon Singapore and is a keen advocate for mental health awareness within Singapore. She has also been involved in providing mental health related talks for school counsellors and teachers. Apart from her clinical work, Nishta has worked as an Adjunct Lecturer for locally conducted overseas psychology courses. Her key interests are in mood and anxiety disorders, personality disorders, eating disorders, psychosis, autism, ADHD and intellectual disability. Nishta is also a member of the Singapore Psychological Society.

Dr. Ranjani UTPALA, BSc. Psy., PG. Dip. Psy., D. Clin. Psy.

Lecturer, National University of Singapore
Manager, Clinical Health & Psychology Centre

Ranjani has over ten years of clinical experience in both public and private sectors in Singapore, Australia and the UK. Her area of interest and clinical expertise lies in the treatment of eating disorders for adults and adolescents. In addition to treatment of eating disorders, she also has experience and interest in the drug and alcohol field, having worked in this field in both Sydney and London. In working with adolescents, she is trained in the current evidence-based treatment of choice, Family Based Therapy for treatment of eating disorders (also known as FBT/Maudsley), and also supervises clinicians using this approach. In her work with adults, she uses cognitive behavioural therapy (CBT), Acceptance and Commitment Therapy (ACT) as well as mindfulness based approaches. She is a registered Psychologist in Australia and is endorsed as a Clinical Psychologist by the Psychology Board of Australia and the APS College of Clinical Psychologists.

A/Prof Munidasa WINSLOW, MBBS, MMed (Psych), FAMS.

Executor Director and Senior Consultant Psychiatrist, Promises Healthcare Pte Ltd

Muni is a Psychiatrist who specializes in addictions (e.g. alcohol, substances, gambling, gaming and sexual compulsivity). His last appointment was as Chief of the Addiction Medicine Department, Institute of Mental Health. He was one of the pioneers responsible for the setting up and development of addiction services both in Woodbridge Hospital and in the community; and a pioneer in Addiction and Impulse-Control Disorders in the Asia-Pacific region. He is a certified master addiction counsellor and a certified clinical supervisor.

He founded Promises in 2008 and started Winslow Clinic in 2011. His passion is to help therapists develop and hone their skills to effect real change in those they seek to help. He has been the chairman of the Asia-Pacific Certification Board since its inception which certifies Addictions & Mental Health therapists in the Asia-Pacific region.

Eunice YAP-WONG, MA. Clin. Psy.

Senior Clinical Psychologist, Department of Psychological Medicine, Khoo Teck Puat Hospital

Eunice oversees the provision of psychotherapy and psychological assessments to children and their families with developmental and mental health issues. A firm believer in outreach work, she also conducts talks and workshops to equip people with the knowledge and skills to understand and deal with children. Her area of interest and expertise is in Autism Spectrum Disorders (ASDs). She has worked extensively with this population, including conducting assessments for individuals with ASD. She has also conducted research into the parenting characteristics of Singapore parents.

RESOURCES

The following resources are collated by our authors and pertain directly to the content of their chapters. The resources include lists of local organisations for assessment and treatment, support groups for clients and their families, and relevant online resources and treatment manuals. Resources for education, assessment and treatment of psychological issues develop rapidly—both locally and internationally—and we do not intend this section to be all-inclusive or even a comprehensive list. Rather, these resources provide a starting point for readers with further interest.

CHAPTER 1. EATING DISORDER (ANOREXIA NERVOSA)

Local organisations for assessment and treatment

- Eating Disorders Program at Singapore General Hospital (SGH): http://www.sgh.com.sg/Clinical-Departments-Centers/EDUnit/Pages/ eatingdisorders-programme.aspx

- KK Women and Children's Hospital (KKH): http://www.kkh.com.sg/Pages/ Home.aspx

Support groups

- Support for eating disorders Singapore (SEDS) run by Singapore Association for Mental Health and SGH: http://www.samhealth.org.sg/support-for-eating- disorderssingapore-seds/

Online resources

- The Maudsley Parents website includes information and videos about ED and treatment specifically about FBT for both parents and professionals: http://www.maudsleyparents.org/

- Families Empowered and Supporting Treatment of Eating Disorders (FEAST-ED) http://members.feast-ed.org/

- The Butterfly Foundation: http://thebutterflyfoundation.org.au/

- Training Institute for Child and Adolescent Eating Disorders:
  http://train2treat4ed.com/

- Centre for Eating and Dieting Disorders (CEDD): http://cedd.org.au/

- The Victorian Centre for Excellence in Eating Disorders (CEED):
  http://ceed.org.au/

CHAPTER 2. ENCEPHALITIS AND CHALLENGING BEHAVIOURS

Local organisations for assessment and treatment

- Individualised neuropsychological and multidisciplinary care for development
  disorders is provided at KK Hospital, http://www.kkh.com.sg/Services/Children/
  ChildDevelopment/Pages/Home.aspx

Online resources

- The Ministry of Social and Family Development Child Protection and Welfare
  website provides information about Children and Young Persons Homes:
  http://app.msf.gov.sg/Policies/Strong-and-Stable-Families/NurturingProtecting-the-
  Young/Child-Protection-Welfare/Children-and-Young-PersonsHomes

Local resources for ANE appear to be limited. International resources also tend to
emphasise generic encephalitis resources and information, such as the two websites
below:

- UK-based encephalitis resource: http://www.encephalitis.info/

- International discussion forum: https://www.inspire.com/groups/encephalitis-
  global/

CHAPTER 3. ADHD AND OPPOSITIONAL DEFIANT DISORDER

Local organisations for assessment and treatment

- Child Guidance Clinic (CGC, Institute of Mental Health): http://www.imh.com.sg/
  page.aspx?id=140

- Child Development Unit (KK Women's and Children's Hospital):
  http://www.kkh.com.sg/Services/Children/ChildDevelopment/Pages/Home.aspx

- The Children's Specialist Clinic (CSC) & Child Development Unit (CDU, National
  University Hospital)

- The Response, Early Intervention and Assessment in Community Mental Health

- (REACH) program falls under the Singapore National Mental Health Blueprint and is a collaboration with the Ministry of Social and Family Development, IMH, KKH, NUH and other hospitals for provision of specialised care for child development issues including ADHD.

Support groups

- Society for the Promotion of ADHD Research and Knowledge (SPARK), an independent, voluntary welfare organization which promotes ADHD awareness and runs a support group for parents who have children with ADHD/ADD. It holds monthly Parent Support Group meetings and talks relating to ADHD, treatment methods and coping strategies: http://www.spark.org.sg

- YouthReach (YR, Singapore Association for Mental Health), a specialised community youth mental health service for children and youths with emotional and psychological problems: http://www.youthreach.org.sg

Online resources

- Online Portal by Health Promotional Board on ADHD: https://www.roc-n-ash.com/imheportal/welcome/

- Institute of Mental Health educational video on ADHD: http://www.imh.com.sg/clinical/page.aspx?id=249

- Living with ADHD (English and Chinese versions) by Dr Cai Yiming (IMH): http://www.imh.com.sg/uploadedfiles/apps/eShop/Attachment/Living%20with%20ADHD c_634813298766410324.pdf

- 'Pay Attention, Alex' by Ms Carolyn Kee: http://www.imh.com.sg/page.aspx?id=689

- A Parent's Guide to Children's Behaviour by the DCAP Research Team http://www.imh.com.sg/uploadedfiles/apps/eShop/Attachment/

CHAPTER 4. ANXIETY AND AUTISM SPECTRUM DISORDER

Local organisations for assessment and treatment

- Child Development Unit (KK Women's and Children's Hospital): http://www.kkh.com.sg/Services/Children/ChildDevelopment/Pages/Home.aspx

- Child Development Unit (National University Hospital): http://www.nuh.com.sg/ktp-nucmi/clinical-care/facilities/clinics-and-centres/child-development-unit-jurong-medical-centre-level-2.html

- Neuro-Behavioural Clinic (Autism Services), Child Guidance Clinic (CGC,

Institute of Mental Health): http://www.imh.com.sg/clinical/page.aspx?id=283 & http://www.imh.com.sg/clinical/page.aspx?id=267

- Developmental & Behavioural Paediatric Services, National University Hospital: http://www.nuh.com.sg/ktp-nucmi/clinical-care/facilities/clinics-and-centres/ developmental-and-behavioural-paediatric-services-nuhs-childrens-clinic-2-onlevel-4.html

- Child and Adolescent Psychiatry and Psychology Service, Khoo Teck Puat Hospital:

- http://www.ktph.com.sg/main/specialties_n_services/4/16/psychological_medicine

- Autism Resource Centre: http://www.autism.org.sg/main/index.php

- Adult Neuro-Developmental Services (ANDS), IMH includes inpatient consultancy, outpatient clinics and outreach services targeted at patients with an intellectual disability and/or autism spectrum disorder/pervasive developmental disorder between the ages of 19–64, for further assessment and management of psychiatric as well as behavioural issues.

Online resources

- Autism Resource Centre: http://www.autism.org.sg/main/index.php

- Autism Association Singapore: http://autismlinks.org.sg/main/

- We CAN: http://www.wecaneip.com/arc/web/

- Autism Spectrum Disorders in Pre-School Children. AMS-MOH Clinical Practice Guidelines 1/2010: http://www.moh.gov.sg/content/moh_web/home/Publications/ guidelines/cpg.html

CHAPTER 5. SELECTIVE MUTISM

Local organisations for assessment and treatment

- Selective Mutism Anxiety Research and Treatment Centre: http://www.selectivemutismcenter.org/

Online resources

- ChildMind Institute mental health guide on selective mutism: http://www.childmind.org/en/health/disorder-guide/selective-mutism

- Selective Mutism Foundation: http://www.selectivemutismfoundation.org/

- Selective Mutism Group—Childhood Anxiety Network: http://www.selectivemutism.org/

- Selective Mutism Information & Research Association: http://www.smira.org.uk/

Treatment manuals

- McHolm, A.E., Cunningham, C.E., & Vanier, M.K. (2005). *Helping your child overcome selective mutism or a fear of speaking: A parent's guide.* Oakland, California: New Harbinger Publications, Inc.

- Johnson, M., & Wintgens, A. (2001). *The selective mutism resource manua*l. London, UK: Speechmark Publishers.

- Bryson, C. (2009). *Why Dylan doesn't talk: A real-life look at selective mutism through the eyes of a child.* USA: Sweet Greetings, Inc.

- Kearney, C. (2010). *Helping children with selective mutism and their parents: A guide for school-based professionals.* USA: Oxford University Press.

CHAPTER 6. GENERALIZED ANXIETY DISORDER

Local organisations for assessment and treatment

- Response Early Intervention and Assessment in Community Mental Health (REACH)—a community mental healthcare service that is set up to work closely with schools to help students with emotional or behavioural problems: http://reachforstudents.com/

- Community Health Assessment Team (CHAT)—a national youth mental health team that provides mental health assessment for young people aged 16 to 30: http://www.youthinmind.sg

- Child Guidance Clinic (CGC) of the Institute of Mental Health (IMH) treats young clients (up to the age of 19 years old) who are facing emotional or behavioural problems: http://www.imh.com.sg/clinical/ page.aspx?id=283

- Child and Adolescent Psychiatry and Psychology Service of Khoo Teck Puat Hospital (KTPH) treats children of all ages for anxiety, emotional, behavioural problems and other psychiatric conditions: https://www.ktph.com.sg/psychmed

- Child and Adolescent Psychiatry Clinic of National University Hospital (NUH) provides outpatient diagnostic and consultation services for children and adolescents under stress: https://www.nuh.com.sg/umc/about-us/about-us/ department-of-psychological-medicine/clinical-services/outpatient-services/ childand-adolescent-psychiatry-clinic.html

Support groups

- YouthReach—community recovery program for children and youth identified with emotional and/or psychological issues: http://www.samhealth.org.sg/youthreach/

CHAPTER 7. FRONTAL LOBE EPILEPSY

Online Resources

For ADHD and Child Behaviour:

- Children and Adults with Attention-Deficit/Hyperactivity Disorder: www.chadd.org

- Kids Health from Nemours: www.kidshealth.org

- Raising Children, The Australian Parenting Website: raisingchildren.net.au

For Epilepsy:

- International League Against Epilepsy: http://www.ilae.org

- Singapore Epilepsy Foundation: http://www.epilepsy.com.sg

- Epilepsy Care Singapore: http://www.epilepsycare.org

- Epilepsy Action Plan: http://www.kkh.com.sg/AboutUs/PressRelease/Pages/28–08–2013.aspx

CHAPTER 8. POST-TRAUMATIC STRESS DISORDER

Online resources

- The National Child Traumatic Stress Network (NCTNS): http://www.nctsnet.org/

- TF-CBT Web Learning: http://tfcbt.musc.edu/

- Ministry of Social and Family Development website for information on child abuse: http://www.msf.gov.sg

- Emotional and Psychological Trauma: http://www.helpguide.org/mental/emotional_psychological_trauma.htm

- KK Women's and Children's Hospital, Psychosocial Trauma Support Service: www.kkh.com.sg

- Trauma Recovery & Corporate Solutions: www.traumarecovery.com.sg

Local organisations for assessment and treatment

For conduct-related problems:

- Central Youth Guidance Office (CYGO) (http://app.msf.gov.sg/): An inter-ministry central agency that coordinates programs and services targeting the needs of at-risk youth

- Child Guidance Clinic (CGC) (http://www.imh.com.sg): Provides medical consultation and psychological assessment and intervention services for young persons (up to 19 years of age) who are facing emotional/behavioural problems

- Beyond Social Services (http://www.beyond.org.sg): A voluntary welfare organisation that aims to help curb delinquency among disadvantaged youth

- Singapore Children's Society (http://www.childrensociety.org.sg/): Runs ten service centres island-wide providing services to children, youth and families in need

For domestic violence:

- Promoting Alternatives to Violence (PAVE) (http://www.pave.org.sg/): A voluntary welfare organisation that provides casework, group work and community work services to individuals and families experiencing intra/interpersonal violence

Treatment manuals

- "Seeing Red—Help Your Child Deal with Anger at Home and in Public" by Dr. Rebecca Ang, A/Prof Daniel Fung and contributors, Carolyn Kee and Geraldine Wong. Seeing Red gives an excellent perspective on understanding and managing anger in children. Dr Ang and Dr Fung provide tested techniques based on their vast experience helping parents develop effective strategies to teach their children important life skills of anger management.

CHAPTER 10. PYROMANIA

Local organisations for assessment and treatment

- Child Guidance Clinic (CGC): https://www.imh.com.sg/page.aspx?id=140

- Institute of Mental Health (IMH): https://www.imh.com.sg

- Clinical and Forensic Psychology Branch (CFPB). The CFPB only considers referrals by Ministry of Social Family Development, Guidance Programme agencies, Police, and Attorney General's Chambers on case-by-case basis.

Local organisations for assessment and treatment

Whilst many psychologists in Singapore work with people with Borderline Personality Disorder and have completed training in therapies such DBT, we are not aware of any mental health clinics in Singapore currently specialising specifically in the assessment and treatment of BPD. The following organisations are the two primary providers for the assessment and treatment of mental health disorders, including, but not specific to personality disorders:

- Institute of Mental Health (IMH) provides a range of assessment and psychological treatment for adults with various types of mental health problems: http://www.imh.com.sg

- Singapore Association for Mental Health (SAMH) provides counselling services for individuals with psychiatric, psychological, emotional, or relationship issues and their families: http://www.samhealth.org.sg/

Online resources

- Behavioural Tech, LLC, founded by Dr Marsha Linehan, provides a comprehensive range of information on DBT. Training, resources, and products related to DBT: www.behavioraltech.org/

- DBT Self Help website was created by a non-clinicians who have been treated with DBT. It provides detailed information on the various DBT skills, coupled with personal experiences on the application of the skills: http://www.dbtselfhelp.com/index.html

CHAPTER 12. AUTISM SPECTRUM DISORDER

Local organisations for assessment and treatment

- St. Andrew's Adult Autism Services: http://www.saac.org.sg/saaas.html

- Eden Centre for Adults: http://autismlinks.org.sg/programme/adults-centre.php

- Adult Neurodevelopmental Service at IMH: https://www.imh.com.sg/clinical/page.aspx?id=265

- Autism Clinic at the Child Guidance Clinic IMH (for children and adolescents): https://www.imh.com.sg/page.aspx?id=267

If an adult suspects that they or another adult family member may have undiagnosed ASD, they can seek an adult psychiatrist who will discuss with them the available options for establishing a diagnosis of ASD in adulthood.

Online resources

- Autism Resource Centre (ARC): http://www.autismresourcecentre.com

- Autism Association Singapore: http://www.autismlinks.org.sg/main/index.php

- National Institute of Mental Health UK guidelines on recognition, assessment and interventions for adults with ASD: http://www.nice.org.uk/nicemedia/live/13774/59685/59685.pdf

- Autism Speaks: http://www.autismspeaks.org/family-services/resource-library/adults-autism

- The National Autistic Society, UK: http://www.autism.org.uk/living-with-autism/adults-with-autism-or-asperger-syndrome.aspx

- The National Healthcare Service, Adults with Autism: http://www.nhs.uk/Livewell/Autism/Pages/Diagnosisinadults.aspx

CHAPTER 13. DEVIANT SEXUAL BEHAVIOUR

Online resources

- Singapore Statutes Online (http://statutes.agc.gov.sg/aol/home.w3p) provides Acts and Constitutional Documents. The legal clauses pertaining to the Mandatory Treatment Order can be found in the Criminal Procedure Code 2010, Section 339.

- Sex and Love Addicts Anonymous: http://www.sg-slaa.com

- Health Promotion Board's Page on Sexual Health: http://www.hpb.gov.sg/HOPPortal/healthtopic/Sexual%20Health

Treatment manuals

- For psychological treatment techniques for sexual offending (e.g covert sensitization), *see* Laws & O'Donohue.

- For relapse prevention strategies, including those for sexual offenders *see* Witkiewitz, K., & Marlatt, G. A., *Therapist guide to evidence-based relapse prevention* (2007), Burlington, MA: Elsevier.

CHAPTER 14. MAJOR DEPRESSION AND PARANOID PERSONALITY DISORDER

Local organisations for assessment and treatment

- Samaritans of Singapore (SOS) is a non-profit organization that assists individuals in distress. Their services include a 24-hour hotline (1800–221–4444) manned by

volunteers, an email befriending service (pat@samaritans.org.sg), face-to-face
counselling, a suicide bereavement support group: http://www.samaritans.org.sg

For individuals seeking help upon release from prison:

- Family Service Centres: http://app.msf.gov.sg/Policies/StrongandStableFamilies/
  SupportingFamilies/FamilyServiceCentres.aspx.

- Singapore Corporation of Rehabilitative Enterprises (SCORE), Industrial &
  Services Cooperative Society Ltd., Singapore Aftercare Association (SACA) and
  Singapore

- Anti-Narcotics Association (SANA): www.carenetwork.org.sg

CHAPTER 15. GAMBLING DISORDER

Local organizations for assessment and treatment

- National Council on Problem Gambling (NCPG): http://www.knowtheline.sg/;
  Helpline: 1800-6-668-668

- National Addictions Management Service (NAMS), Institute of Mental
  Health: http://www.nams.sg/addictions/gambling/Pages/Gambling-Overview.aspx.
  The following programs are available at NAMS: Gambling Addiction Management
  through Education (GAME), Families in Recovery through Education and
  Empowerment on Problem Gambling (FREE-PG), Continual Recovery through
  Education and Skills Training (CREST), and Women in Recovery through Support,
  Education and Empowerment (WISE)

- Tanjong Pagar Family Service Centre (family and debt counselling services for
  problem gamblers): https://www.gamblingtherapy.org/tanjong-pagar-familyservice-
  centre-fsc

- Thye Hua Kwan Problem Gambling Recovery Centre: http://www.thkmc.org.sg/
  thk-problem-gambling-recovery-centre/

- Ang Mo Kio Family Service Centre Group—Ang Mo Kio, Cheng San and
  Sengkang branches/Nexus Family Resource Centre

- Marine Parade Family Service Centre Group

- Tampines Family Service Centre

- Thye Hua Kwan Moral Society Family Service Centre Group—Tanjong Pagar and
  Bukit Panjang branches/Centre for Family Harmony

Support groups

- Gamblers Anonymous: https://www.gamblingtherapy.org/singapore-gamblersanonymous

- Gam-Anon: Help for Family and Friends: http://www.gam-anon.org/

Online resources

- Types of Psychotherapy for Pathological Gamblers: http://www.ncbi.nlm.nih.gov/pmc/articles/PMC3000184/pdf/PE_2_5_32.pdf

- National Addictions Management Service (NAMS), Institute of Mental Health resources website provides videos with psychologists and counsellors, educational materials and self-assessment tools: http://www.nams.sg/addictions/gambling/Pages/Gambling-Overview.aspx

- The Victorian Responsible Gambling Foundation website: http://www.professionals.problemgambling.vic.gov.au/stages-of-gambling/stages–of-change

- The Problem Gambling Institute of Ontario website: http://www.problemgambling.ca/en/resourcesforprofessionals/pages/treatmentforproblemgambling.aspx

- DSM-5 changes to Pathological Gambling: http://www.responsiblegambling.org/rgnews-research/newscan/newscan-item/2012/06/01/pathological-gambling-changesin-the-dsm-5

Treatment manuals

- Ladouceur, R. & Lachance, S. (2006). *Overcoming your pathological gambling: Therapist guide (Treatments that work)*. USA: Oxford University Press.

- Ladouceur, R. & Lachance, S. (2006). *Overcoming your pathological gambling:Workbook (Treatments that work)*. USA: Oxford University Press.

- Wong, K.E., Anantha, S., Lim, R. & Lee, T.K.M. (2010). *Don't gamble your life away! Help for pathological gamblers*. Singapore: Strait Times Press.

CHAPTER 16. PANIC DISORDER

Online resources

- An overview of and resources for anxiety disorders, by the Agency of Integrated Care: https://careinmind.aic.sg/conditions/

Support groups

- Singapore support group for anxiety and panic attacks: http://www.meetup.com/
  Singapore-Support-Group-for-Anxiety-and-Panic-Attacks/

CHAPTER 17. OBSESSIVE-COMPULSIVE DISORDER

Online resources

- Institute of Mental Health (IMH) psychoeducation on
  OCD: https://www.imh.com.sg/clinical/ page.aspx?id=256

- National University Hospital (NUH) psychoeducation: http://www.nuh.com.sg/
  umc/patients-andvisitors/diseases-and-conditions/head/obsessivecompulsive-
  disorder-ocd.html

- The psychology tools website provides a range of CBT forms and assessment
  questionnaires which are useful in the treatment and intervention for
  OCD: http://psychology.tools/obssessive-compulsive-disorder.html

- The Oxford Cognitive Therapy Centre describes and provides questionnaires for
  assessing and monitoring therapy progress of patients with OCD:
  http://www.octc.co.uk/resources

- The International OCD Foundation provides brochures, fact sheets, articles and
  books both for people with OCD and for practitioners:
  http://www.ocfoundation.org/

CHAPTER 18. NEUROPSYCHOLOGICAL ASSESSMENT OF FINANCIAL
DECISION MAKING

Online resources

- Mental Capacity Act Code of Practice (Singapore: Office of the Public Guardian,
  Ministry of Community Development, Youth & Sports; 2010) provides guidance on
  the rights and responsibilities of caregivers and those who act or make decisions on
  behalf of individuals who lack mental capacity.

- The Office of the Public Guardian ("OPG") works towards protecting the dignity
  and interests of individuals who lack mental capacity and are vulnerable as well as
  encouraging proactive planning for an eventuality of losing one's mental capacity:
  http://www.publicguardian.gov.sg

Local organisations for assessment and treatment

- Alexandra Hospital Geriatric Medicine Clinic: https://www.alexhosp.com.sg

- Changi General Hospital Geriatric Clinic: https://www.cgh.com.sg

- Institute of Mental Health Psychogeriatric Clinic: https://www.imh.com.sg

- Khoo Teck Puat Hospital: https://www.ktph.com.sg

- Neuroscience Institute, Alzheimer's Disease and Dementia: https://www.nni.com.sg

- National University Hospital Neuroscience Clinic: https://www.nuh.com.sg

- Singapore General Hospital, Dept of Neurology/Geriatric Medicine: https://www.sgh.com.sg

- Tan Tock Seng Hospital Geriatric Medicine Clinic: https://www.ttsh.com.sg

Community-based care:

- Aged Psychiatry Community Assessment and Treatment Service (APCATS)

- Department of Geriatric Psychiatry, Institute of Mental Health

- Community Psychogeriatric Programme (CPGP), Psychological Medicine Division, Changi General Hospital, email: CPGP@cgh.com.sg

- Geriatric Psychiatry Out-Reach Assessment, Consultation and Enablement (GRACE), Department of Psychological Medicine, National University Hospital, email: g_race@nuhs.edu.sg

Dementia Day Care Centres:

- Alzheimer's Disease Association: New Horizon Centre: Toa Payoh, Bukit Batok, Tampines, Jurong Point

- Apex Harmony Lodge: https://www.apexharmony.org.sg

- Peacehaven Bedok Multi-service Centre: https://www.salvationarmy.org.sg

Support groups

- Alzheimer's Disease Association, Caregiver Support Centre: https://www.alz.org.sg

- Referral Services Helpline (Agency For Integrated Care): https://www.aic.sg

- Dementia Helpline (Alzheimer's Disease Association): 6377 0700 (Monday to Friday, 9 am to 6 pm)

Local organisations for assessment and treatment

- Functional Gastrointestinal Disorders (FGID) Unit at National University Hospital Singapore (NUHS) provides a multidisciplinary functional gastrointestinal disorders clinic: http://www.singhealth.com.sg/PatientCare/ConditionsAndTreatments/Pages/Irritable-Bowel-Syndrome.aspx

Support groups

- Singapore IBS Support Group Facebook Page: https://www.facebook.com/pages/IBS-Support-Group-Singapore/112089335524301

Online resources

- Singapore General Hospital psychoeducation: http://www.singhealth.com.sg/PatientCare/ConditionsAndTreatments/Pages/Irritable-Bowel-Syndrome.aspx

- Singapore Health Promotion Board: http://www.hpb.gov.sg/HOPPortal/dandcarticle/10450

- National University Hospital Singapore psychoeducation: http://www.nuh.com.sg/usc/patients-and-visitors/diseases-and-conditions/bowel/irritable-bowel-syndrome-ibs.html

INDEX